Resuscitation

Antonino Gullo · Giuseppe Ristagno
Editors

Resuscitation

Translational Research, Clinical
Evidence, Education, Guidelines

Foreword by Massimo Antonelli

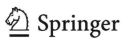 Springer

Editors
Antonino Gullo
UCO di Anestesia e Rianimazione
Azienda Ospedaliero-Universitaria
  Policlinico Vittorio Emanuele
Catania
Italy

Giuseppe Ristagno
Department of Cardiovascular Research
IRCCS—Istituto di Ricerche
  Farmacologiche "Mario Negri"
Milan
Italy

ISBN 978-88-470-5506-3   ISBN 978-88-470-5507-0   (eBook)
DOI 10.1007/978-88-470-5507-0
Springer Milan Heidelberg New York Dordrecht London

Library of Congress Control Number: 2013953232

Printed on acid-free paper

Springer is part of Springer Science+Business Media (www.springer.com)

Foreword

State-of-the-Art in Resuscitation represents a good example of careful attention given to the evidence and guidelines coherent with a modern approach to the clinical Intensive Care Medicine, and of an open-minded approach to translational research, as a means to link the laboratory to the bedside. The main topics of cardiopulmonary resuscitation have been treated and updated with the current knowledge. The present textbook is an essential educational tool for training in intensive care medicine.

The vast and solid scientific and clinical experience of Antonino Gullo and Giuseppe Ristagno made them the perfect Editors of a work inspired to the teaching of an unrivalled master as Max Harry Weil, the father of "Critical Medicine."

Following in the footsteps of this giant of Medicine, and in collaboration with distinguished international researchers and intensivists, the Editors prepared a work of great professional value, thoughtfully analyzing the various aspects of cardiopulmonary intensive care and going into the details of most of the problems inherent in the cardiovascular and cerebral monitoring and treatment, with special attention to the application of new techniques and criteria of advanced life support.

The analysis of the cellular microcosm opens a window toward future scientific developments and offers a new opportunity of interpretation of the clinical and pharmacological phenomena in the field of cardiovascular resuscitation.

More experienced intensivists as well as intensivists in training will certainly benefit by this state-of-art guide to a discipline that has many implications that are difficult to master.

I am confident of the success of this textbook, thanks to the contributions coordinated by two mentors as Antonino Gullo and Giuseppe Ristagno, whose motivation and competence are internationally well known and eloquently expressed in this work.

Rome, Italy, 13 November 2013   Massimo Antonelli

Preface

Three years have passed since the last guidelines for Cardiopulmonary Resuscitation and Emergency Cardiovascular Care and the new one is underway and expected to be released during 2015. Thus, this volume has the purpose to assemble updates on *Resuscitation* science from international experts in the field and to explore the current state-of-the-art in this important, continuously developing, and controversial area. The different contributions will stimulate improved clinical resuscitation practices through the translation of laboratory and clinical research into routine practice, in prehospital and in-hospital populations.

Indeed, the authors of the different chapters are international experts on CPR, shock states, and trauma who participated in the first "Weil Conference" in Milan, in September 2012. Max Harry Weil was one of the world's leading clinicians, educators, and researchers in the field of critical care medicine and resuscitation science. He was a pioneer in this field, and was considered the "father" of critical care. Dr. Weil's effort contributed to a long list of seminal insights that led to dramatic improvement in survival of people with "circulatory failure" caused by sepsis, septic shock, heart failure, cardiac arrest, and trauma.

Being most of the experts contributing to this volume either a Dr. Weil former fellow or one of his professional colleagues and scientific collaborators, this book on *Resuscitation* is an occasion to honor Dr. Weil's memory and life spent "saving lives," through providing updated experimental and clinical perspectives to scientists, physicians, researchers, and fellows in the specialty of intensive and critical care medicine.

Antonino Gullo
Giuseppe Ristagno

Contents

Resuscitation Science: From the Beginning to the Present Day

1

Carmelina Gurrieri, Giuseppe Ristagno and Antonino Gullo

1.1 Introduction

Cardiovascular disease remains the leading cause of death in the Western world, with 350,000 Americans and 700,000 Europeans sustaining cardiac arrest each year [1]. Indeed, cardiopulmonary resuscitation (CPR) is an emergency procedure to be performed as soon as possible after collapse in the attempt to restore spontaneous circulation and respiration. Resuscitation is a relatively modern science, although its roots extend back in the centuries. The earliest report of a resuscitation attempt, in fact, has been described in the Bible, in the Old Testament, where "the life of a boy was restored by placing a mouth in the boy mouth" [2]. However, until the nineteenth century, routine resuscitation from death was not viewed as feasible. Yet, as early as the nineteenth century, resuscitation by delivery of an electrical shock was demonstrated. Indeed, modern CPR emerged only during the latter half of the twentieth century. A sequence of interventions was established in the 1960s under the acronym ABCD [3], namely airway, breathing, chest compression, and defibrillation. Although to some extent now modified to take into account priorities of chest compression over the airway, breathing, and defibrillation, the ABCD acronym continues to have a determinant role and practical utility.

C. Gurrieri · A. Gullo
Dipartimento di Anestesia e Rianimazione, Universita' degli studi di Catania, Catania, Italy

G. Ristagno (✉)
Department of Cardiovascular Research, IRCCS—Istituto di Ricerche Farmacologiche "Mario Negri", via La Masa 19, 20156, Milan, Italy
e-mail: gristag@gmail.com

A. Gullo and G. Ristagno (eds.), *Resuscitation*,
DOI: 10.1007/978-88-470-5507-0_1, © Springer-Verlag Italia 2014

1.2   History

Indeed, it was in 1874 when the pathophysiology of the direct cardiac compression was explained by Dr. Moritz Schiff. He noted the presence of carotid pulsations closely corresponding to the ejection of blood produced by directly squeezing the canine heart in an open-chest dog model. This led to the term "open chest cardiac massage." Friedrich Maass is credited with the first successful human closed-chest cardiac massage that was performed in 1891 [4]. However, all these initial trials remained anecdotal. Consequently, during the first half of the twentieth century, cardiac resuscitation was restricted to the operating room or closely proximal in-hospital settings. In 1958, however, Dr. Kouwenhoven and his coworkers, Drs. Jude and Knickerbocker [5], reawakened the potential value of chest massage when they observed that coincidental with the positioning of paddles on the anterior chest for delivery of an electrical shock, an arterial pulse was produced. External compression could therefore be performed without surgical expertise or equipment and now became widely taught and used, and open-chest cardiac massage became obsolescent except for intraoperative or post traumatic resuscitation. A combination of closed-chest compression and mechanical ventilation thereupon formed the platform after the 1960s and remains as the present-day CPR.

The modern resuscitation achieved its consistency in the 1950s, thanks to the experiments of doctors James Elam, Peter Safar, and Archer S. Gordon. Dr. Elam was the father of *rescue breathing* [6]. His experiments were soon joined by Dr. Safar who proved the efficacy of exhaled air ventilation without adjuncts and airway patency by backward tilt of the head with jaw thrust. The S-shaped oropharyngeal airway, which continues to be used in the present, was utilized by Safar, together with the now routine positions of the forehead and mandible with which a patient airway is secured in unconscious victims [7]. Correct patency of the airway was described by Dr. Safar who observed in anesthetized, breathing patients, the return of inflated gas into a bag which was connected to the endotracheal tube. In 1954, the mouth-to-mask ventilation for resuscitation was proposed by Elam which achieved arterial oxygen saturations of more than 90 % [8]. Safar, instead, reproposed mouth-to-mouth ventilation as an effective ventilation method during resuscitation because it required no instrumentation [9]. Subsequently, the self-refilling bag introduced by Ruben [10] in 1958 followed by the addition of the oxygen gas-powered pneumatic demand valve resuscitator in 1964 added importantly to support breathing in emergency settings. Concurrently, the valve mask bag became the primary manual emergency ventilation device for resuscitation and it continues to be in active use to the present day [11]. Mouth-to-mouth ventilation was then further improved by Dr. Gordon's clinical observation on children population. As for mechanical ventilation, the Drinker respirator or "iron lung" paved the way for prolonged mechanical ventilation, especially for patients afflicted with neuromuscular failure of breathing, including cervical spinal cord injury and, most of all, paralytic poliomyelitis. Intermittent positive pressure ventilation, instead, first evolved in Europe when cuffed tracheotomy tubes became available. In 1952, Bjørn Ibsen [12] utilized manual positive pressure ventilation during the Danish polio epidemics with the participation of hundreds of medical students breathing for victims who had a tracheostomy tube attached to a vented rubber bag for delivery of air or oxygen.

The first demonstration that ventricular fibrillation could be terminated by an electrical current was in 1899, when Prevost and Battelli [13] observed that directly delivered low voltage AC currents induced ventricular fibrillation in dogs and higher voltage currents terminated ventricular fibrillation. Dr. Paul Zoll subsequently recorded the first successful closed-chest human defibrillation in 1955 in a man with recurrent syncope which terminated in ventricular fibrillation [14]. In 1979, the first portable external defibrillator was developed, the precursor to automatic external defibrillators.

1.3   Introduction of CPR Guidelines

Under the auspices of the National Academy of Science National Research Council, James Elam, Archer Gordon, James Jude, and Peter Safar formed a working committee. This committee developed the first national guidelines for what to teach to whom and how, which was published in 1966 [15]. The first CPR guidelines were established. Guidelines were also developed under the auspices of the World Federation of Societies of Anesthesiologists, which expanded guidelines for advanced life support (ALS), including cerebral resuscitation. In the decade that followed, the first National Conference on Standards for CPR and Emergency Cardiac Care (ECC) was organized under the auspices of the American Heart Association (AHA), which thereafter assumed increasing responsibility for professional leadership in the field both nationally and later internationally. In 1973, the second National Conference on CPR was held under the auspices of the AHA [16]. At the end of the 1970s Advanced Cardiovascular Life Support (ACLS) was developed. Ten years later the AHA introduced the first pediatric basic life support (BLS) and ALS and neonatal resuscitation guidelines. In the 1990s, Public Access Defibrillation (PAD) programs were developed and the International Committee on Resuscitation (ILCOR) was founded. The importance of early cardiac arrest recognition and activation of emergency system, early CPR, early defibrillation, and early ALS was addressed by Cummins and colleagues, who first introduced the concept of the "Chain of Survival" [17, 18]. Today a new link has been added to the chain, the so-called "post-resuscitation care" [19]. The implementation of the fifth link provided significant and important improvements in favorable neurological outcome and survival and became more and more emphasized in the 2010 guidelines [20]. The 2005 and, even more, 2010 guidelines stressed also the importance of high-quality CPR in order to achieve better outcome of cardiac arrest [21].

1.4   Utstein Style

Despite the large amount of literature focusing on out-of-hospital cardiac arrest outcome, a comparison of data among different emergency medical service systems was almost impossible until two decades ago, due to the lack of consensus and uniformity in data recordings and reporting. Thus, in order to establish uniform terms and recommendations for the evaluation and reporting of data from cardiac arrest, in 1991 a task force developed the **Utstein style** [22]. Member representatives of different organizations, i.e., AHA, European Resuscitation Council, European Society of Cardiology, European Academy of Anesthesiology, and European Society for Intensive Care Medicine, attended an international resuscitation meeting hosted at the Utstein Abbey, in Norway. It represented a starting point for a more effective registration of data and information from a cardiac arrest event and a better understanding of the elements of resuscitation practice. Thereafter, the term "Utstein style" was adopted to indicate the uniform reporting of data from prehospital cardiac arrests [23]. Moreover, the international meeting addressed the importance and the potential value of bystander CPR which demonstrated to reduce the mortality of cardiac arrest. The need for easy accessibility to training and CPR education was another topic of interest. Many other Utstein style international consensus statements have been published over the past 20 years, including the uniform reporting of pediatric ALS, laboratory CPR research, in-hospital resuscitation, neonatal life support, CPR registries, and trauma data. The standardized definitions established by the Utstein scientific statements enabled comparative analysis between resuscitation studies and healthcare systems. Nevertheless, there is still confusion in the scientific literature due to a persisting lack of uniformity in reporting some specific data. For example, differences in terms referring to defibrillation success or in the different survival outcomes chosen to report the effect of a specific treatment/intervention [24–27]. Moreover, the likelihood of survival from cardiac arrest patients may depend also on sociodemographic factors as well as biological and clinical characteristics. There are, for example, some areas with higher cardiac arrest risk population and consequently higher risk of poor outcome; thus the estimation of cardiac arrest and outcome may be subject to potential external bias [24]. Other factors to be taken into consideration are the local emergency response organization and post-resuscitation care after hospital admission [24, 26]. Thus, knowledge of regional variations in outcome after cardiac arrest could guide identification of effective interventions to be undertaken, such as appropriate public health initiatives, community support, high-quality pre and posthospital emergency care, and good education in CPR skills.

1.5   Translational Research

The translation of basic science into the clinical practice may be difficult and remains a major issue in contemporary medicine. For this purpose, a new discipline has been created, the *translational research*, which tries to assess the discrepancies between research and clinical needs. Translational research is a continuum loop in which basic science discovering is integrated into clinical application and clinical observations are used to generate scientific topics to be studied by basic science [28]. This integration is extremely important for medicine improvement. Translation science deals with health policy, health economy, and it should have a holistic approach. However, about three-quarters of the basic science promises have not been tested yet in randomized clinical trials and only few of the basic science promises have had a major impact on current medical practice [29]. This result may represent a failure of translational medicine to match basic science advances. Many explanations might account for this "failure," such as lack of sufficient fundings, high cost and slow results, inadequate samples, conflict of interest, fragmented infrastructures, shortage of qualified investigators, shortage of willing participants, incompatible databases, and lack of congressional and public supports [29–32]. Health systems should consider translational science as a cornerstone of modern health which can have a strong impact on the well-being of society and on clinical practice. Only educational interventions may implement translational science for improving collaboration among scientists, clinicians, researchers, and healthcare systems.

1.6   Resuscitation Science

Advances in resuscitation science have improved survival rate of cardiac arrest. Resuscitation science was first defined by the Post-resuscitative and initial Utility in Life Saving Efforts (PULSE) Conference, an initiative taken by leaders of the international scientific community to improve clinical outcomes after CPR [33]. This conference defined *resuscitation science* as the study of pathophysiology, mechanisms, and management of sudden states of illness, in particular of the states of whole body oxygen deprivation. Resuscitation science includes five principal domains which are: basic science, pharmacology, translational studies, bioengineering, and clinical evaluative research. All of the above domains focus their attention on scientific research which might ameliorate resuscitation care. For example, different studies have shown that therapeutic hypothermia is an effective treatment for comatose adults resuscitated from cardiac arrest [34–37]. It requires a multidisciplinary team approach and comprehensive targeted temperature protocols, which include shivering assessment and seizure management. However, despite the strong evidence of efficacy and apparent simplicity of intervention, recent surveys show that therapeutic hypothermia is delivered inconsistently, incompletely, and often with delay. This is a case of difficulty in translation research into clinical practice. Different reasons might be listed, such as lack of awareness of recommended practice, of standard protocols for applying hypothermia, and staff shortages. To overcome these, standardized protocols, educational sessions, reminders, audit feedbacks, and education of clinicians are mandatory.

1.7 Education

The quality of education, training programs, and frequency of retraining are critical factors in improving the effectiveness of resuscitation. Resuscitation programs should systematically monitor cardiac arrests, the quality of resuscitation care provided, and the outcome. These informations are necessary to optimize resuscitation care and improve the resuscitation performance [38]. Survival rates after cardiac arrest depend, in fact, not only on the validity and reliability of guidelines and a well-functioning Chain of Survival, but also on the quality of education. These factors interact with each other. Unfortunately, less than 15 % of adult out-of-hospital cardiac arrest victims survive to hospital discharge despite the progress on resuscitation care [1].

Training courses on resuscitation are now well-established worldwide. Many courses provide combined training in BLS and ACLS skills. Training organized in small groups is advantageous and more interactive. Scenario-based teaching allows for useful repetition of sequence and items and should be a central part of the course. Teaching strategies should be evaluated and compared on the basis of how well attendees achieve predefined teaching goals [38]. Patient simulation could be an ideal tool for teaching and lets attendees to be actively engaged in their learning process. By definition, in fact, simulation places trainers in a similar realistic scenario created with a simulator that replicates the real environment. Unfortunately, there is not a single method suitable for all circumstances. Thus, audit for evaluation of training methods, instructors' skills, acquired knowledge, and effectiveness of courses should be mandatory. Mass education and television campaigns are other examples of educational tools in CPR training [39]. Another example of a potential good teaching method might be the "virtual technology" which includes computer games and videogames. This method has been efficiently experimented in schools [40]; it is feasible, reliable, and it could represent an alternative starting point for teaching CPR to young laypersons.

1.8 A Tribute to Dr. Weil

Finally, we cannot conclude this chapter without a tribute to the "father of the critical care" and pioneer of resuscitation science, Dr. Max Harry Weil [41]. He, in fact, first introduced the term critical care medicine in the late 1950s at the University of Southern California Medical Center. In 1961, Dr Weil cofounded, together with Dr. Shubin "The Institute of Critical Care Medicine," a nonprofit public foundation at the University of Southern California, recognized as a comprehensive international center for medical and biomedical engineering research in critical care and resuscitation medicine. Indeed, together with Dr. Safar, he signed a progress in understanding the pathophysiology of sudden death and in recognizing the importance of early cardiopulmonary and cerebral resuscitation maneuvers. These concepts were considered a real challenge to achieve by continuous refining of guidelines and their popularization, including widespread programs of training. In 1967, Safar, Shoemaker, and Weil had an impromptu meeting on the Boardwalk of Atlantic City in conjunction with an annual meeting of the American Physiological Society. They subsequently corresponded regularly, and Dr. Weil then invited 28 medical leaders from different specialties representing internal medicine, cardiology, surgery, anesthesiology, and pediatrics to propose a multidisciplinary organization to implement and guide the field which evolved into the "Society of Critical Care Medicine." Dr. Weil's effort contributed to a long list of insights that led to the dramatic improvement in survival of people suffering "circulatory failure" due to sepsis, septic shock, heart failure, cardiac arrest, and trauma. He realized that in the absence of real-time measurements of vital signs and alarms, professional providers were either not aware of immediate life threats or they could not define with sufficient precision the immediate events that led to the fatal outcome. The assumption was that immediately life-endangered patients, the critically ill and injured, may have substantially better chances of survival if provided with professionally advanced minute-to-minute objective measurements. Thus, Dr. Weil was prompted to implement continuous monitoring of the electrocardiogram, blood pressure, pulse, breathing, and other vital signs complemented by arterial and central venous pressures, urine output, central, and peripheral temperatures, and by intermittent measurements of blood gases from vascular sites. That concept was pioneered in a four-bed unit called the "Shock Ward" that became the prototype of the early intensive care unit (ICU) [42]. Thereafter, progress in the management of the acutely life-threatened patient has been accelerated by rapid advances in both monitoring and measurement technologies and the interventions today routinely used worldwide in modern ICUs.

References

1. Nolan JP, Soar J, Zideman DA et al (2010) European Resuscitation Council guidelines for Resuscitation 2010 Section 1. Executive summary. Resuscitation 81:1219–1276
2. Cooper JA, Cooper JD, Cooper JM (2006) Cardiopulmonary resuscitation: history, current practice, and future direction. Circulation 114(25):2839–2849
3. Nakagawa Y, Weil MH, Tang W (1999) The history of CPR. In: Weil MH, Tang W (eds) Resuscitation of the arrested heart. WB Saunders, Philadelphia, pp 1–12
4. Eisenberg MS, Baskett P et al (2007) A history of cardiopulmonary resuscitation. In: Paradis NA, Halperin HR, Kern KB, Wenzel V, Chamberlain D (eds) Cardiac arrest: the science and practice of resuscitation medicine, 2nd edn. Cambridge University Press, Cambridge, pp 2–25

5. Kouwenhoven WB, Jude JR, Knickerbocker GG (1960) Closed-chest cardiac massage. JAMA 173:1064–1067
6. Sands RP Jr, Bacon DR (1998) An inventive mind: the career of James O. Elam, M.D. (1918–1995). Anesthesiology 88(4):1107–1112
7. Safar P, Escarraga LA, Chang F (1959) Upper airway obstruction in the unconscious patient. J Appl Physiol 14:760–764
8. Elam JO, Brown ES, Elder JD (1954) Artificial respiration by mouth to mask method: a study of the respiratory gas exchange of paralyzed patient ventilated by operator's expired air. N Engl J Med 250(18):749–754
9. Safar P (1958) Ventilatory efficacy of mouth to mouth artificial respiration. JAMA 167(3):335–341
10. Ruben H (1958) Combination resuscitator and aspirator. Anesthesiology 19(3):408–409
11. Pearson JW, Redding JS (1964) Equipment for respiratory resuscitation. 2. Anesthesiology 25:858–859
12. Ibsen B (1954) The anaesthesist's viewpoint on the treatment of respiratory complications in poliomyelitis during epidemic in Copenhagen, 1952. Proc R Soc Med 47(1):72–74
13. Prevost JL, Battelli F (1899) La mort par les courants electriques-courants alternatifs a haute tension. J Physiol Pathol Gen 1:427–442
14. Zoll PM, Linenthal AJ, Gibson W et al (1956) Termination of ventricular fibrillation in man by externally applied electric countershock. N Engl J Med 254(16):727–732
15. American Heart Association (AHA) and National Academy of Sciences-National Research Council (NAS-NRC) (1996) Standards for cardiopulmonary resuscitation (CPR) and emergency cardiac care (ECC). JAMA 198:372–379
16. JAMA (1974) Standards for cardiopulmonary resuscitation (CPR) and emergency cardiac care (ECC). JAMA 227(7):833–868
17. Cummins RO, Ornato JP, Thies WH et al (1991) Improving survival from sudden cardiac arrest: the "chain of survival" concept: a statement for health professionals from the Advanced Cardiac Life Support Subcommittee and the Emergency Cardiac Care Committee, American Heart Association. Circulation 3(5):1832–1847
18. Ristagno G, Fumagalli F, Gullo A (2011) The 'take home message' from the 'Take Heart America' program: strengthen the chain! Crit Care Med 39(1):194–196
19. Peberdy MA, Callaway CW, Neumar RW et al (2010) Part 9: post-cardiac arrest care: 2010 American Heart Association guidelines for cardiopulmonary resuscitation and emergency cardiovascular care. Circulation 122(18 Suppl 3):S768–S786
20. Tagami T, Hirata K, Takeshige T et al (2012) Implementation of the fifth link of the chain of survival concept for out-of-hospital cardiac arrest. Circulation 126(5):589–597
21. Travers AH, Rea TD, Bobrow BJ et al (2010) Part 4: CPR overview: 2010 American Heart Association guidelines for cardiopulmonary resuscitation and emergency cardiovascular care. Circulation 122(18 Suppl 3):S676–S684
22. Chamberlain DA, Hazinski MF et al (2003) Education in resuscitation: an ILCOR symposium: Utstein Abbey: Stavanger, Norway: June 22–24. Circulation 108(20):2575–2594
23. Peberdy MA, Cretikos M, Abella BS (2007) Recommended guidelines for monitoring, reporting, and conducting research on medical emergency team, outreach, and rapid response systems: an Utstein-style scientific statement: a scientific statement from the International Liaison Committee on Resuscitation (American Heart Association, Australian Resuscitation Council, European Resuscitation Council, Heart and Stroke Foundation of Canada, Inter American Heart Foundation, Resuscitation Council of Southern Africa, and the New Zealand Resuscitation Council); the American Heart Association Emergency Cardiovascular Care Committee; the Council on Cardiopulmonary, Perioperative, and Critical Care; and the Interdisciplinary Working Group on Quality of Care and Outcomes Research. Circulation 116(21):2481–2500

24. Nichol G, Thomas E, Callaway CW et al (2008) Regional variation in out-of-hospital cardiac arrest incidence and outcome. JAMA 300(12):1423–1431

25. Vukmir RB (2004) The influence of urban, suburban, or rural locale on survival from refractory prehospital cardiac arrest. Am J Emerg Med 22(2):90–93

26. Yasunaga H, Miyata H, Horiguchi H et al (2011) Population density, call-response interval, and survival of out-of-hospital cardiac arrest. Int J Health Geogr 10:26

27. Grmec S, Krizmaric M, Mally S et al (2007) Utstein style analysis of out-of-hospital cardiac arrest–bystander CPR and end expired carbon dioxide. Resuscitation 72(3):404–414

28. Keramaris NC, Kanakaris NK, Tzioupis C et al (2008) Translational research: from benchside to bedside. Injury 39(6):643–650

29. Ioannidis JP (2004) Materializing research promises: opportunities, priorities and conflicts in translational medicine. J Transl Med 2(1):5

30. Littman BH, Di Mario L, Plebani M et al (2007) What's next in translational medicine? Clin Sci (Lond) 112(4):217–227

31. Fontanarosa PB, DeAngelis CD, Hunt N (2005) Medical research—state of the science. JAMA 294(11):1424–1425

32. Cohen JJ, Siegel EK (2005) Academic medical centers and medical research: the challenges ahead. JAMA 294(11):1367–1372

33. Becker LB, Weisfeldt ML, Weil MH et al (2002) The PULSE initiative: scientific priorities and strategic planning for resuscitation research and life saving therapies. Circulation 105(21):2562–2570

34. Safar P, Xiao F, Radovsky A et al (1996) Improved cerebral resuscitation from cardiac arrest in dogs with mild hypothermia plus blood flow promotion. Stroke 27:105–113

35. Maze R, Le May MR, Hibbert B et al (2013) The impact of therapeutic hypothermia as adjunctive therapy in a regional primary PCI program. Resuscitation 84(4):460–464

36. Ristagno G, Tantillo S, Li Y (2012) Should we be afraid of mild hypothermia? Not at all! Just do not underestimate risk factors and optimize post-resuscitation care. Crit Care Med 40(3):1029–1031

37. Hypothermia after Cardiac Arrest Study Group (2002) Mild therapeutic hypothermia to improve the neurologic outcome after cardiac arrest. N Engl J Med 346(8):549–556

38. Chamberlain DA, Hazinski MF, European Resuscitation Council et al (2003) Education in resuscitation: an ILCOR symposium: Utstein Abbey: Stavanger, Norway: June 22–24, 2001. Circulation 108(20):2575–2594

39. Nielsen AM, Isbye DL, Lippert FK et al (2013) Can mass education and a television campaign change the attitudes towards cardiopulmonary resuscitation in a rural community? Scand J Trauma Resusc Emerg Med 21:39

40. Creutzfeldt J, Hedman L, Heinrichs L et al (2013) Cardiopulmonary resuscitation training in high school using avatars in virtual worlds: an international feasibility study. J Med Internet Res 15(1):e9

41. Kette F, Pellis T, Ristagno G (2011) Max Harry Weil: a tribute from the Italian research fellows. J Crit Care 26(6):626–633

42. Weil MH, Shubin H (1969) Critical care medicine I: the "VIP" approach to the bedside management of shock. JAMA 207:337–340

From Experimental and Clinical Evidence to Guidelines

2

Jerry P. Nolan

2.1 Introduction

Clinical guidelines should be evidence based and in this respect cardiopulmonary resuscitation (CPR) guidelines should be at least as robust as any other guidelines that support our practice. Guidelines improve the quality of care received by patients by closing the gap between what clinicians do and what scientific evidence supports. Guidelines provide a point of reference for auditing performance of clinicians or hospitals. The steps involved in the process for developing evidence-based guidelines have been outlined by the Grades of Recommendation Assessment, Development and Evaluation (GRADE) Working Group (Table 2.1) [1–3].

This chapter will review the process involved in reviewing experimental and clinical evidence in CPR and steps taken to translate this into clinical practice.

2.2 The History of International CPR Consensus and Guideline Development

The modern approach to cardiopulmonary resuscitation (CPR)—rescue breathing and closed-chest compression—was described in the late 1950s and early 1960s [4, 5]. Although this was undoubtedly the birth of CPR, the challenge was to spread the word and educate the healthcare workers and lay people throughout the world. This same challenge faces us today whenever CPR guidelines are modified and updated.

J. P. Nolan (✉)
Royal United Hospital, Bath, BA1 3NG, UK
e-mail: jerry.nolan@btinternet.com

A. Gullo and G. Ristagno (eds.), *Resuscitation*,
DOI: 10.1007/978-88-470-5507-0_2, © Springer-Verlag Italia 2014

Table 2.1 Steps involved in translating science into clinical guidelines according to the GRADE process (adapted from [1])

Establish the guideline development group
Define the scope of the guidelines
Prioritize the problems
Ask precise clinical questions using the population intervention comparator outcome (PICO) format
Decide on the relative importance of outcomes
Identify the existing evidence for every clinical question
Develop evidence profiles
Grade the quality of existing evidence for each outcome separately
Determine the overall quality of available evidence across outcomes
Decide on the balance between desirable and undesirable consequences
Decide on the strength of recommendation
Formulate the recommendation reflecting its strength
Write the guideline
Disseminate the guideline

In 1966, the National Academy of Sciences' National Research Council convened an ad hoc conference on CPR. This was the first conference to review specifically the evidence and recommend standard CPR techniques; more than 30 national organizations were represented [6]. International awareness was enhanced in the following year, when an International Symposium on Emergency Resuscitation was held in Oslo, Norway. The American Heart Association (AHA) sponsored subsequent conferences in 1973 and 1979 [7, 8]. Parallel efforts occurred internationally as other resuscitation organizations faced a growing demand for CPR training [9]. Inevitably, variations in resuscitation techniques and training methods began to emerge from individual countries and regions of the world.

Increasing awareness of international variations in resuscitation practices generated interest in the possibility of gathering international experts at a single location with the aim of achieving consensus in resuscitation techniques. The AHA invited resuscitation leaders from many countries to observe its 1985 review of standards and guidelines for CPR and emergency cardiovascular care (ECC) [10]. These international guests played a major role in discussions and disseminated the findings and recommendations to their own countries.

In June 1990, representatives from the AHA, European Resuscitation Council (ERC), Heart and Stroke Foundation of Canada (HSFC), and the Australian Resuscitation Council (ARC) held a meeting at Utstein Abbey on the island of Mosteroy, Norway. The lack of standardized terminology in reports relating to adult out-of-hospital cardiac arrest was highlighted. At a follow-up meeting in

December 1990 in Surrey, England, the term "Utstein-style" was adopted for the uniform reporting of data from out-of-hospital cardiac arrests (OHCAs) [11]. Many other "Utstein-style" international consensus statements have been published over the last 22 years, including the uniform reporting of pediatric advanced life support [12], laboratory CPR research [13], in-hospital resuscitation [14], neonatal life support [15], drowning [16], post-resuscitation care [17], medical emergency teams [18], and dispatch [19]. The original Utstein statements on OHCA and in-hospital cardiac arrest (IHCA) were merged and updated in a single statement on resuscitation registries in 2004 [20]. Following meetings in 2012 and 2013, an update of the 2004 Utstein reporting document is being written.

The Fifth National Conference on CPR and ECC was held in Dallas, Texas, in 1992. More than 40 % of the participants were from outside the United States, representing 25 countries and 53 international organizations [10]. Concepts discussed at this meeting included the creation of a permanent infrastructure for international cooperation and the desirability of common international guidelines and an international conference on CPR and ECC.

2.3   The International Liaison Committee on Resuscitation

The first international conference held by the ERC took place in Brighton, England in 1992 [21]. At the end of the conference, representatives from the guidelines-producing organizations (AHA, ERC, HSFC, ARC, and the Resuscitation Council of Southern Africa (RCSA)) held the first meeting of the International Liaison Committee [22]. The founding member organizations of The International Liaison Committee on Resuscitation (ILCOR) were the AHA, the ERC, the Heart and Stroke Foundation of Canada, the Resuscitation Council of Southern Africa (RCSA), and the Australian Resuscitation Council (ARC). These organizations were later joined by the Consejo Latino-Americano de Resuscitatión (now part of the Inter-American Heart Foundation), the New Zealand Resuscitation Council (which now forms part of the Australia and New Zealand Committee on Resuscitation—ANZCOR), and the Resuscitation Council of Asia (RCA).

Since its formation, ILCOR has coordinated international systematic reviews of the evidence to support resuscitation standards and guidelines. To date, ILCOR has published 23 scientific advisory statements with the goal of endorsing evidence-based resuscitation science that can be adopted by regional councils to formulate resuscitation guidelines [11, 13, 16, 23–42]. While some regional differences in guidelines are inevitable because of varying implementation issues or resources, the ultimate goal of ILCOR is to provide a unified consensus on the science of resuscitation and on the science of resuscitation education/implementation. This goal defined the international CPR evidence evaluation conferences held in 2000, 2005, and 2010, as well as several other international consensus statements [37, 43, 44]. The 2000 Guidelines Conference [45], the first major assembly coordinated by ILCOR, used a sophisticated process for gathering and assessing evidence; this process evolved further in 2005 [46] and was refined for 2010 [47].

The goal of a single best set of international CPR guidelines has not yet been achieved. Broadly, consensus on resuscitation science has been reached, but local variations in treatment recommendations are inevitable because of differences in epidemiology, model of care, implementation, culture, or economic factors. These variations will be reflected by some subtle differences in regional and national resuscitation guidelines. Reasons for failure to achieve truly universal guidelines include:

1. For many interventions, high-level evidence in the form of randomized clinical trials is not available.
2. The evidence may be inconsistent or contradictory.
3. Resuscitation has evolved over 50 years and many of the practices originally recommended were based on the best available evidence and the opinions of experts at the time. In some cases, this evidence was minimal or difficult to interpret.

2.4 Implementation

Failure to translate research findings into daily practice is a well-recognized problem [48, 49]. The development of good guidelines does not ensure that they will be adopted in clinical practice and passive methods of disseminating and implementing guidelines (e.g., publication in journals) are unlikely to change professional behavior [50]. Recent evidence suggests that full implementation of new resuscitation guidelines can range from 18 months up to 5 years [51, 52]. Resuscitation organizations have a primary responsibility for disseminating and implementing resuscitation guidelines; this will require significant resources. Resuscitation guidelines can be disseminated effectively through the Internet, through national scientific meetings, and by local meetings held in hospitals and in the community. Resuscitation training materials should be updated as rapidly as possible to reflect the new guidelines. Standardized courses play a crucial role in disseminating resuscitation guidelines. Evaluation and verification of the implementation of new guidelines is achieved through audit.

The science of resuscitation is evolving rapidly. It would not be in the best interests of patients if resuscitation experts were to wait 5 or more years to inform healthcare professionals of therapeutic advances in this field. Some groups have advocated reviewing guidelines as frequently as every 2 years [53]. However, frequent changes in recommendations that do not have a major impact on outcome might undermine the process, because teaching and learning new guidelines takes time and resources. New science must be reviewed continually; if major new research evidence is published, groups such as ILCOR should publish interim consensus advisory statements to update treatment guidelines. Large, multicenter registries that use Utstein-style consensus definitions of the process of care and outcomes following resuscitation will track the dissemination of new techniques and interventions from science to guidelines and to practice, and lead to further refinements in the guidelines [37, 54–56]. Ideally, important interventions and practices could be taught and reviewed rapidly, giving feedback on quality of performance for all healthcare providers. The interface between resuscitation research and continuous quality improvement (audit) is becoming more blurred.

ILCOR and international collaboration has continued to mature. The quest for a single set of universal guidelines is idealistic: many problems in resuscitation require local modifications and solutions. The common goals of the resuscitation community are to reduce the rates of morbidity and mortality from cardiovascular disease. The consensus statements and treatment recommendations in this publication are based on the most comprehensive review of resuscitation science ever undertaken, and this has been achieved by active and effective international collaboration.

2.5 The 2010 International Consensus on Cardiopulmonary Resuscitation and Emergency Cardiovascular Care Science with Treatment Recommendations

The 2010 International Consensus Conference involved 313 experts from 30 countries [42]. A total of 277 specific resuscitation questions, each in PICO format, were considered by 356 worksheet authors who reviewed thousands of relevant, peer-reviewed publications. Many of these worksheets were presented and discussed at monthly or semimonthly task force international web conferences. The evidence review and summary portions of the evidence evaluation worksheets, with worksheet author conflict of interest (COI) statements, were posted on the ILCOR Website (www.ilcor.org). Journal advertisements and emails invited public comment. Public comments were sent to the appropriate ILCOR task force chair and worksheet author for consideration.

2.5.1 The Evidence Evaluation Process for the 2010 International Consensus on CPR and ECC Science

Evidence-based medicine is now a fundamental component of clinical practice. The evidence evaluation process used in preparation for the 2010 International Consensus on CPR and ECC Science with Treatment Recommendations (2010 CoSTR) has been described in detail and was updated from the approach that had been used in 2005 [47].

The specific questions for systematic review were drawn up by each of six ILCOR specialty task forces (BLS, ALS, acute coronary syndromes, PLS, NLS, and education, implementation and teams (EIT)), from the ILCOR member resuscitation councils and from the knowledge gaps that had been identified after the 2005 conference [57]. Questions structured in a PICO format were allocated to worksheet authors by the relevant task forces. Each author had to complete a

Table 2.2 Levels of evidence used in the 2010 Consensus on CPR Science (reproduced from [47])

2A. Levels of Evidence for Studies on Therapeutic Interventions

LOE 1: Randomized Controlled Trials (or meta-analyses of RCTs)

LOE 2: Studies using concurrent controls without true randomization (e.g., pseudo randomized)

LOE 3: Studies using retrospective controls

LOE 4: Studies without a control group (e.g., case series)

LOE 5: Studies not directly related to the specific patient/population (e.g., different patient/ population, animal models, mechanical models, etc.)

2B. Levels of Evidence for Prognostic Studies

LOE P1: Inception (prospective) cohort studies (or meta-analyses of inception cohort studies), or validation of Clinical Decision Rule (CDR)

LOE P2: Follow-up of untreated control groups in RCTs (or meta-analyses of follow-up studies), or derivation of CDR, or validated on split-sample only

LOE P3: Retrospective cohort studies

LOE P4: Case series

LOE P5: Studies not directly related to the specific patient/population (e.g., different patient/ population, animal models, mechanical models, etc.)

2C. Levels of Evidence for Diagnostic Studies

LOE D1: Validating cohort studies (or meta-analyses of validating cohort studies), or validation of Clinical Decision Rule (CDR)

LOE D2: Exploratory cohort study (or meta-analyses of follow-up studies), or derivation of CDR, or a CDR validated on a split-sample only

LOE D3: Diagnostic case–control study

LOE D4: Study of diagnostic yield (no reference standard)

LOE D5: Studies not directly related to the specific patient/population (e.g., different patient/ population, animal models, mechanical models, etc.)

rigorous conflict of interest (COI) assessment [58]. Instructions were provided on the search strategy and the databases to be searched. The minimum electronic databases to be searched included the Cochrane database for systematic reviews and the Central Register of Controlled Trials (http://www.cochrane.org/), MED-LINE (http://www.ncbi.nlm.nih.gov/PubMed/), EMBASE (www.embase.com), and the EndNote (www.endnote.com) reference library collated by the AHA.

Abstracts obtained from the search were reviewed so that all relevant articles could be identified. For the 2010 process a simplified list of five levels of evidence (LOE) was used. Specific LOEs based on the likelihood for bias were developed for therapeutic interventions, diagnostic questions, and prognosis (Table 2.2). The principles of allocation for studies related to therapeutic interventions were based on the likelihood of eliminating bias in the control group: true randomization (LOE 1), concurrent (LOE 2) versus historic (LOE 3) controls, absence of controls

(LOE 4), or studies that were related to the worksheet question but that did not directly answer it (LOE 5). LOE 5 studies included studies in related populations, animal studies, and bench and mathematical models [47].

Using predefined criteria, the reviewers assessed the quality of research design and methods and allocated each study to one of three categories: good, fair, and poor. Studies were designated as good if they had most or all of the relevant quality items, fair if they had some of the relevant quality items, and poor if they had only a few of the relevant quality items but sufficient quality to include for further review [47]. All of the evidence identified was placed in one of three tables: supportive, neutral, or opposing. Authors formulated a consensus on science statement, which summarized the relevant evidence and then proposed a treatment recommendation. These science statements and treatment recommendations were reviewed and edited by the relevant task before being posted online for public comment. In general, the treatment recommendations were intentionally broad and lacking the detail that would be required for implementation in clinical practice. This final step—the generation of detailed guidelines for clinical practice—was the responsibility of regional resuscitation organizations such as the AHA [59] and the ERC [60]. The ERC and the AHA guidelines can be downloaded at www.erc.edu and http://circ.ahajournals.org/content/122/18_suppl_3.toc, respectively.

2.5.2 Controversies Associated with the 2010 International Consensus on CPR Science

Although the 2010 CoSTR was a major success, there are always aspects that can be improved. The process was highly time-consuming and very expensive. Inevitably, some authors failed to complete their reviews on time, or even at all. In some areas, there was failure to reach consensus, usually because data were lacking or there was disagreement on interpretation. Dealing with late-breaking science is problematic—important science should be included but there is a danger that it is not treated with the same rigor as other studies. Since the 2010 conference, many discussions have taken place on the best way forward for reviewing resuscitation science and the plans for 2015 are discussed below.

2.5.3 The Formula for Survival

The ILCOR Advisory Statement on Education and Resuscitation in 2003 included a hypothetical formula—"the formula for survival (FfS)"—whereby three interactive factors, guideline quality (science), efficient education of patient caregivers (education), and a well-functioning chain of survival at a local level (local implementation), form multiplicands in determining survival from resuscitation [36] (Fig. 2.1 and Table 2.3). In May 2006, a symposium was held to discuss the validity of the formula for survival hypothesis and to investigate the influence of each of the multiplicands on survival. A summary of this symposium is in press.

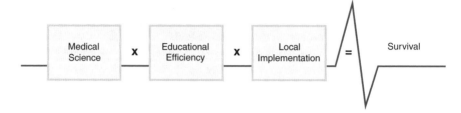

Fig. 2.1 The formula for survival

Table 2.3 Components of the formula for survival (adapted from Chamberlain et al. [36] with permission)

	1. Guideline quality	2. Efficient education of patient caregivers	3. A well-functioning local chain of survival	Patient survival relative to theoretical potential (factors multiplied)
Utopia	1	1	1	=1.00
Ideal	0.9	0.9	0.9	=0.72
Attainable	0.8	0.9	0.5	=0.36
Actual	0.8	0.5	0.5	=0.20

The components that were considered to optimize local implementation, the third multiplicand in the FfS, included:

- Local champion and effective team to steer the process [61–63].
- Simple protocol and an approved order set crossing all departments and disciplines involved in the care process [64].
- Identify and target site-specific barriers to routine implementation (political, legislative, cultural, or professional) [65].
- Buy-in through personal, group, and organizational ownership and partnership with the required resources to make it happen at the local level.
- Constant feedback based on goal-directed benchmarks. An effective implementation strategy must appeal to the majority of individuals regardless of speed of adoption to optimally affect the outcome.
- Constant measuring of quality and outcome. Participants should be engaged in the process and encouraged to perform research and publish their findings in local publications, media, as well as in peer-reviewed journals.

2.6   The Future for Consensus Development in Resuscitation

The science of resuscitation is evolving rapidly. It would not be in the best interests of patients if resuscitation experts were to wait 5 or more years to inform healthcare professionals of therapeutic advances in this field. New science must be reviewed continually; if major new research is published, groups such as ILCOR should publish interim consensus advisory statements to update treatment guidelines. The planning for a consensus conference on resuscitation in 2015 is well underway. The intention is to design a process that enables continual review and updating online. Ultimately, the resource for evidence reviews, consensus on CPR science statements, and treatment recommendations will be a website instead of conventional journal publications. The 2015 evidence review is following the GRADE process [1–3], which will bring it into line with most other international guideline-producing organizations. One of the advantages of the GRADE system is that it is possible to make a "strong" recommendation (most clinicians would use the intervention in most circumstances and most well-informed patients would accept it) even if the quality of the evidence is low [66].

References

1. Brozek JL, Akl EA, Alonso-Coello P et al (2009) Grading quality of evidence and strength of recommendations in clinical practice guidelines. Part 1 of 3. An overview of the GRADE approach and grading quality of evidence about interventions. Allergy 64:669–677
2. Brozek JL, Akl EA, Compalati E et al (2011) Grading quality of evidence and strength of recommendations in clinical practice guidelines. Part 3 of 3. The GRADE approach to developing recommendations. Allergy 66:588–595
3. Brozek JL, Akl EA, Jaeschke R et al (2009) Grading quality of evidence and strength of recommendations in clinical practice guidelines. Part 2 of 3. The GRADE approach to grading quality of evidence about diagnostic tests and strategies. Allergy 64:1109–1116
4. Safar P (1958) Ventilatory efficacy of mouth-to-mouth artificial respiration; airway obstruction during manual and mouth-to-mouth artificial respiration. JAMA 167:335–341
5. Kouwenhoven WB, Jude JR, Knickerbocker GG (1960) Closed-chest cardiac massage. JAMA 173:1064–1067
6. National Research Council (1966) Cardiopulmonary resuscitation: statement by the Ad Hoc Committee on Cardiopulmonary Resuscitation, of the Division of Medical Sciences. JAMA 198:372–379
7. JAMA (1974) Standards for cardiopulmonary resuscitation (CPR) and emergency cardiac care (ECC). Advanced life support. JAMA 227:(Suppl);852–860
8. American Heart Association (1980) Standards and guidelines for cardiopulmonary resuscitation (CPR) and emergency cardiac care (ECC). JAMA 244:453–509
9. Chamberlain D (1992) Editorial introducing ERC guidelines. Resuscitation 24:99–101
10. JAMA (1992) Guidelines for cardiopulmonary resuscitation (CPR) and emergency cardiac care (ECC). JAMA 286:2135–2302
11. Cummins RO, Chamberlain DA, Abramson NS et al (1991) Recommended guidelines for uniform reporting of data from out-of-hospital cardiac arrest: the Utstein style. A statement for health professionals from a task force of the American Heart Association, the European Resuscitation Council, the Heart and Stroke Foundation of Canada, and the Australian Resuscitation Council. Circulation 84:960–975
12. Zaritsky A, Nadkarni V, Hazinski MF et al (1995) Recommended guidelines for uniform reporting of pediatric advanced life support: the pediatric Utstein style. A statement for healthcare professionals from a task force of the American Academy of Pediatrics, the American Heart Association, and the European Resuscitation Council. Resuscitation 30:95–115
13. Idris AH, Becker LB, Ornato JP et al (1996) Utstein-style guidelines for uniform reporting of laboratory CPR research. A statement for healthcare professionals from a task force of the American Heart Association, the American College of Emergency Physicians, the American

College of Cardiology, the European Resuscitation Council, the Heart and Stroke Foundation of Canada, the Institute of Critical Care Medicine, the Safar Center for Resuscitation Research, and the Society for Academic Emergency Medicine. Resuscitation 33:69–84

14. Cummins RO, Chamberlain D, Hazinski MF et al (1997) Recommended guidelines for reviewing, reporting, and conducting research on in-hospital resuscitation: the in-hospital 'Utstein style'. A statement for healthcare professionals from the American Heart Association, the European Resuscitation Council, the Heart and Stroke Foundation of Canada, the Australian Resuscitation Council, and the Resuscitation Councils of Southern Africa. Resuscitation 34:151–183

15. Kattwinkel J, Niermeyer S, Nadkarni V et al (1999) Resuscitation of the newly born infant: an advisory statement from the pediatric working group of the international liaison committee on resuscitation. Resuscitation 40:71–88

16. Idris AH, Berg RA, Bierens J et al (2003) Recommended guidelines for uniform reporting of data from drowning: the "Utstein style". Resuscitation 59:45–57

17. Langhelle A, Nolan J, Herlitz J et al (2005) Recommended guidelines for reviewing, reporting, and conducting research on post-resuscitation care: the Utstein style. Resuscitation 66:271–283

18. Peberdy MA, Cretikos M, Abella BS et al (2007) Recommended guidelines for monitoring, reporting, and conducting research on medical emergency team, outreach, and rapid response systems: an Utstein-style scientific statement. A Scientific Statement from the International Liaison Committee on Resuscitation; the American Heart Association Emergency Cardiovascular Care Committee; the Council on Cardiopulmonary, Perioperative, and Critical Care; and the Interdisciplinary Working Group on Quality of Care and Outcomes Research. Resuscitation 75:412–433

19. Castren M, Bohm K, Kvam AM et al (2011) Reporting of data from out-of-hospital cardiac arrest has to involve emergency medical dispatching—taking the recommendations on reporting OHCA the Utstein style a step further. Resuscitation 82:1496–1500

20. Jacobs I, Nadkarni V, Bahr J et al (2004) Cardiac arrest and cardiopulmonary resuscitation outcome reports: update and simplification of the Utstein templates for resuscitation registries. A statement for healthcare professionals from a task force of the International Liaison Committee on Resuscitation (American Heart Association, European Resuscitation Council, Australian Resuscitation Council, New Zealand Resuscitation Council, Heart and Stroke Foundation of Canada, Inter American Heart Foundation, Resuscitation Council of Southern Africa). Resuscitation 63:233–249

21. Nolan JP, Nadkarni VM, Billi JE et al (2010) 2010 International Consensus on cardiopulmonary resuscitation and emergency cardiovascular care science with treatment recommendations. Part 2: international collaboration in resuscitation science. Resuscitation 81:e26–e31

22. Chamberlain D (2005) The International Liaison Committee on Resuscitation (ILCOR)—past and present: compiled by the Founding Members of the International Liaison Committee on Resuscitation. Resuscitation 67:157–161

23. Chamberlain D, Cummins RO (1993) International emergency cardiac care: support, science, and universal guidelines. Ann Emerg Med 22(pt 2):508–511

24. Zaritsky A, Nadkarni V, Hazinski M et al (1995) Recommended guidelines for uniform reporting of pediatric advanced life support: the pediatric Utstein style. Circulation 92:2006–2020

25. Cummins RO, Chamberlain DA (1997) Advisory statements of the International Liaison Committee on Resuscitation. Circulation 95:2172–2173

26. Handley AJ, Becker LB, Allen M, van Drenth A, Kramer EB, Montgomery WH (1997) Single-rescuer adult basic life support: an advisory statement from the basic life support working group of the International Liaison Committee on Resuscitation. Circulation 95:2174–2179

27. Kloeck W, Cummins RO, Chamberlain D et al (1997) The universal advanced life support algorithm: an advisory statement from the Advanced Life Support Working Group of the International Liaison Committee on Resuscitation. Circulation 95:2180–2182

28. Kloeck W, Cummins RO, Chamberlain D et al (1997) Early defibrillation: an advisory statement from the Advanced Life Support Working Group of the International Liaison Committee on Resuscitation. Circulation 95:2183–2184

29. Nadkarni V, Hazinski MF, Zideman D et al (1997) Pediatric resuscitation: an advisory statement from the pediatric working group of the International Liaison Committee on Resuscitation. Circulation 95:2185–2195

30. Kloeck W, Cummins RO, Chamberlain D et al (1997) Special resuscitation situations: an advisory statement from the International Liaison Committee on Resuscitation. Circulation 95:2196–2210

31. Cummins RO, Chamberlain D, Hazinski MF et al (1997) Recommended guidelines for reviewing, reporting, and conducting research on in-hospital resuscitation: the in-hospital 'Utstein style' American Heart Association. Circulation 95:2213–2239

32. Kattwinkel J, Niermeyer S, Nadkarni V et al (1999) ILCOR advisory statement: resuscitation of the newly born infant. An advisory statement from the pediatric working group of the International Liaison Committee on Resuscitation. Circulation 99:1927–1938

33. American Heart Association (2000) American Heart Association in collaboration with International Liaison Committee on Resuscitation. Guidelines for cardiopulmonary resuscitation and emergency cardiovascular care. Circulation 102(suppl):I1–I384

34. Nolan JP, Morley PT, Vanden Hoek TL et al (2003) Therapeutic hypothermia after cardiac arrest: an advisory statement by the advanced life support task force of the International Liaison Committee on Resuscitation. Circulation 108:118–121

35. Samson R, Berg R, Bingham R, Pediatric Advanced Life Support Task Force ILCoR (2003) Use of automated external defibrillators for children: an update. An advisory statement from the pediatric advanced life support task force, International Liaison Committee on Resuscitation. Resuscitation 57:237–243

36. Chamberlain DA, Hazinski MF (2003) Education in resuscitation. Resuscitation 59:11–43

37. Jacobs I, Nadkarni V, Bahr J et al (2004) Cardiac arrest and cardiopulmonary resuscitation outcome reports: update and simplification of the Utstein templates for resuscitation registries: a statement for healthcare professionals from a task force of the International Liaison Committee on Resuscitation (American Heart Association, European Resuscitation Council, Australian Resuscitation Council, New Zealand Resuscitation Council, Heart and Stroke Foundation of Canada, Inter-American Heart Foundation, Resuscitation Councils of Southern Africa). Circulation 110:3385–3397

38. Proceedings of the 2005 international consensus on cardiopulmonary resuscitation and emergency cardiovascular care science with treatment recommendations. Resuscitation 67:157–341

39. Gazmuri RJ, Nadkarni VM, Nolan JP et al (2007) Scientific knowledge gaps and clinical research priorities for cardiopulmonary resuscitation and emergency cardiovascular care identified during the 2005 international consensus conference on ECC (corrected) and CPR science with treatment recommendations: a consensus statement from the International Liaison Committee on Resuscitation (American Heart Association, Australian Resuscitation Council, European Resuscitation Council, Heart and Stroke Foundation of Canada, InterAmerican Heart Foundation, Resuscitation Council of Southern Africa, and the New Zealand Resuscitation Council); the American Heart Association Emergency Cardiovascular Care Committee; the Stroke Council; and the Cardiovascular Nursing Council. Circulation 116:2501–2512

40. Peberdy MA, Cretikos M, Abella BS et al (2007) Recommended guidelines for monitoring, reporting, and conducting research on medical emergency team, outreach, and rapid response systems: an Utstein-style scientific statement: a scientific statement from the International Liaison Committee on Resuscitation (American Heart Association, Australian Resuscitation

Council, European Resuscitation Council, Heart and Stroke Foundation of Canada, InterAmerican Heart Foundation, Resuscitation Council of Southern Africa, and the New Zealand Resuscitation Council); the American Heart Association Emergency Cardiovascular Care Committee; the Council on Cardiopulmonary, Perioperative, and Critical Care; and the Interdisciplinary Working Group on Quality of Care and Outcomes Research. Circulation 116:2481–2500

41. Neumar RW, Nolan JP, Adrie C et al (2008) Post-cardiac arrest syndrome: epidemiology, pathophysiology, treatment, and prognostication. A consensus statement from the International Liaison Committee on Resuscitation (American Heart Association, Australian and New Zealand Council on Resuscitation, European Resuscitation Council, Heart and Stroke Foundation of Canada, Inter American Heart Foundation, Resuscitation Council of Asia, and the Resuscitation Council of Southern Africa); the American Heart Association Emergency Cardiovascular Care Committee; the Council on Cardiovascular Surgery and Anesthesia; the Council on Cardiopulmonary, Perioperative, and Critical Care; the Council on Clinical Cardiology; and the Stroke Council. Circulation 118:2452–2483

42. Nolan JP, Hazinski MF, Billi JE et al (2010) Part 1: executive summary: 2010 International consensus on cardiopulmonary resuscitation and emergency cardiovascular care science with treatment recommendations. Resuscitation 81(Suppl 1):e1–e25

43. Chamberlain DA, Hazinski MF (2003) Education in resuscitation: an ILCOR symposium: Utstein Abbey: Stavanger, Norway: June 22–24, 2001. Circulation 108:2575–2594

44. Nolan JP, Morley PT, Vanden Hoek TL, Hickey RW (2003) Therapeutic hypothermia after cardiac arrest. An advisory statement by the advancement life support task force of the International Liaison Committee on Resuscitation. Resuscitation 57:231–235

45. Anonymous (2000) Guidelines 2000 for cardiopulmonary resuscitation and emergency cardiovascular care—an international consensus on science. Resuscitation 46:1–447

46. Morley PT, Zaritsky A (2005) The evidence evaluation process for the 2005 international consensus conference on cardiopulmonary resuscitation and emergency cardiovascular care science with treatment recommendations. Resuscitation 67:167–170

47. Morley PT, Atkins DL, Billi JE et al (2010) Part 3: evidence evaluation process: 2010 international consensus on cardiopulmonary resuscitation and emergency cardiovascular care science with treatment recommendations. Resuscitation 81(Suppl 1):e32–e40

48. Grimshaw J, Eccles M, Tetroe J (2004) Implementing clinical guidelines: current evidence and future implications. J Contin Educ Health Prof 24(Suppl 1):S31–S37

49. Toma A, Bensimon CM, Dainty KN, Rubenfeld GD, Morrison LJ, Brooks SC (2010) Perceived barriers to therapeutic hypothermia for patients resuscitated from cardiac arrest: a qualitative study of emergency department and critical care workers. Crit Care Med 38:504–509

50. Feder G, Eccles M, Grol R, Griffiths C, Grimshaw J (1999) Clinical guidelines: using clinical guidelines. BMJ 318:728–730

51. Berdowski J, Schmohl A, Tijssen JG, Koster RW (2009) Time needed for a regional emergency medical system to implement resuscitation guidelines 2005—The Netherlands experience. Resuscitation 80:1336–1341

52. Binks AC, Murphy RE, Prout RE et al (2010) Therapeutic hypothermia after cardiac arrest—implementation in UK intensive care units. Anaesthesia 65:260–265

53. Raine R, Sanderson C, Black N (2005) Developing clinical guidelines: a challenge to current methods. BMJ 331:631–633

54. Meaney PA, Nadkarni VM, Kern KB, Indik JH, Halperin HR, Berg RA (2010) Rhythms and outcomes of adult in-hospital cardiac arrest. Crit Care Med 38:101–108

55. Iwami T, Nichol G, Hiraide A et al (2009) Continuous improvements in "chain of survival" increased survival after out-of-hospital cardiac arrests: a large-scale population-based study. Circulation 119:728–734

56. Lund-Kordahl I, Olasveengen TM, Lorem T, Samdal M, Wik L, Sunde K (2010) Improving outcome after out-of-hospital cardiac arrest by strengthening weak links of the local chain of survival; quality of advanced life support and post-resuscitation care. Resuscitation 81:422–426

57. Gazmuri RJ, Nolan JP, Nadkarni VM et al (2007) Scientific knowledge gaps and clinical research priorities for cardiopulmonary resuscitation and emergency cardiovascular care identified during the 2005 international consensus conference on ECC and CPR science with treatment recommendations. A consensus statement from the international liaison committee on resuscitation; the American Heart Association Emergency Cardiovascular Care Committee; the Stroke Council; and the Cardiovascular Nursing Council. Resuscitation 75:400–411

58. Shuster M, Billi JE, Bossaert L et al (2010) Part 4: conflict of interest management before, during, and after the 2010 international consensus conference on cardiopulmonary resuscitation and emergency cardiovascular care science with treatment recommendations. Resuscitation 81(Suppl 1):e41–e47

59. Field JM, Hazinski MF, Sayre MR et al (2010) Part 1: executive summary: 2010 American heart association guidelines for cardiopulmonary resuscitation and emergency cardiovascular care. Circulation 122:S640–S656

60. Nolan JP, Soar J, Zideman DA et al (2010) European resuscitation council guidelines for resuscitation 2010 section 1 executive summary. Resuscitation 81:1219–1276

61. Brooks SC, Morrison LJ (2008) Implementation of therapeutic hypothermia guidelines for post-cardiac arrest syndrome at a glacial pace: seeking guidance from the knowledge translation literature. Resuscitation 77:286–292

62. Grol R, Grimshaw J (2003) From best evidence to best practice: effective implementation of change in patients' care. Lancet 362:1225–1230

63. Bradley EH, Holmboe ES, Mattera JA, Roumanis SA, Radford MJ, Krumholz HM (2001) A qualitative study of increasing beta-blocker use after myocardial infarction: why do some hospitals succeed? JAMA 285:2604–2611

64. Berwick DM (2003) Disseminating innovations in health care. JAMA 289:1969–1975

65. Grol R (1997) Personal paper. Beliefs and evidence in changing clinical practice. BMJ 315:418–421

66. Guyatt G, Oxman AD, Akl EA et al (2011) GRADE guidelines: 1. Introduction—GRADE evidence profiles and summary of findings tables. J Clin Epidemiol 64:383–394

Trauma Systems and Trauma Care

3

Kelly N. Vogt, Philip D. Lumb and Demetrios Demetriades

3.1 Introduction

Trauma systems are designed to care optimally for a population and its injured members. These systems extend far beyond in-hospital care of the injured patient. They must also include injury prevention, prehospital care, hospital care, education, and research, as well as long-term rehabilitation and recovery. Trauma systems require coordination between hospitals, physicians, nurses, allied health professionals, policy makers, governing bodies, community leaders, and many others to be successful. This review will describe the history and development of trauma systems, the key components of such systems, and the impact that trauma systems have on a population.

K. N. Vogt · D. Demetriades (✉)
Trauma & Surgical Critical Care, LA County/University of Southern California,
2051 Marengo Street, Los Angeles, CA 90033, USA
e-mail: demetria@usc.edu

K. N. Vogt
e-mail: Kelly.vogt@gmail.com

P. D. Lumb
Department of Anaesthesiology, Keck School of Medicine and the University of Southern
California, 1520 San Pablo Street, Los Angeles, CA 90033, USA
e-mail: lumb@med.usc.edu

A. Gullo and G. Ristagno (eds.), *Resuscitation*,
DOI: 10.1007/978-88-470-5507-0_3, © Springer-Verlag Italia 2014

3.2   History of Trauma Systems and the Development of the American Trauma System

Although the foundations arose from military conflicts, the American College of Surgeons Committee on Trauma was instrumental in the creation of the modern day trauma system in America. In 1966, the Committee on Shock and the Committee on Trauma of the Division of Medical Sciences of the National Academy of Science/National Research Council published the landmark "Accidental Death and Disability: The Neglected Disease of Modern Society" [1]. In this report, injury was identified as the "neglected epidemic," and leadership to overcome this epidemic was encouraged. The focus of this document was on research, education, and training for those involved in the care of the injured patient from the prehospital phase to the acute care institution. As such, the initial trauma systems in this country were focused primarily on the prevention of unnecessary death in the severely injured patient [2]. The "Accidental Death and Disability" report laid the groundwork for what would eventually become trauma center designations, as well as the emergence of the specialty of Emergency Medicine [1]. The concept of trauma registries and quality improvement can also be traced back to this report, with a brief mention also made on the need for research, education, and regulations aimed at injury prevention.

After the publication of "Accidental Death and Disability," regionalized trauma systems began to emerge throughout the US, starting in Maryland, Illinois, and Virginia [3]. These efforts were furthered in the late 1970s by the American College of Surgeons Committee on Trauma publication "Optimal Hospital Resources for the Care of the Seriously Injured" [4]. This document provided a framework not only for care, but also for evaluation of care, and for the first time, suggested criteria for the categorization of hospitals based on the ability to provide varying degrees of trauma care. There have been multiple revisions of this document since its initial publication, and references can be found in the operating procedures of many American trauma centers.

In the early 1980s, in response to the personal tragedy of an orthopedic surgeon, the American College of Surgeons Committee on Trauma initiated the Advanced Trauma Life Support (ATLS) Course [5]. The ATLS course is designed to train all providers in the initial stabilization and life-saving techniques vital in the early management of the critically injured patient. Training in the standardized initial assessment and management of the injured patient has been shown to improve knowledge of what to do in an emergency situation [6], as well as outcomes [7], and has become an important part of many trauma systems.

Finally, as trauma systems have evolved, so has the understanding that the focus must expand from the immediate care of the injured patient to include prevention, education, and long-term recovery [2]. The National Research Council published a document entitled "Injury in America: A Continuing Health Care Problem" in 1985 [8]. This report outlined the progress to date on the development of trauma systems, and, while recognizing the importance of the trauma systems present at the time, the overall progress toward organization was felt to be limited. Further, the importance of research on epidemiology and injury prevention was again stressed in this document, coinciding with a decision to identify the Centers for Disease Control as the coordinating body for American injury research.

Today, both the American College of Surgeons Committee on Trauma and the American College of Emergency Physicians work with a goal of improving the care of the injured patient [9]. The foundations laid have contributed to the ongoing development of trauma systems and, though the process continues to be in evolution, have educated the involved parties on the importance of such systems.

3.3   Components of a Trauma System

3.3.1   Prehospital Care

Efficient and effective identification, management, and transportation of patients from the scene of injury to specialized trauma centers are essential components of any trauma system. For those sustaining injury, prehospital personnel will be the first point of contact with the trauma system, and these personnel, along with the system in which they work, can have a direct impact on the patient's outcome. A comprehensive trauma system requires easy access to the system in the prehospital setting. Further, both the training of the prehospital personnel and the mechanisms in place to safely and expeditiously transport patients are vital.

Trained Emergency Medical personnel deliver the majority of prehospital care. Providers are typically Emergency Medical Technicians (EMTs), trained and certified for varying degrees including basic and advanced life support [9]. The job of these EMTs extends beyond the clinical patient care provided to include important roles in triage and prioritization, as well as education and safety. Triage in the prehospital setting can be a complex process, and includes adequately determining the appropriate facility to which to transport a given patient to, as well as determining which patients to prioritize when faced with a multiple casualty situation. EMTs work within a system that requires coordinated transportation systems, as well as access to remote backup from experienced EMTs and physician medical directors [9]. In extreme circumstances, it may even be necessary for trained medical personnel, including physicians, to travel to the prehospital setting to assist with triage or medical care of patients who cannot be evacuated, and an effective prehospital system will have a mode to facilitate this process.

In the presence of highly trained EMTs, the question arises as to whether or not time should be spent stabilizing the patient in the field, or if it is better to "scoop and run" to the nearest hospital or trauma center. Despite the clinical skills of many EMTs, procedures and interventions beyond the level of basic life support in urban centers have not been shown to improve outcomes, and in fact may worsen outcomes compared to patients who are simply removed from the scene and rapidly transported to more definitive care [10, 11]. A similar strategy of minimal intervention applies to prehospital fluid resuscitation, with evidence supporting restriction of fluid administration prior to hospital arrival [12]. Delays in transport to a trauma center, even when patients are transported quickly to hospital, appear to be associated with an increased mortality [13].

Much has been written on the most efficient way to transport the injured patient. The most common modes discussed include ground transportation, helicopter, and fixed wing aircraft. Though helicopter transport was considered by many to be ideal, the importance of location is paramount in the discussion of the ideal mode of transportation, as are local factors including weather and traffic. Further, identification of the severely injured patient most likely to benefit from helicopter transport is essential [14, 15]. Heterogeneity in the literature surrounding the impact of helicopter transport on the outcomes for trauma patients makes definitive conclusions difficult. A recent Cochrane review of this topic concluded that an accurate composite estimate of the benefits of helicopter emergency medical services could not be made based on the available evidence, and that further research is required in this area [16]. What appears clear from the literature is that the most rapid form of transport is likely the best [9]. Therefore, for patients in urban areas at the time of injury, there may be little benefit to air transportation over traditional ground transportation [15]. Additionally, in this setting, there may be an increased risk associated with the risk of crash during air transportation. For patients in rural settings at the time of trauma, this risk is outweighed by the benefit of expedited transport to specialized care that is typically some distance away.

3.3.2 Hospital Care

Of all the components of a trauma system, the hospital care of the injured patient is the most discussed, and therefore the most established. As previously mentioned, the initial foundations of trauma systems focused on the in-hospital care of the injured patient, from the initial resuscitation to the operative management to the post-injury convalescence and prevention of secondary insult. The importance of a coordinated effort in response to the arrival of a trauma patient cannot be understated, and will be discussed further below.

To better delineate a given hospital's capabilities to manage the acute trauma patient, the concept of trauma center verification was introduced. This process involves evaluating a given center in five key areas: institution commitment to trauma care; injury volume and acuity; facility layout, dedicated material, and human resources; operation of the clinical trauma team; and the trauma performance improvement program [17]. Verification of these components and designation of a trauma center level are performed in many places by the American College of Surgeons, though it is important to recognize that this task may fall to other bodies as well. Trauma centers are designated from level I to level IV based on available resources and involvement in trauma systems. Level I trauma centers are leaders in the trauma field, and are the specialists in trauma care. Level IV trauma centers are typically found in small rural areas, and focus only on initial stabilization of the patient prior to transfer to a larger facility for definitive management. The American College of Surgeons recently recommended that all level I trauma centers admit at least 1,200 patients per year, with at least 240 of these being severely injured, while others suggest a threshold of 915 patients, irrespective of injury severity [18]. Though the exact number of patients required appears to remain unknown, it is clear that level I trauma centers should be high-volume centers to maximize patient outcomes.

Triage, though traditionally thought of in the prehospital setting, also has an important role to play in in-hospital care. Some patients will be initially triaged to a hospital without the expertise or resources required for their care, while others will develop complications requiring more specialized care. In such circumstances, a rapid method for identification and transfer of such patients to an appropriate center must exist. The risks of patient transport should be balanced against the need for more specialized care [19, 20]. Further, even within a specialized trauma center, multiple patients may require care with limited resources. In such circumstances, physicians must decide how best to share these limited resources for the best possible care of all patients.

3.3.3 Rehabilitation

In recent years, more recognition is being given to the importance of post-injury rehabilitation. The majority of trauma patients are young, previously healthy, productive members of society. As such, the importance of rehabilitation to the previous level of functioning is paramount.

The process of rehabilitation includes both physical and psychological components, and should begin as early as possible in the patient's injury course [21]. A recent retrospective review by Clark and colleagues compared trauma and burn intensive care unit patients before and after implementation of an early mobility program [22]. Early mobilization was associated with a decrease in pulmonary and vascular complications without an increase in adverse events. In recovery from brain injury, active high-intensity rehabilitation programs have been shown to lead to improved functional outcomes particularly in those with injury due to trauma [23]. With admission to acute inpatient rehabilitation, the majority of patients with even severe traumatic brain injury will be able to achieve independent ambulation [24], an outcome of significant importance post-injury. The importance of psychosocial support must also be recognized post-injury. Strategies shown to be effective to assist in psychosocial rehabilitation and coping with post-injury include inpatient counseling, acute rehabilitation, and telephone-based community counseling [25–27]. Such strategies should be in place for a successful trauma system. Further, up to 32 % of patients may develop posttraumatic stress disorder after trauma, and early identification and psychological intervention should be considered for successful prevention and recovery [28, 29].

3.3.4 Injury Prevention, Education, and Research

It is estimated that over 50 % of deaths due to trauma are preventable in the preinjury phase [30], and as such, the importance of strategies to prevent injury in the first place cannot be overestimated. In fact, prevention may be considered the most important part of any trauma system, though it is often overlooked in favor of the management of the injured patient. A recent policy review published by Kone and colleagues highlighted some of the Centers for Disease Control and Prevention's injury prevention success stories from the last decade [31]. These include the impact of laws for maximum blood alcohol concentration while operating a motorized vehicle, the use of child restraints, and programs aimed at the prevention of shaken baby syndrome. This review also highlighted the ongoing need for not only research, but also for outcome evaluation and knowledge translation. On the twentieth anniversary of the establishment of the National Center for Injury Prevention and Control of the Centers for Disease Control and Prevention, Greenspan and colleagues published an additional review of the Center's injury prevention work [32]. The Injury Center focus lies in four areas: Motor vehicle-related injury, traumatic brain injury, violence against children and youth, and prescription drug overdose. Despite these identified foci, however, the Injury Center attempts to apply the public health model to any injury pattern to identify prevention strategies and assist in the implementation of such strategies [32].

One important component of both research and quality improvement is the trauma database or registry. Many individual institutions maintain databases of prospectively collected demographic, injury, management, and outcome data on all admitted patients during the acute phase after injury [33, 34]. State-wide registries, with both mandatory and voluntary reporting, also exist [33]. The National Trauma Databank is maintained by the American College of Surgeons, and contains data voluntarily contributed by level I and II trauma centers throughout the country [35]. Trauma registries can be linked to population-level administrative databases to further improve their inclusiveness [36]. Trauma registries have numerous applications, including quality improvement, evaluation of clinical interventions, identifying areas for prevention, and assessment of both pre and posthospital care [33]. Further, despite the limitations of database-driven research, these registries provide a rich dataset for conducting retrospective research, and for identifying areas for prospective research.

3.3.5 Quality Improvement

The ongoing assessment of the structure and function of a trauma system is imperative to its success. Although quality improvement initiatives should exist at all levels of a trauma system, perhaps the most recognized is at the level of the trauma center itself. Quality improvement initiated at the trauma center can reach to all levels of the system and intervene when required. Bailey and colleagues outline the quality indicators for trauma center performance in their 2012 review [17]. The first is phases of care, including the prehospital, hospital, posthospital, and secondary prevention phases. Second is the structure, including triage, information sharing, rehabilitation referral, and prevention such as alcohol screening. Third is the process, including response times of EMS, wait times in the ED and hospital, and alcohol recidivism. Fourth, and finally, is outcome, including not only mortality, but also admission to long-term care and the incidence of recurrent injury. It is important to recognize that this is just one scheme through which to approach quality improvement, as there is a paucity of evidence to support any particular scheme as it relates to outcomes. Nonetheless, a scheme should remain in place to allow ongoing improvement in any trauma system.

At the level of an individual hospital, even a well-established level I trauma center will have preventable or potentially preventable mortalities and morbidities [30, 37]. A system must therefore be in place to identify and learn from these cases to aid in future prevention [37]. This typically occurs in the form of a regularly scheduled morbidity and mortality conference, designed to provide a forum for open discussion and review of complicated patient encounters [38, 39]. Beyond the individual hospital level, an informative analysis highlighting ongoing quality improvement at the system level was published by Cryer and colleagues in 2010 [40]. Their analysis focused on two train mass-casualty incidents in Los Angeles. After the first crash in 2005, a problem with triage to trauma centers was identified. The majority of patients were triaged to community hospitals as opposed to the trauma centers, and this was felt to have been related to suboptimal patient outcomes. As such, a task force was convened to address the system-wide issues, and to develop a new disaster policy in Los Angeles County. With this new policy in place, a second train crash in 2008 was handled with greater ease, and the vast majority of patients were taken directly to a trauma center. On an even bigger scale, the Trauma Quality Improvement Program was recently created by the American College of Surgeons [17, 41]. This program is the first of its kind, designed to provide a risk-adjusted outcome assessment for participating institutions, and a benchmark to compare to other similar institutions [17, 41]. Although in its infancy, programs such as this can be expected to contribute to the ongoing quality improvement of trauma centers and systems.

3.4 The Impact of Trauma Systems

The development of trauma systems has impacted favorably on patient outcomes. Although it is difficult to measure the improvements made in injury prevention, it is somewhat easier to identify the metric associated with system-wide change. For example, it has been shown repeatedly that the American College of Surgeons Committee on Trauma verification process has led to improved outcomes. The reasons for this are certainly multifactorial, but the role that the system plays in this improvement must be recognized. As suggested by Bailey and colleagues in their review of trauma systems, the commitment of a facility to the resources for trauma care, as well as the synergy spanning from the highest levels of leadership to the staff, play an important role [17].

Shackford and colleagues were among the first to assess the impact of trauma systems on outcome, and found that, compared to an index population, those triaged to trauma centers after both blunt and penetrating trauma had survival rates much higher than predicted [42]. The authors attributed this improved survival to the integration of prehospital and hospital care, and to rapid surgical intervention. In 1995, Demetriades and colleagues reported on the impact of a dedicated trauma program after implementation at the Los Angeles County-University of Southern California Medical Center [43]. This before–after study demonstrated a 43 % reduction in mortality after penetrating trauma, and a 33 % reduction after blunt trauma, supporting continued investment in the development of dedicated trauma programs.

More recently, Durham and colleagues assessed the impact of a mature trauma system in the state of Florida in 2006 [44]. Results from this study demonstrated an 18 % reduction in the risk of death associated with appropriate triage to a trauma center.

Similarly, the National Study on the Cost and outcomes of Trauma demonstrated a 25 % lower risk of death for those cared for in a level I trauma center [45]. Further, data from this same study were used to demonstrate management in a level I trauma center to be cost-effective based on quality adjusted life years gained, particularly for more severely injured and younger patients [46]. In an analysis of the Glue Grant Trauma Database, Nirula and colleagues demonstrated that patients who were initially triaged to a non-trauma hospital had a 3.8 times higher odds of death than those triaged to a trauma center [13]. The impact of trauma center verification has also been shown for centers that have not achieved level I status. Piontek and colleagues published a before–after study looking at the impact of achieving level II status in a community hospital, and demonstrated a reduction in mortality and cost as well as a reduction in length of hospital stay [47]. Beyond verification, trauma system processes also appear to have a beneficial impact. The importance of a dedicated trauma inpatient service to oversee the complexities of multidisciplinary patient care was highlighted by Davis and colleagues [48]. This study demonstrated that, despite an increase in clinical volume, system efficiency increased significantly with the introduction of a dedicated trauma team. Ryb and colleagues recently assessed the impact of a delay in activation of the in-hospital trauma team for patients meeting activation criteria, and found this delay to be associated with increased morbidity, including length of hospital stay and associated need for rehabilitation after discharge [49].

3.5   The Current State of US Trauma Systems

By 2011, 90 % of the states in America had a state-wide trauma system [17]. Although systems vary widely, the adoption of recommendations for creating a framework for the care of the community and of the injured patient is encouraging. Experts in the field value trauma systems, including leadership, evaluation, research, and formalized operations and procedures [50]. Less encouraging is the fact that, of these state trauma systems, only 60 % are funded at present [17]. A lack of funding for a trauma system suggests questionable sustainability, and may lead to a lapse in the quality of care provided within that system. As such, funding needs to be aggressively pursued to maintain quality trauma care.

3.6   Conclusions

Trauma systems have an extremely important role to play in a community, and the development of such systems continues to evolve. A controlled and integrated response to trauma that is subject to critical review and quality improvement initiatives improves outcomes for the community and its victims of trauma. Continued work should focus on the adequate funding of such systems, and ongoing assessment of emerging strategies for prevention, acute management, and rehabilitation of the trauma patient.

References

1. National Academy of Sciences (1966) Accidental death and disability: the neglected disease of modern society. National Academy of Sciences, Washington
2. Mullins RJ (1999) A historical perspective of trauma system development in the United States. J Trauma Acute Care Surg 47:S8
3. Boyd DR (1973) A symposium on the Illinois trauma program: a systems approach to the care of the critically injured. Introduction: a controlled systems approach to trauma patient care. J Trauma 13:275–276
4. Optimal hospital resources for care of the seriously injured (Bull Am Coll Surg. 1976)—PubMed—NCBI. libproxy.usc.edu (cited Apr 23, 2013). https://libproxy.usc.edu/login?url= http://www.usc.edu/libraries/services/remote_access/
5. Jayaraman S, Sethi D (2009) Advanced trauma life support training for hospital staff, Cochrane Database of Systematic Reviews 2009, Issue 2, American College of Surgeons Advanced Trauma Life Support. http://www.facs.org/trauma/atls. pp 1–7
6. Jayaraman S, Sethi D (2010) Advanced trauma life support training for hospital staff, Cochrane Database of Systematic Reviews 2009, Issue 2, American College of Surgeons Advanced Trauma LIfe Support. http://www.facs.org/trauma/atls. pp 1–17
7. Ali J, Adam R, Butler AK et al (1993) Trauma outcome improves following the advanced trauma life support program in a developing country. J Trauma 34:890–898; (discussion 898–899)
8. National Research Council (1985) Injury in America: a continuing health care problem. National Academy Press, Washington

9. Blackwell T, Kellam JF, Thomason M (2003) Trauma care systems in the United States. Injury 34:735–739
10. Smith RM, Conn AK (2009) Prehospital care–scoop and run or stay and play? Injury 40:S23–S26
11. Haas B, Nathens AB (2008) Pro/con debate: is the scoop and run approach the best approach to trauma services organization? Critical care (London, England) 12:224
12. Cotton BA, Jerome R, Collier BR et al (2009) Guidelines for prehospital fluid resuscitation in the injured patient. J Trauma 67:389–402
13. Nirula R, Maier R, Moore E et al (2010) Scoop and run to the trauma center or stay and play at the local hospital: hospital transfer's effect on mortality. J Trauma 69:595–601
14. Bledsoe BE, Wesley AK, Eckstein M et al (2006) Helicopter scene transport of trauma patients with nonlife-threatening injuries: a meta-analysis. J Trauma 60:1257–1266
15. Talving P, Teixeira PGR, Barmparas G et al (2009) Helicopter evacuation of trauma victims in Los Angeles: does it improve survival? World J Surg 33:2469–2476
16. Galvagno SM Jr, Thomas S, Stephens C, Haut ER, Hirshon JM, Floccare D, Pronovost P (2012) Helicopter emergency medical services for adults with major trauma. Wiley, New York, pp 1–51
17. Bailey J, Trexler S, Murdock A, Hoyt D (2012) Verification and regionalization of trauma systems. Surg Clin N Am 92:1009–1024
18. Diggs BS, Mullins RJ, Hedges JR et al (2008) Proportion of seriously injured patients admitted to hospitals in the US with a high annual injured patient volume: a metric of regionalized trauma care. J Am Coll Surg 206:212–219
19. Andrews PJ, Piper IR, Dearden NM et al (1990) Secondary insults during intrahospital transport of head-injured patients. Lancet 335:327–330
20. Olson CM, Jastremski MS, Vilogi JP et al (1987) Stabilization of patients prior to interhospital transfer. Am J Emerg Med 5:33–39
21. Browne AL, Appleton S, Fong K et al (2012) A pilot randomized controlled trial of an early multidisciplinary model to prevent disability following traumatic injury. Disabil Rehabil 1–15
22. Clark DE, Lowman JD, Griffin RL et al (2013) Effectiveness of an early mobilization protocol in a trauma and burns intensive care unit: a retrospective cohort study. Phys Ther 93:186–196
23. Katz DI, Polyak M, Coughlan D et al (2009) Natural history of recovery from brain injury after prolonged disorders of consciousness outcome of patients admitted to inpatient rehabilitation with 1–4 year follow-up. Elsevier, Berlin
24. Katz DI, White DK, Alexander MP et al (2004) Recovery of ambulation after traumatic brain injury. Arch Phys Med Rehabil 85:865–869
25. Heinemann AW, Wilson CS, Huston T et al (2012) Relationship of psychology inpatient rehabilitation services and patient characteristics to outcomes following spinal cord injury: the SCIRehab project. J Spinal Cord Med 35:578–592
26. Aitken LM, Chaboyer W, Schuetz M et al (2012) Health status of critically ill trauma patients. J Clin Nurs. doi: 10.1111/jocn.12026
27. Dorstyn DS, Mathias JL, Denson LA (2011) Psychosocial outcomes of telephone-based counseling for adults with an acquired physical disability: a meta-analysis. Rehabil Psychol 56:1–14
28. Holbrook TL, Hoyt DB, Stein MB et al (2001) Perceived threat to life predicts posttraumatic stress disorder after major trauma: risk factors and functional outcome. J Trauma 51:287–292; (discussion 292–293)
29. Malcoun E, Houry D, Arndt-Jordan C et al (2010) Feasibility of identifying eligible trauma patients for posttraumatic stress disorder intervention. West J Emerg Med 11:274–278
30. Stewart RM, Myers JG, Dent DL et al (2003) Seven hundred fifty-three consecutive deaths in a level I trauma center: the argument for injury prevention. J Trauma 54:66–70; (discussion 70–71)

31. Koné RG, Zurick E, Patterson S et al (2012) Injury and violence prevention policy: celebrating our successes, protecting our future. J Saf Res 43:265–270
32. Greenspan AI, Noonan RK (2012) Twenty years of scientific progress in injury and violence research and the next public health frontier. J Saf Res 43:249–255
33. Moore L, Clark DE (2008) The value of trauma registries. Injury 39:686–695
34. Pollock DA, McClain PW (1989) Trauma registries. Current status and future prospects. JAMA, J Am Med Assoc 262:2280–2283
35. Goble S, Neal M, Clark DE et al (2009) Creating a nationally representative sample of patients from trauma centers. J Trauma 67:637–644
36. Clark DE, Anderson KL, Hahn DR (2004) Evaluating an inclusive trauma system using linked population-based data. J Trauma 57:501–509
37. Teixeira PGR, Inaba K, Hadjizacharia P et al (2007) Preventable or potentially preventable mortality at a mature trauma center. J Trauma 63:1338–1347
38. Taylor M, Tesfamariam A (2012) Conducting a multidisciplinary morbidity and mortality conference in the trauma-surgical intensive care unit. Crit Care Nurs Q 35:213–215
39. Stewart RM, Corneille MG, Johnston J et al (2006) Transparent and open discussion of errors does not increase malpractice risk in trauma patients. Ann Surg 243:645–651
40. Cryer HG, Hiatt JR, Eckstein M et al (2010) Improved trauma system multicasualty incident response: comparison of two train crash disasters. J Trauma 68:783–789
41. PhD ABNM (2012) MD HGC, MD JF: the american college of surgeons trauma quality improvement program. Surg Clin NA 92:441–454
42. Shackford SR, Mackersie RC, Hoyt DB et al (1987) Impact of a trauma system on outcome of severely injured patients. Arch Surg 122:523–527
43. Demetriades D, Berne TV, Belzberg H et al (1995) The impact of a dedicated trauma program on outcome in severely injured patients. Arch Surg 130:216–220
44. Durham R, Pracht E, Orban B et al (2006) Evaluation of a mature trauma system. Ann Surg 243:775–785
45. MacKenzie EJ, Rivara FP, Jurkovich GJ et al (2006) A national evaluation of the effect of trauma-center care on mortality. N Engl J Med 354:366–378
46. MacKenzie EJ, Weir S, Rivara FP et al (2010) The value of trauma center care. J Trauma 69:1–10
47. Piontek FA, Coscia R, Marselle CS et al (2003) Impact of American College of Surgeons verification on trauma outcomes. J Trauma 54:1041–1047
48. Davis KA, Cabbad NC, Schuster KM et al (2008) Trauma team oversight improves efficiency of care and augments clinical and economic outcomes. J Trauma 65:1236–1244
49. Ryb GE, Cooper C, Waak SM (2012) Delayed trauma team activation. J Trauma Acute Care Surg 73:695–698
50. Mann NC, MacKenzie E, Teitelbaum SD et al (2005) Trauma system structure and viability in the current healthcare environment: a state-by-state assessment. J Trauma 58:136–147

Part II

Advances in Cardiopulmonary Resuscitation (CPR) and Defibrillation

Compression-Only CPR Versus CPR with Ventilations

4

Maaret K. Castrén

4.1 Introduction

Interventions for restoring blood circulation during cardiac arrest were a development of the 1960s, when a sequence of interventions was established under the acronym ABCD: Airway, Breathing, Chest compression, and Defibrillation. Although to some extent, now modified to take into account priorities of chest compression over the airway, breathing, and defibrillation, the ABCD acronym continues to have practical utility, especially for other than primary cardiac causes of cardiac arrest, such as in newborns, children, and younger adults. Since the 1970s, it has been known that bystander cardiopulmonary resuscitation (CPR) is beneficial for the patient. After the landmark article by Hallström et al. in 2000 [1], many groups have vigorously tried to find the right answer to the question of what kind of CPR should be offered when telephone instructions in a case of cardiac arrest are given by the dispatcher to the caller. Hallström et al. reported a similar outcome for instructions to give both compression-only and compression with ventilations. Of course, here we have to remember that we do not know what kind of CPR the bystander actually gave to the victim, we only know what kind of instructions the dispatchers in a randomized way gave to the caller during the emergency call. This study was terminated earlier than planned and many researchers felt that it did not give the final answer to the question. In this chapter, the clinical evidence on chest compression-only or chest compression plus ventilation CPR are summarized.

M. K. Castrén (✉)
Department of Clinical Science and Education, Karolinska Institutet, Södersjukhuset,
Sjukhusbacken 10, 11883, Stockholm, Sweden
e-mail: Maaret.castren@ki.se

A. Gullo and G. Ristagno (eds.), *Resuscitation*,
DOI: 10.1007/978-88-470-5507-0_4, © Springer-Verlag Italia 2014

4.2   Clinical Evidence

Many registry studies were published in the following years with almost the same result. In a Swedish study with 11,275 patients receiving bystander CPR (years 1990–2005), the ambulance personnel reported the way in which this CPR was given on scene when they arrived. In 73 % of the cases the patient received standard CPR and in only 10 % chest compression-only CPR. From the survival data on these patients in the Swedish Cardiac Arrest Registry no difference between these two groups could be seen in the amount of survivors after 1 month from the cardiac arrest [2]. In a letter to the editor, Ristagno and Gullo pointed out that the ambulance response time reported by Bohm et al. was only 6 min in patients treated with chest compression-only CPR, an interval that was significantly shorter than that for victims treated with standard CPR [3]. This detail had them still advocate for standard CPR.

The same year, 2007, Iwami et al. published their retrospective study on 4,902 witnessed cardiac arrests of which 783 received standard CPR and 544 chest compression-only CPR. Both groups had similar survival, though all were very low; 4.3 % versus 4.1 % after 1 year from cardiac arrest [4]. Lederer and Wiedemann responded to this article and argued that since willingness of bystanders to initiate CPR depends on a variety of factors, of which distaste for rescue breathing is not the most important, it could be that only taking away the ventilations would not necessarily increase willingness to resuscitate [5].

The study with the most publicity that year, 2007, was the prospective SOS-KANTO study [6]. The study included 4,068 patients of which 439 received chest compression-only CPR, 712 standard CPR, and 2917 no CPR at all. The survival when any CPR was given was twice as high as with no CPR given. They showed no survival benefit from mouth-to-mouth ventilation, in any of the subgroups and in their conclusion they state that the preferable CPR for adult witnessed cardiac arrest patients is chest compression-only CPR. Perkins et al. tried to give these results an explanation. Minutes after the onset of ventricular fibrillation, a rapid right-ventricular dilatation takes place and left-ventricular volume falls. Left-ventricular myocyte stretch is reduced and the heart is unable to generate an effective contraction. Chest compressions decompress the ventricles, allowing the opportunity for defibrillation to restore a spontaneous circulation. Even brief interruptions in compression allow rapid recurrence of ventricular dilatation. This might contribute to the improved outcomes seen in the study [7]. As a reply to Lancet for the SOS-KANTO study, Gordon Ewy writes that a major flaw with all previous guidelines for resuscitation is that they "recommend the same approach for two entirely different clinical conditions: primary cardiac arrest where the arterial blood is well oxygenated at the time of the cardiac arrest, and respiratory arrest when the arterial blood is so severely desaturated that it contributes to hypotension and secondary cardiac arrest." He urges in his letter to continue with standard CPR for respiratory arrest, for example drowning and children, but to change the guidelines to chest compression-only for witnessed sudden collapse [8].

Inspired by the Hallström study in 2000, we started planning for a study in Sweden and Finland. The aim was to confirm the results in a large enough trial. Unfortunately, the young researcher from Finland himself was a victim of an unsuccessful resuscitation of a sudden cardiac arrest, so the study presents only the Swedish results. In the TANGO study, we enrolled 1,276 patients with the exclusion criteria of children, trauma, and respiratory arrest. They got help by the caller getting telephone CPR instructions in a randomized way. In the final analyses, we had 282 in the chest compression-only group and 297 in the standard CPR group.This study was also stopped early. It is difficult and hard to perform a study of such magnitude and it was not possible to continue. The result showed that 19 % survived in the compression-only group and 15 % in the standard CPR group [9]. These studies were meant for the ILCOR guidelines group, but the results had not come out yet. The 2010 guidelines stated that there is limited evidence regarding the survival benefit of telephone CPR instructions and that the standard method was the way of teaching laypersons.

In a meta-analyses, looking at the three prospective studies with the same aim Hupfl et al. could show that with chest compression-only the number needed to treat was 41 and the absolute increase in survival was 2.4 % [10]. In the discussion, after the meta-analyses were published, the European Resuscitation Council stated that marketing chest compression-only CPR could decrease survival rates. The authors of the article wrote also that they at no point suggested that chest compression-only CPR should become the new standard method of CPR to bystanders. They claimed that readers had misinterpreted and oversimplified the article. They also wrote that the media was only interested in catchy headlines. Also, in many professional contexts it was clear that this was how the article and its results were read; abandon mouth-to-mouth ventilation.

Inspired by the articles, Deakin studied 17 patients in cardiac arrest during chest compression-only CPR in the emergency department (ED). All the patients were intubated and a LUCAS was applied on arrival to the ED. LUCAS was modified to only give passive chest recoil as in manual compressions. All patients were in a late stage of cardiac arrest. Gas flow and volumes, airway pressures, and CO_2 concentration were measured. The median inspiratory tidal volume in passive ventilation per compression was 41.5 ml. This was less than the measured anatomical dead space, 162.7 ml. What can be said as a conclusion is that passive ventilation at least in late stage cardiac arrest does not seem to maintain adequate gas exchange, only the dead space moves in and out [11].

I have wondered if we really use all the possibilities we have to help our patients. We hear a lot of talk of how bystanders don't want to give mouth-to-mouth ventilation and how difficult it is to instruct via the telephone. Not wanting should not be such a problem since most of the cardiac arrests occur at home, and mostly it is not the laypersons but the professionals who state that they are not willing to give mouth-to-mouth to a stranger [12]. No one has yet made a study on mouth-to-nose in a setting where the dispatcher gives telephone instructions in cardiac arrest, but a study is made on anesthetized patients. Jiang and colleagues studied in total 24 patients in general anesthesia. They randomized them into two groups and were given mouth-to-nose or mouth-to-mouth ventilations. The result showed that mouth-to-nose breathing was more effective than mouth-to-mouth in these adult patients. It would be interesting to find out if this mode of ventilation can produce better patient outcomes after CPR [13]. At least it should be easier to perform than mouth-to-mouth ventilation by an untrained bystander.

A survey in three different Norwegian hospitals with 3- and 6-h basic life support courses showed (N = 361) that only 10.8 % of the participants had attended a CPR course in the last 6 months, of nurses and physicians 15.5 % versus 12.5 %. Only 32.7 % had taken an active part in a real cardiac arrest situation with resuscitation. Only 14 % had acted in more than one resuscitation [14]. These results show that a cardiac arrest is a frightening situation also for healthcare professionals, and they rarely have real-life experience in resuscitation. So, we need to do it as simple as possible. But, is doing it too simple decreasing survival of some of the important patient groups, like children?. Ogawa et al. showed in their very large registry study with 20,707 patients a better outcome for young patients and patients in cardiac arrest of noncardiac origin when they were given standard CPR. This means that they benefited from getting ventilations, not only chest compressions [15].

As a conclusion, we need two kinds of instructions: those for adult CPR with chest compression-only CPR, and those for children and patients with hypoxia with chest compressions combined with ventilations.

References

1. Hallstrom A, Cobb L, Johnson E, Copass M (2000) Cardiopulmonary resuscitation by chest compression alone or with mouth-to-mouth ventilation. N Engl J Med 342(21):1546–1553
2. Bohm K, Rosenqvist M, Herlitz J, Hollenberg J, Svensson L (2007) Survival is similar after standard treatment and chest compression only in out-of-hospital bystander cardiopulmonary resuscitation. Circulation 116(25):2908–2912 (Epub 10 Dec 2007)
3. Ristagno G, Gullo A (2008) Letter by Ristagno and Gullo regarding article, "Survival is similar after standard treatment and chest compression only in out-of-hospital bystander cardiopulmonary resuscitation". Circulation 117(17):e325. doi:10.1161/CIRCULATIONAHA.107.763250
4. Iwami T, Kawamura T, Hiraide A, Berg RA, Hayashi Y, Nishiuchi T, Kajino K, Yonemoto N, Yukioka H, Sugimoto H, Kakuchi H, Sase K, Yokoyama H, Nonogi (2007) Effectiveness of bystander-initiated cardiac-only resuscitation for patients with out-of-hospital cardiac arrest. Circulation 116(25):2900–2907 (Epub 10 Dec 2007)
5. Lederer W, Wiedermann FJ (2008) Letter by Lederer and Wiedermann regarding article, "effectiveness of bystander-initiated cardiac-only resuscitation for patients with out-of-hospital cardiac arrest". Circulation. 117(25):e508; author reply e509. doi: 10.1161/CIRCULATIONAHA.107.761551
6. SOS-KANTO study group (2007) Cardiopulmonary resuscitation by bystanders with chest compression only (SOS-KANTO): an observational study. Lancet 369(9565):920–926
7. Perkins GD, Chamberlain DA, Frenneauxc M (2007).Correspondence. Chest-compression-only or full cardiopulmonary resuscitation? Lancet 369(9577):1926
8. Ewy GA (2007) Cardiac arrest–guideline changes urgently needed. Lancet 369(9565): 882–884

9. Svensson L, Bohm K, Castrèn M, Pettersson H, Engerström L, Herlitz J, Rosenqvist M (2010) Compression-only CPR or standard CPR in out-of-hospital cardiac arrest. N Engl J Med 363(5):434–442
10. Hüpfl M, Selig HF, Nagele P (2010) Chest-compression-only versus standard cardiopulmonary resuscitation: a meta-analysis. Lancet 376(9752):1552–1557
11. Deakin CD, O'Neill JF, Tabor T (2007) Does compression-only cardiopulmonary resuscitation generate adequate passive ventilation during cardiac arrest? Resuscitation. 75(1):53–59 (Epub 15 May 2007)
12. Taniguchi T, Sato K, Fujita T, Okajima M, Takamura M (2012) Attitudes to bystander cardiopulmonary resuscitation in Japan, 2010. Circ J 76(5):1130–1135. (Epub 2012 Mar 2)
13. Jiang Y, Bao FP, Liang Y, Kimball WR, Liu Y, Zapol WM, Kacmarek RM (2011) Effectiveness of breathing through nasal and oral routes in unconscious apneic adult human subjects: a prospective randomized crossover trial. Anesthesiology 115(1):129–135
14. Hopstock LA (2008) Cardiopulmonary resuscitation; use, training and self-confidence in skills. A self-report study among hospital personnel. Scand J Trauma Resusc Emerg Med 16(16):18
15. Ogawa T, Akahane M, Koike S, Tanabe S, Mizoguchi T, Imamura T (2011) Outcomes of chest compression only CPR versus conventional CPR conducted by lay people in patients with out of hospital cardiopulmonary arrest witnessed by bystanders: nationwide population based observational study. BMJ 27(342):c7106

Ventricular Fibrillation and Defibrillation: State of Our Knowledge and Uncertainities

5

Roger D. White

5.1 Defibrillation and Resuscitation

We know it when we see it, yet despite decades of experimental and clinical investigations, the mechanisms that evolve and sustain ventricular fibrillation (VF) are still not fully clarified. Defining, describing, and understanding VF continue to be daunting tasks [1, 2]. A description of what we now know as VF was discovered on Egyptian papyri around 1534 BC: "If the heart trembles, has little power and sinks, the disease is advancing….and death is near" [1, 3]. Despite these limitations in our understanding of VF, what we do know is that it can be terminated by delivering electrical current with defined waveform morphologies and timing to fibrillating myocardial cells [4–7]. Because of the inexorable degenerative course untreated VF follows, the timing of defibrillation shock delivery becomes a critical determinant of the likelihood of achieving a favorable outcome [8]. This chapter will discuss some of the areas of controversy in defibrillation.

Defibrillation is an electrophysiologic event that occurs within 100–500 ms of shock delivery (Fig. 5.1). Examination of the rhythm at 5 s after a shock is accepted as a time-point to assess the efficacy of the shock without distortion of the electrocardiogram (ECG) by the voltage offset. Figure 5.2 depicts a successful shock followed by recurrence of VF 9 s later. Resuscitation is a composite of all interventions, and a useful end-point is restoration of a spontaneous circulation (ROSC). This distinction between defibrillation and resuscitation is necessary in order to understand the role and contribution of defibrillation in an overall effort to restore return of ROSC.

R. D. White (✉)
Anesthesiology, Internal Medicine (Cardiovascular Diseases), Emergency Medicine (Pre-Hospital division), Mayo Clinic, 200 1st St. SW, Rochester, MN 55905, USA
e-mail: White.roger@mayo.edu

A. Gullo and G. Ristagno (eds.), *Resuscitation*,
DOI: 10.1007/978-88-470-5507-0_5, © Springer-Verlag Italia 2014

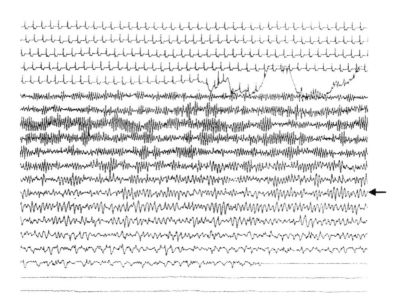

Fig. 5.1 Progressive degeneration of VF over time. The amplitude, frequency, and VF waveform upstroke velocity all decline. From: Valderrabano [2]

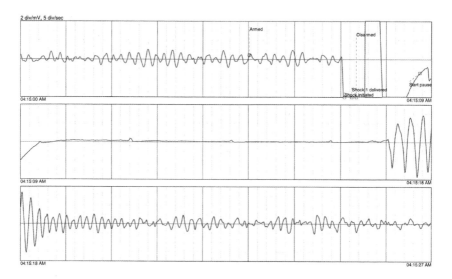

Fig. 5.2 Ventricular fibrillation was terminated by a shock. Nine seconds later VF recurred after a short burst of polymorphic ventricular tachycardia (PVT). *P* waves are visible during the period following the shock. This is an example of a successful defibrillation shock

5.2   Cardiopulmonary Resuscitation First or Shock First

Many studies have been reported assessing the question of whether or not defibrillation shocks should be preceded by a period of CPR [9–13]. At this time there is no evidence that supports one approach over the other. A recent detailed review and meta-analysis of randomized trials concluded that deferring the initial shock until a short period of CPR has been performed did not show a survival-to-discharge benefit over immediate defibrillation irrespective of response time. There is no evidence of harm in deferring the first shock until a period of CPR has been done [14]. Most EMS systems will make decisions on this unresolved question with a strong consideration of response time. The definitive resolution of this question will very likely be determined by algorithms capable of analyzing the initial VF with sufficient sensitivity and specificity to predict the outcome of the shock (Figs. 5.3, 5.4).

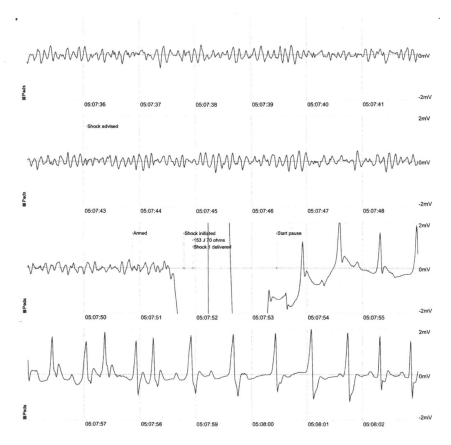

Fig. 5.3 The VF morphology is characterized by high amplitude and frequency and sharp VF waveform upstroke velocity. The shock quickly restored an organized rhythm and ROSC

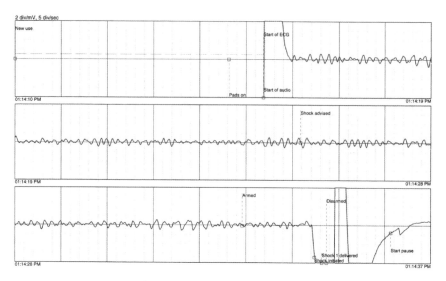

Fig. 5.4 Compared with the VF in Fig. 5.3 the VF here is of relatively low and varying amplitude but the frequency is sufficient to warrant a shock, which was followed by an organized rhythm during post-shock CPR

5.3 Termination of Recurrent VF

Recurrence of VF after a successful shock is common. Recurrence at least once was observed in 52–61 % of patients while in the care of Basic Life Support First Responders [15, 16]. In patients during both Basic and Advanced Life Support, VF was observed to occur in 74–80 % of patients [17–19]. Frequent refibrillation was also observed in 67 % of patients in an earlier study describing post-shock rhythms [20]. The 2005 Guidelines recommended immediate resumption of CPR after a shock without regard to the post-shock rhythm and continuation of the CPR for 2 min before re-analysis of the rhythm [21]. With this approach persistent or recurrent VF can continue for at least 2 min after a shock (Fig. 5.5); the implications of this post-shock CPR period warrant a reconsideration. (1) A recent experimental study documented the high oxygen demands of VF [22]. In that study VF was shown to impair restoration of creatine-phosphate levels during simulated CPR. (2) It is assumed that CPR will be performed with such high quality that this high oxygen demand will be met for periods of two or more minutes. (3) The median duration of VF was shorter with shocks that were followed by ROSC. This observation was applied to both initial and recurrent VF [23]. These investigators concluded that detection of VF during ongoing chest compressions might be helpful because of this relationship between shorter duration of VF episodes and ROSC. Their recommendation was that recurring VF should be shocked as soon as

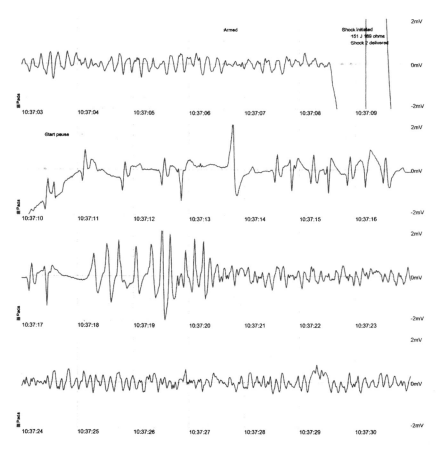

Fig. 5.5 After a successful shock VF resumed at 10:35:08. At 10:37:09, a shock was delivered. Nine seconds later at 10:37:18, PVT was followed by recurrent VF

possible. (4) Chest compressions can induce VF quickly after resumption of post-shock chest compressions and thus permit VF to continue for nearly 2 min before re-analysis of the rhythm and delivery of a shock [24–27]. Berdowski and colleagues reported that time in recurrent VF is associated with worse outcomes and it is thus desirable to terminate recurrent VF as soon as possible because survival decreases with every minute that the next shock is postponed [24]. An analysis of the performance of the amplitude spectral area and slope to predict defibrillation in out-of-hospital cardiac arrest concluded that for recurrent VF a shock should be delivered immediately upon detection [28]. What then can be considered for modification in terminating recurrent VF? Certainly the well-established benefit of minimally interrupted CPR must be weighed against any modification of the 2 min CPR period after a shock. As resuscitation progresses in time the role of CPR becomes increasingly crucial. (Figs. 5.6, 5.7).

In 2001 Blouin and colleagues reported their experience with recurrent VF [29]. Using tape-recorded ECG data in 376 shocks, in 96 patients there were 22 shocks with recurrence of VF in 3 min or less. In their experience VF recurred within 6 s after a shock in only 20 % of recurrences, and in 73 % at 60 s. They suggested performing CPR for 30 s after a shock in order to capture the largest number of recurrences. Yet their conclusion was that recurring VF should be acted on rapidly [29].

An action plan proposal to confront recurrent VF was described and illustrated in an editorial in response to the Blouin study [30]. Amplification of that approach might be a basis for change. During the first several minutes of intervention in VF, recurrent VF should be recognized by the algorithm or operator quickly after onset and a shock delivered as soon as possible (Fig. 5.8). After 2–3 shocks, if VF continues to recur, other measures, including minimally interrupted CPR and anti-arrhythmic therapy, will be necessary. Advances in algorithm design and function will provide accurate recognition of shockable VF without distortion of ECG interpretation by chest compression artifact. Already major improvements in algorithm performance are being reported, such as faster times to a shock advisory following cessation of chest compressions and the optimal timing of defibrillation

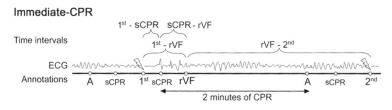

Fig. 5.6 At *A*, rhythm analysis was commenced, followed by CPR (sCPR). The first shock terminated VF but VF resumed after a few chest compressions. Two minutes of CPR then continued with ongoing VF before the next rhythm analysis. Adapted from: Berdowski et al. [24]

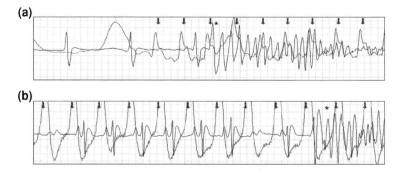

Fig. 5.7 *Red arrows* indicate chest compressions in two patients (**a** and **b**). In both patients VF resumed at the *asterisk*, shortly after compressions were resumed. In the patient depicted in (a) the third compression occurred during ventricular repolarization. From: Osorio et al. [27]

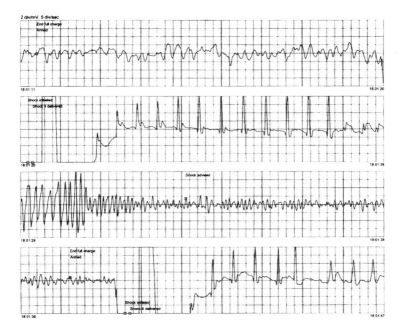

Fig. 5.8 Recurrent VF was detected quickly after the first shock and 12 s after onset of recurrent VF a shock restored an immediate organized rhythm. From: (2001) Ann Emerg Med 38(3):278–281 [30]

by waveform analysis during CPR [3–32]. Sensitivity of over 90 % has been shown to be feasible in recognition of noise-free VF during CPR [33]. Suppression of CPR artifacts using the chest compression rate extracted from the thoracic impedance recording acquired from the defibrillation pads has been demonstrated to be as accurate as methods based on information acquired from CPR feedback data [34]. Continued enhancement of sensitivity and specificity is needed to separate CPR artifact from the ECG to eliminate unacceptable interruptions in CPR. These very recent studies make it evident that we are moving rapidly in that direction. Then prolonged periods of recurrent VF will be minimized with the prospect of more frequent return of an organized rhythm and probably ROSC [13].

5.4 Conclusions

Advances in the treatment of VF, both in defibrillation waveform design and in clinical practice, have contributed significantly to improved outcomes from out-of-hospital cardiac arrest with VF as the initial rhythm. Areas of uncertainty and controversy remain and continue to be subject to ongoing discussion and study. These areas include the appropriate application of CPR first or defibrillation first. For this decision it is very likely that algorithms with high sensitivity and specificity will continue to evolve that will separate VF likely to benefit from a shock first or from CPR first. Because of the very high incidence of recurrent VF and the high oxygen demand of this arrhythmia there is considerable agreement that recurrent VF should be terminated as soon as it is recognized. Again, algorithms that separate chest compression artifact from the underlying rhythm will enable this to occur without unduly compromising ongoing CPR. This is most likely to be clinically applicable in the first several minutes of resuscitation when VF recurs frequently.

References

1. Karagueuzian HS (2004) Ventricular fibrillation: an organized delirium or uncoordinated reason? Heart Rhythm 1:24–26
2. Valderrabano M (2011) Deciphering the electrogram in ventricular fibrillation to extract physiological information. Heart Rhythm 8(5):750–751
3. Breasted JH (1930) The Edwin Smith surgical papyrus. University of Chicago Press, Chicago
4. White RD (2002) New concepts in transthoracic defibrillation. Emerg Med Clin N Am 20:785–807
5. Chen B, Yin C, Ristagno G, Quan W, Tan Q, Freeman G, Li Y et al (2012) Retrospective evaluation of current-based impedance compensation defibrillation in out-of-hospital cardiac arrest. Resuscitation doi:10.1016/j.resuscitation.2012.09.017 (Epub ahead of print)
6. Daubert JP, Sheu SS (2008) Mystery of biphasic defibrillation waveform efficacy. JACC 52(10):836–838
7. Darragh KM, Manoharan G, Maio R et al (2012) A low tilt waveform in the transthoracic defibrillation of ventricular arrhythmias during cardiac arrest. Resuscitation 83:1438–1443
8. Chen PS, Wu TJ, Ting CT et al (2003) A tale to two fibrillations. Circulation 108:2298–2303
9. Cobb LA, Fahrenbruch CE, Walsh TR et al (1999) Influence of cardiopulmonary resuscitation prior to defibrillation in patients with out-of-hospital ventricular fibrillation. JAMA 281(13):1182–1188
10. Wik L, Hansen TB, Fylling F et al (2003) Delaying defibrillation to give basic cardiopulmonary resuscitation to patients with out-of-hospital ventricular fibrillation. JAMA 289(11):1389–1395
11. Jacobs IG, Finn JC, Oxer HF, Jelinek GA (2005) CPR before difibrillation in out-of-hospital cardiac arrest: A randomized trial. Emerg Med Australas 17:39–45
12. Baker PW, Conway J, Cotton C et al (2008) Defibrillation or cardiopulmonary resuscitation first for patient with out-of-hospital cardiac arrests found by paramedics to be in ventricular fibrillation? A randomized control trial. Resuscitation 79:424–431
13. Koike S, Tanabe S, Ogawa T et al (2011) Immediate defibrillation or defibrillation after cardiopulmonary resuscitation. Prehosp Emerg Care 15:393–400
14. Simpson PM, Goodger MS, Bendall JC (2010) Delayed versus immediate defibrillation for out-of-hospital cardiac arrest due to ventricular fibrillation: a systematic review and meta-analysis of randomized controlled trials. Resuscitation 81:925–931
15. White RD, Russell JK (2002) Refibrillation, resuscitation and survival in out-of-hospital sudden cardiac arrest victims treated with biphasic automated external defibrillators. Resuscitation 55:17–23
16. Hess EP, White RD (2004) Recurrent ventricular fibrillation in out-of-hospital cardiac arrest after defibrillation by police and firefighters: implications for automated external defibrillator users. Crit Care Med 32(9) Suppl:S436-S439
17. van Alem AP, Post J, Koster RW (2003) VF recurrence: characteristics and patient outcome in out-of-hospital cardiac arrest. Resuscitation 59:181–188

18. Koster RW, Walker RG, Chapman FW (2008) Recurrent ventricular fibrillation during advanced life support care of patients with prehospital cardiac arrest. Resuscitation 78:252–257

19. Hess EP, Agarwal D, Myers LA et al (2011) Performance of a rectilinear biphasic waveform in defibrillation of presenting and recurrent ventricular fibrillation: a prospective multicenter study. Resuscitation 82:685–689

20. Gliner BE, White RD (1999) Electrocardiographic evaluation of defibrillation shocks delivered to out-of-hospital sudden cardiac arrest patients. Resuscitation 41:133–144

21. American Heart Association guidelines for cardiopulmonary resuscitation and emergency cardiovascular care, part 3: defibrillation. 2005 Circulation 112:III17–III24

22. Hoogendijk MG, Schumacher CA, Belterman CNW et al (2012) Ventricular fibrillation hampers the restoration of creatine-phosphate levels during simulated cardiopulmonary resuscitations. Europace 14:1518–1523

23. Eilevstjonn J, Kramer-Johansen J, Sunde K (2007) Shock outcome is related to prior rhythm and duration of ventricular fibrillation. Resuscitation 75:60–67

24. Berdowski J, Tijssen JGP, Koster RW (2010) Chest compressions cause recurrence of ventricular fibrillation after the first successful conversion by defibrillation in out-of-hospital cardiac arrest. Circ Arrhythm Electrophysiol 3:72–78

25. Berdowski J, ten Haaf M, Tijssen JGP et al (2010) Time in recurrent ventricular fibrillation and survival after out-of-hospital cardiac arrest. Circulation 122:1101–1108

26. Osorio J, Dosdall DJ, Robichaux RP Jr et al (2008) In a swine model, chest compressions cause ventricular capture and, by means of a long-short sequence, ventricular fibrillation. Circ Arrhythmia Electrophysiol 2008:282–289

27. Osorio J, Dosdall DJ, Tabereaux PB et al (2012) Effect of chest compressions on ventricular activation. Am J Cardiol 109:670–674

28. Shanmugasundaram M, Valles A, Kellum MJ et al (2012) Analysis of amplitude spectral area and slope to predict defibrillation in out of hospital cardiac arrest due to ventricular fibrillation (VF) according to VF type: recurrent versus shock-resistant. Resuscitation 83:1242–1247

29. Blouin D, Topping C, Moore S et al (2001) Out-of-hospital defibrillation with automated external defibrillations: postshock analysis should be delayed. Ann Emerg Med 38(3):256–261

30. White RD (2001) To shock or not to shock: that is the question. Ann Emerg med 38(3):278–281

31. Didon JP, Krasteva V, Menetre S (2011) Shock advisory system with minimal delay triggering after end of chest compressions: accuracy and gained hands-off time. Resuscitation 82S:S8–S15

32. Li Y, Tang W (2012) Optimizing the timing of defibrillation: the role of ventricular fibrillation waveform analysis during cardiopulmonary resuscitation. Crit Care Clin 28:199–210

33. Krasteva V, Jekova I, Dotsinsky I, Didon JP (2010) Shock advisory system for heart rhythm analysis during cardiopulmonary resuscitation using a single ECG input of automated external defibrillators. Ann Biomed Eng 38(4):1326–1336

34. Aramendi E, Ayala U, Irusta U et al (2012) Suppression of the cardiopulmonary resuscitation artifacts using the instantaneous chest compression rate extracted from the thoracic impedance. Resuscitation 83:692–698

Amplitude Spectrum Area to Predict the Success of Defibrillation

6

Giuseppe Ristagno and Francesca Fumagalli

6.1 Introduction

In victims of cardiac arrest due to ventricular fibrillation (VF) or pulseless ventricular tachycardia (VT), cardiopulmonary resuscitation (CPR) in conjunction with electrical defibrillation (DF) has the potential of re-establishing the return of spontaneous circulation (ROSC). During cardiac arrest, coronary blood flow ceases, leading to a progressive and severe energy imbalance. Intra-myocardial hypercarbic acidosis is associated with depletion of high energy phosphates and correspondingly severe global myocardial ischemia [1, 2]. The ischemic left ventricle becomes contracted ushering in the stone heart [3, 4]. After onset of contracture, the probability of successful DF is remote. Early CPR, accounting for a partial restoration of coronary perfusion pressure (CPP) and myocardial blood flow, delays onset of ischemic myocardial injury and facilitates DF [5]. Accordingly, VF is characterized by three time-sensitive electrophysiological phases: The electrical phase of 0–4 min; the circulatory phase of 4–10 min; and the metabolic phase of > 10 min. During the electrical phase, immediate DF is likely to be successful. As ischemia progresses, the success of attempted DF diminishes without CPR. This phase is characterized by transition to slow VF wavelets during accumulation of ischemic

G. Ristagno (✉)
Department of Cardiovascular Research, IRCCS—Istituto di Ricerche Farmacologiche "Mario Negri", Via La Masa 19, 20156, Milan, Italy
e-mail: gristag@gmail.com

F. Fumagalli
Department of Cardiovascular Research, IRCCS—Istituto di Ricerche Farmacologiche "Mario Negri", Via La Masa 19, 20157, Milan, Italy
e-mail: francesca.fumagalli@marionegri.it

A. Gullo and G. Ristagno (eds.), *Resuscitation*,
DOI: 10.1007/978-88-470-5507-0_6, © Springer-Verlag Italia 2014

metabolites in the myocardium. In the metabolic phase, there is no likelihood of successful restoration of a perfusing rhythm [6].

Conventional manual chest compressions (CC) are often performed ineffectively and with frequent interruptions, affecting outcome of cardiac arrest [7, 8]. In addition, CCs create artifacts on the electrocardiographic (ECG) signal such that pauses in CPR are mandatory for rhythm analysis prior to a DF attempt [9, 10]. Prolonged and frequent interruptions of CPR for rhythm analysis and delivery of the shock can translate into major compromises in the success of resuscitation efforts and outcome [11, 12]. Finally, it has now been recognized that the severity of post-resuscitation myocardial dysfunction is also related to the magnitude of the electrical energy delivered with DFs [13]. Decision of interrupting CPR for delivering an electrical shock might be therefore controversial and may lead to repetitive unnecessary DF attempts and ultimately to worse outcome.

The development of a non invasive and real-time monitoring that allows for prediction of whether or not a shock would achieve ROSC would be important to prioritize rescuers' intervention (CC or DF), reducing the number of failed DF attempts and CPR interruptions. Electrocardiographic analysis of VF waveform might represent the best non invasive approach to guide the priority of interventions, namely CC or DF. The initial approaches to ECG analysis included measurements of VF amplitude and frequency [14, 15]. To improve sensitivity and specificity of the ECG predictors for ROSC, more sophisticated methods of VF waveform analysis were introduced and investigated, including wavelet decomposition, nonlinear dynamics methods, and a combination of different ECG parameter analyses [16–18]. Indeed, many quantitative techniques have been developed to analyze VF waveform in order to obtain more information about the state of the myocardium vitality and thereby optimizing DF and CPR maneuvres [19]. Among them, one of the most accurate is the "Amplitude Spectrum Area" (AMSA). AMSA analysis algorithm can be summarized as follows [20–24]. In brief, the ECG signal is filtered between 4 and 48 Hz to minimize low-frequency artifacts produced by CC and to exclude the electrical interference of ambient noise at frequencies greater than 48 Hz. Analog ECG signals are digitalized and converted from a time to a frequency domain by fast Fourier transformation. AMSA is calculated as the sum of the product of individual frequency and its amplitude (Fig. 6.1), i.e., AMSA $= \sum$ Ai · Fi, where Ai represents the amplitude at ith frequency Fi.

6.2 AMSA to Predict DF Success

AMSA has been extensively demonstrated to be one of the most accurate predictors for successful DF, in numerous animal models of cardiac arrest and CPR [20, 21, 24, 25]. Clinically, the accuracy of AMSA as a tool to predict DF success was initially confirmed in a retrospective analysis of ECG traces, including 108 DF attempts with an automated external defibrillator, of 46 victims of cardiac arrest

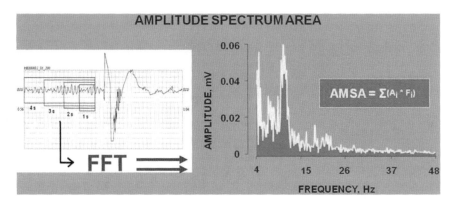

Fig. 6.1 Fast fourier transformation (FFT) with AMSA calculation

due to VF [22]. An AMSA value of 13 mV-Hz predicted successful DF, with a sensitivity of 91 % and a specificity of 94 %. AMSA, therefore, predicted the success of electrical DF with high specificity and appeared as a tool to minimize interruptions of precordial compression and the myocardial damage caused by delivery of repetitive and ineffective electrical shocks. We have then confirmed the above results in a subsequent retrospective study including 90 out-of-hospital cardiac arrests. AMSA values were significantly greater in successful DFs, compared to unsuccessful ones, 16 and 7 mV-Hz, respectively [23]. A threshold value of AMSA of 12 mV-Hz was able to predict the success of each DF attempt with a sensitivity of 91 % and a specificity of 97 %. The positive predictive value, which refers to the proportion of the shocks that were correctly predicted to restore a perfusing rhythm, was 95 %. The negative predictive value, which instead refers to the proportion of the shocks that were predicted to fail and actually failed to restore a perfusing rhythm, was 97 %.

We are continuing our studies for assessing the accuracy of AMSA on predicting DF success with two concurrent retrospective analyses of two large datasets, one from US, including 609 out-of-hospital cardiac arrests, and another from Italy including more than 818 patients.

Study 1: AMSA and DF success on 609 US out-of-hospital cardiac arrest patients [26, 27].

More in detail, a 1024 point, or 4.1 s, ECG window ending at 0.5 s before DF was analyzed and AMSA calculated prior to first DF attempts and subsequent DF delivered in cases of DF-resistant VF. Successful DF was defined as return of an organized rhythm within 60 s from the attempt. For first and subsequent DFs, AMSA threshold values were analyzed with regard to their ability to discriminate among successful and not successful DFs. Sensitivity, specificity, accuracy, and positive predictive values (DF success rate) of an AMSA-based decision algorithm were calculated. The DF performance was then compared between two DF decision algorithms with and without AMSA threshold, respectively. Before the first DF, mean AMSA was 16.8 mV-Hz when shocks were successful, while it was

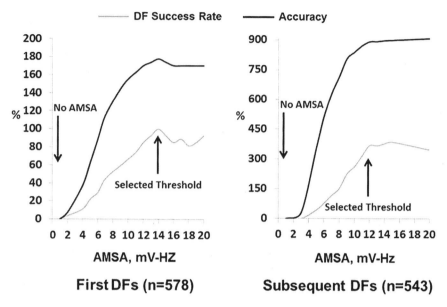

Fig. 6.2 Improvements in DF performance as a function of AMSA thresholds

11.4 ($p < 0.0001$) in those that were not. After the first DF, AMSA significantly decreased, but remained higher in successful shock episodes (15.0 vs. 7.4 mV-Hz, $p < 0.0001$). For the DF decision algorithm without AMSA, the DF success rate and accuracy were 27 %/27 % for the first DFs, and 9 %/9 % for the subsequent DFs, respectively. An optimized AMSA threshold was found to be 14 mV-Hz for first DFs, and 12 mV-Hz for subsequent ones. Incorporation of these AMSA thresholds into a DF decision algorithm increased both DF success rate and accuracy. The first DF achieved a DF success rate of 54 % and an accuracy of 75 %, while subsequent DF attempts achieved 42 % in DF success rate and 89 % in accuracy. These results translated into an increase in DF success rate and accuracy by 100 and 180 % for the first DFs and 360 and 880 % for the subsequent DFs (Fig. 6.2). Moreover, considering lower AMSA values, with an AMSA threshold of 7.5 mV-Hz, a large amount of unnecessary DFs (35 % for the first DF and 50 % for the subsequent DFs) were avoided by using AMSA with the accuracy of 93 % for the first DF and 95 % for the subsequent DFs (Fig. 6.3).

Study 2: AMSA and DF success on 818 Italian out-of-hospital cardiac arrest patients [28].

In a highly populated area of northern Italy, we evaluated the capability of AMSA to predict DF outcome in out-of-hospital cardiac arrests. We hypothesized that threshold values of AMSA could be identified such to be used as a guide for CPR intervention, i.e., CC or DF. ECG data recorded by automated external defibrillators from different manufactures were obtained from 8.419 cardiac arrest events occurring in seven cities in Lombardia Region, Italy, between 2008 and 2009.

Prediction of Non-successful Defibrillations

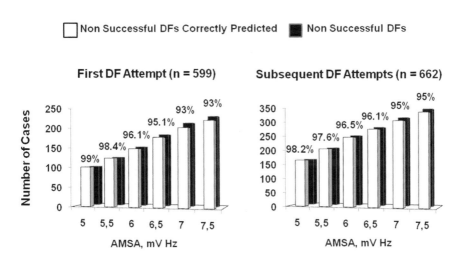

Fig. 6.3 Percentage of avoided unnecessary defibrillation attempts for different AMSA thresholds, with an AMSA-based algorithm

Among these events, only VF/VT cardiac arrests receiving DFs were selected (n = 984). A 2 s ECG window ending at 0.5 s before DF was analyzed and AMSA calculated. DF was defined as successful in the presence of spontaneous rhythm >40 bpm starting within 60 s from the shock. Threshold values of AMSA able to discriminate among successful and not successful DFs were individuated and sensitivity, specificity, accuracy, positive, and negative predictive values (PPV, NPV) of the AMSA-based decision algorithm were calculated. Finally, area under the receiver operating characteristic (ROC) curve was measured. A total of 1,969 quality DF events, including 818 first attempts and 1151 subsequent ones, from 818 out-of-hospital cardiac arrests were included in the analyses. DF success rates were 26.9, 27.7, and 26.4 % for all, first, and subsequent DFs, respectively. AMSA was significantly greater prior to successful DFs compared to that preceding unsuccessful ones (13.8 vs. 6.9 mV-Hz, and 13.9 vs. 6.8 mV-Hz, and 13.7 vs. 7 mV-Hz, for all, first, and subsequent DFs, respectively, $p < 0.0001$). Intersection of sensitivity, specificity, and accuracy curves identified a threshold value of AMSA of approximately 9.5 mV-Hz able to predict DF outcome, with a balanced sensitivity, specificity, and accuracy of 80 %, for all, first, and subsequent DFs. Moreover, intersection of PPV and accuracy curves identified a threshold value of AMSA of approximately 15 mV-Hz able to predict a successful DF with a PPV and accuracy of 80 %, for all, first, and subsequent DF attempts. AMSA values greater than 27 mV-Hz correctly predicted the success of DF with a PPV value of 100 %. AMSA below 8 mV-Hz correctly predicted the DF failure with an NPV of >95 %, for all, first, and subsequent DFs. Area under ROC curves was 0.872, 0.869, and 0.875 for all, first, and subsequent DFs, respectively, ($p < 0.0001$).

6.3 AMSA to Assess CPR Quality

Existing predictors of successful CPR intervention include CPP, and end-tidal CO_2 (EtCO2) [29, 30]. CPP and EtCO2 values generated during CPR are directly related to the depth of the CCs and threshold levels have been identified as the leading prognosticators of the success of the resuscitative maneuvres. CPP assessment, however, is generally inapplicable in preclinical settings, while portable capnometers are not widely available and require endotracheal intubation. These restraints are in contrast with AMSA analysis, which is a simple parameter easily obtained by routine availability of the ECG available in current external defibrillators.

Since CCs are usually performed without feedback and relatively small changes in the depth of compression profoundly alter hemodynamic effectiveness and outcomes, there is an increasingly recognized need for a monitor of effectiveness of CCs. Thus, compression depth has been estimated by measuring the compression and decompression displacements with force transducers or accelerometers [31]. These approaches with real-time visual and audible feedback during CPR have shown to improve the quality of CPR to more closely conform to guidelines, but no improvements in both ROSC and other clinical outcomes. In addition, CPR feedback devices with accelerometers may overestimate compression depth when compressions are performed on a soft surface [32, 33]. Yet, these techniques do not reflect the physiological effectiveness of CCs. The ECG and in turn AMSA analyses have the advantages of detecting changes in the electrical status of the myocardium during CPR. AMSA indicator would be expected to correlate with measurement of myocardial perfusion.

We have previously [24] reported the possibility of assessing CC depth utilizing AMSA, in a porcine model of cardiac arrest and CPR, in which animals were randomized to optimal or suboptimal depth of mechanical CC. Like threshold value of CPP, AMSA threshold value was achieved contingent on the depth of compressions such that AMSA increased progressively during CCs, and like CPP, predicted the likelihood of successful DF. We are now confirming that AMSA is an indicator of CC depth in human patients. A sub-analysis, in fact, was conducted on DF events obtained from 303 patients, for whom CC depth data were available together with ECG traces. Depth of chest compression was measured from a CPR feedback accelerator sensor output signal and registered by the AEDs. Changes in AMSA values between consecutive DF attempts were analyzed in relation to depth of compression. The average CC depth was below the current recommended depth of at least 2 inch, i.e., 1.3 ± 0.06, 1.5 ± 0.05, and 1.5 ± 0.08 inch, prior to the first, second, and third DF attempt, respectively. The average cutoff value of CC depth of 1.75 inch was therefore considered for the analysis. For patients with an

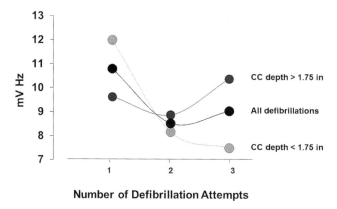

Fig. 6.4 Relationship between chest compression (CC) depth and AMSA

average depth of <1.75 inch, AMSA values decreased by 3.9 mV-Hz between the first and second DF attempt ($p < 0.001$). AMSA further decreased between the second and third DF attempt, when CC depth was <1.75 inch. By contrast, for patients with an average depth >1.75 inch, AMSA was equivalent for the first and second DF attempt ($p = 0.47$) and then increased by 1.7 mV-Hz between the second and third DF attempt (Fig. 6.4). AMSA values therefore decreased within consecutive shocks during shallow CCs, while they increased when CCs were of greater depth. Therefore, when the real-time AMSA value is of insufficient magnitude, the rescuer would be prompted to push harder and perhaps to push faster.

6.4   Conclusions

Indeed, the effectiveness of CCs in relation to the timing of DF has been a subject of major interest. Based on available evidence, the 2005 guidelines for CPR had diminished enthusiasm for early DF in favor of an initial interval of CCs [34]. Nevertheless, the recent 2010 guidelines for CPR have highlighted the insufficient evidence to recommend for or against delaying DF to provide a period of CC and called again for rapid DF [35]. Accordingly, the duration of VF is rarely known, especially in the out-of-hospital setting and thereby it is not reliable to determine the priority of CPR based on the duration of the untreated cardiac arrest. Moreover, there is insufficient evidence to determine the optimal duration of the CPR interval prior to DF. A real-time AMSA analysis would be a useful tool to guide decision for the most appropriate treatment, namely CC or DF, when rescuers arrive at the cardiac arrest scene. AMSA had the additional promise of monitoring the effectiveness of CC together with predicting for the optimal timing of DF.

The capability to measure AMSA without additional instrumentation by augmentation of software in existing AEDs would make this option especially attractive. Moreover, AMSA by reducing futile interruptions in CC for the delivery of a failing DF, would potentially ameliorate also post-resuscitation myocardial dysfunction. Even minimal interruptions of less than 4 s generate declines in myocardial perfusion to near 40 % [36]. Particularly, the duration of interruptions in CC during prehospital CPR for rhythm analysis alone and delivery of a DF have been of more than 20 and 24 s, respectively [37]. Thus, real-time analyses of AMSA, with the potential advantage of not being invalidated by artifacts produced by CC, might be continuously performed during CC thereby reducing further detrimental interruptions. The major limitation of the current studies on this topic was that they included only retrospective analyses. Thus, a prospective study directed to validate the safety and the potential benefit of an AMSA-guided CPR has to be planned and performed. This limitation notwithstanding, there is consistent evidence that AMSA analysis represents a clinically applicable method, which may provide a real-time indication for DF timing and efficacy of CC.

References

1. Johnson BA, Weil MH, Tang W et al (1995) Mechanisms of myocardial hypercarbic acidosis during cardiac arrest. J Appl Physiol 78:1579–1584
2. Kern KB, Garewal HS, Sanders AB et al (1990) Depletion of myocardial adenosine triphosphate during prolonged untreated ventricular fibrillation: effect on defibrillation success. Resuscitation 20:221–229
3. Steen S, Liao Q, Pierre L et al (2003) The critical importance of minimal delay between chest compressions and subsequent defibrillation: a haemodynamic explanation. Resuscitation 58:249–258
4. Klouche K, Weil MH, Sun S et al (2002) Evolution of the Stone Heart After Prolonged Cardiac Arrest. Chest 122:1006–1011
5. Deshmukh HG, Weil MH, Gudipati CV et al (1989) Mechanism of blood flow generated by precordial compression during CPR, I: studies on closed chest precordial compression. Chest 95:1092–1099
6. Chen PS, Wu TJ, Ting CT et al (2003) A tale of two fibrillations. Circulation 108:2298–2303
7. Abella BS, Alvarado JP, Myklebust H et al (2005) Quality of cardiopulmonary resuscitation during in-hospital cardiac arrest. JAMA 293:305–310
8. Wik L, Kramer-Johansen J, Myklebust H et al (2005) Quality of cardiopulmonary resuscitation during out-of-hospital cardiac arrest. JAMA 293:299–304
9. Eftestol T, Sunde K, Steen PA (2002) Effects of interrupting compressions on the calculated probability of defibrillation success during out-of-hospital cardiac arrest. Circulation 105:2270–2273
10. Snyder D, Morgan C (2004) Wide variation in cardiopulmonary resuscitation interruption intervals among commercially available automated external defibrillators may affect survival despite high defibrillation efficacy. Crit Care Med 32:S421–S424
11. Steen S, Liao Q, Pierre L et al (2003) The critical importance of minimal delay between chest compressions and subsequent defibrillation: a haemodynamic explanation. Resuscitation 58:249–258
12. Yu T, Weil MH, Tang W et al (2002) Adverse outcome of interrupted precordial compression during automated defibrillation. Circulation 106:368–372

13. Osswald S, Trouton TG, O'Nunain SS et al (1994) Relation between shock-related myocardial injury and defibrillation efficacy of monophasic and biphasic shocks in a canine model. Circulation 90:2501–2509

14. Weaver MD, Cobb LA, Dennis D et al (1985) Amplitude of ventricular fibrillation waveform and outcome after cardiac arrest. Ann Intern Med 102:53–55

15. Brown CG, Griffith RF, Van Ligten P et al (2004) Median frequency: a new parameter for predicting defibrillation success rate. Ann Emerg Med 20:787–789

16. Watson JN, Uchaipichat N, Addison P et al (2004) Improved prediction of defibrillation success for out-of-hospital VF cardiac arrest using wavelet transform methods. Resuscitation 63:269–275

17. Callaway CW, Sherman LD, Mosesso VN Jr et al (2001) Scaling exponent predicts defibrillation success for out-of-hospital ventricular fibrillation cardiac arrest. Circulation 103:1656–1661

18. Eftestol T, Sunde K, Aase SO et al (2000) Predicting outcome of defibrillation by spectral characterization and nonparametric classification of ventricular fibrillation in patients with out-of-hospital cardiac arrest. Circulation 102:1523–1529

19. Callaway CW, Menegazzi JJ (2005) Waveform analysis of ventricular fibrillation to predict defibrillation. Curr Opin Crit Care 11:192–199

20. Povoas H, Weil MH, Tang W et al (2002) Predicting the success of defibrillation by electrocardiographic analysis. Resuscitation 53:77–82

21. Pernat AM, Weil MH, Tang W et al (2001) Optimizing timing of ventricular defibrillation. Crit Care Med 29:2360–2365

22. Young C, Bisera J, Gehman S et al (2004) Amplitude spectrum area: measuring the probability of successful defibrillation as applied to human data. Crit Care Med 32:S356–S358

23. Ristagno G, Gullo A, Berlot G et al (2008) Prediction of successful defibrillation in human victims of out-of-hospital cardiac arrest: a retrospective electrocardiographic analysis. Anaesth Intensive Care 36:46–50

24. Li Y, Ristagno G, Bisera J et al (2008) Electrocardiogram waveforms for monitoring effectiveness of chest compression during cardiopulmonary resuscitation. Crit Care Med 36:211–215

25. Sun S, Weng Y, Wu X et al (2011) Optimizing the duration of CPR prior to defibrillation improves the outcome of CPR in a rat model of prolonged cardiac arrest. Resuscitation 82:S3–S7

26. Ristagno G, Tan Q, Quan W, et al. (2010) AMSA-based shock decision: a human retrospective analyses during pre-hospital CPR intervention. Circulation 122:A20547 (Abstract)

27. Ristagno G, Quan W, Freeman G. (2012) Amplitude spectrum area to predict defibrillation outcome after recurrent and defibrillation resistant ventricular fibrillation during pre-hospital cardiopulmonary resuscitation. Resuscitation 83:e11–e12 (Abstract)

28. Ristagno G, Fornari C, Li Y, et al. (2012) Amplitude spectrum area-based defibrillation decision during prehospital cardiopulmonary resuscitation in lombardia, Italy. Circulation 126:A143 (Abstract)

29. Paradis NA, Martin GB, Rivers EP et al (1990) Coronary perfusion pressure and the return of spontaneous circulation in human cardiopulmonary resuscitation. JAMA 263:1106–1113

30. Grmec S, Klemen P (2001) Does the end-tidal carbon dioxide (EtCO2) concentration have prognostic value during out-ofhospital cardiac arrest? Eur J Emerg Med 8:263–269

31. Hostler D, Everson-Stewart S, Rea TD et al (2011) Effect of real-time feedback during cardiopulmonary resuscitation outside hospital: prospective, cluster-randomised trial. BMJ 342:d512

32. Perkins GD, Kocierz L, Smith SC et al (2009) Compression feedback devices over estimate chest compression depth when performed on a bed. Resuscitation 80:79–82

33. Nishisaki A, Nysaether J, Sutton R et al (2009) Effect of mattress deflection on CPR quality assessment for older children and adolescents. Resuscitation 80:540–545
34. ECC Committees, Subcommittees, and Task Forces of the American Heart Association. (2005) 2005 American Heart Association guidelines for cardiopulmonary resuscitation and emergency cardiovascular care: part 4. Adult basic life support. Circulation 112:IV-19 –IV-34
35. Berg RA, Hemphill R, Abella BS et al (2010) Part 5: adult basic life support: 2010 American Heart Association Guidelines for Cardiopulmonary Resuscitation and Emergency Cardiovascular Care. Circulation 122:S685–S705
36. Berg RA, Sanders AB, Kern KB et al (2001) Adverse hemodynamic effects of interrupting chest compressions for rescue breathing during cardiopulmonary resuscitation for ventricular fibrillation cardiac arrest. Circulation 104:2465–2470
37. Krarup NH, Terkelsen CJ, Johnsen SP et al (2011) Quality of cardiopulmonary resuscitation in out-of-hospital cardiac arrest is hampered by interruptions in chest compressions–a nationwide prospective feasibility study. Resuscitation 82:263–269

The Importance of Automated External Defibrillation Implementation Programs

7

Fulvio Kette, Yongqin Li, Bihua Chen, Marcella Bozzola, Aldo Locatelli, Guido Villa, Alberto Zoli and Marco Salmoiraghi

7.1 Emphasis on Early Defibrillation: From Clinical Observation to Current Guidelines

The annual incidence of sudden cardiac arrest (CA) is higher than the annual incidence of Alzheimer's disease, diabetes, car accidents, breast cancer, prostate cancer, and house fires combined in the U.S. [1]. In patients who are in ventricular fibrillation (VF), the application of early external electrical countershock has been widely accepted as basic cardiopulmonary resuscitation (CPR) is unlikely to

F. Kette (✉) · M. Bozzola · A. Locatelli · G. Villa · A. Zoli · M. Salmoiraghi
AREU (Azienda Regionale Emergenza Urgenza) – Lombardia Regional Emergency Service,
V. Campanini 6, 20124, Milan, Italy
e-mail: f.kette@areu.lombardia.it

M. Bozzola
e-mail: m.bozzola@areu.lombardia.it

A. Locatelli
e-mail: a.locatelli@areu.lombardia.it

G. Villa
e-mail: gf.villa@areu.lombardia.it

A. Zoli
e-mail: direzione.generale@areu.lombardia.it

M. Salmoiraghi
e-mail: direzione.sanitaria@areu.lombardia.it

Y. Li · B. Chen
School of Biomedical Engineering, Third Military Medical University and Chongqing
University, Chongqing, China
e-mail: leeoken@gmail.com

A. Gullo and G. Ristagno (eds.), *Resuscitation*,
DOI: 10.1007/978-88-470-5507-0_7, © Springer-Verlag Italia 2014

convert VF into a normal rhythm and to guarantee a return of spontaneous circulation (ROSC).

Prehospital defibrillation by ambulance-transported physicians was first established in Belfast in 1966 with an overall significant improvement in the prehospital care. Some notable developments included the tiered response system, training of the general public in CPR, low-energy defibrillators, automatic external defibrillators (AEDs), and 12-lead electrocardiographic telemetry. Unfortunately, emergency medical systems (EMS) with equipped defibrillators sometimes arrive at the scene too late.

Although the deployment of defibrillators is becoming more widespread, it is not as prevalent as one might think. Some estimates suggest that 90 % of ambulances, 10–15% of first-response fire department vehicles, and less than 1% of police vehicles carry defibrillators [2]. Provision of CPR, while waiting for the defibrillator, is of vital importance since it contributes to the preservation of heart and brain function. When performed immediately after collapse from VF, CPR can double or triple the victim's chance of survival, particularly when more than 4–5 min have elapsed from collapse to rescuer intervention [3]. The ILCOR recommendations, converted into the separate American Heart Association (AHA) and European Resuscitation Council (ERC) Guidelines, emphasized the importance of improving chest compressions in terms of depth, rate, and as little interruptions as possible, i.e., the delay from CPR to defibrillation negatively affects the ROSC [4–6].

7.2 The AED Technologies

Created in 1978, AED is a particular lightweight portable device with built-in hardware and software to detect the presence of a shockable rhythm based on ECG sensors placed on the patient's chest. These automated devices have been demonstrated to reduce the training for adequate use and have saved thousands of people's lives since their invention. Advances in AED techniques over the past two decades have made the AEDs more reliable, easy to use, and smarter, such as by adding instrumentations that can monitor the quality of CPR and optimize the timing of defibrillation during CPR.

AEDs were developed for trained emergency medical technicians (EMTs), paramedics, firefighters, polices, securities, and untrained bystander lay persons. The devices therefore must accurately diagnose the lethal arrhythmias without requiring interpretation of the ECG. Their safety largely depends on the automation and quick analysis of ECG to reliably discriminate VF and ventricular tachyarrhythmia (VT) from other rhythms.

Based on the features of diverse nature of the ECG signals (time domain, frequency domain, time frequency analysis), methods with combined parameters were evolved to detect the presence of a shockable rhythm [7]. Although the reliability of the rhythm detection algorithms is convincing, a minimal analysis window of 10 s or more is usually required to accurately detect VF/VT in the current available algorithms. More recently, Li et al. [8] developed a novel continuous wavelet transformation based on morphology consistency evaluation algorithm, which can detect VF in the presence of CPR. The performance of this method was evaluated on both uncorrupted and corrupted ECG signals recorded from AEDs obtained from out-of-hospital victims of CA. Although there was a modest decrease in specificity and accuracy when chest compression artifacts were present, the performance of the proposed method was still superior to other reported methods for VF detection during uninterrupted CPR. However, the developed new algorithms still need to be validated on large patient database to assure high sensitivity for shockable VF/VT and high specificity for non-shockable rhythms.

7.2.1   From Monophasic to Biphasic Waveforms

Earlier AEDs used monophasic waveforms which deliver the current to the patient in a single direction (from one electrode to another). Unlike monophasic waveforms, the biphasic waveforms are more effective than monophasic waveforms due to a lesser tendency to reinitiate VF in regions of residual charge left on the myocardium. The second phase of the biphasic shock is believed to neutralize virtual electrodes and tissue polarization residual from the first phase. The most widely used is the biphasic truncated exponential (BTE) waveform, which was initially developed for implantable cardioverter defibrillator and became the standard for AEDs in the late 1980s. The advantage of this waveform is that it has lower defibrillation threshold compared to monophasic defibrillation and could therefore allow the design of devices that are substantially smaller and lighter than the monophasic waveform.

The rectilinear biphasic waveform (RBW) was developed specifically for external defibrillation and takes into account the high and variable patient impedance levels. It was successfully tested in multicenter, prospective, randomized, transthoracic defibrillator animal, and clinical trials. It has also been proven to have superior efficacy to monophasic damped sine waveforms and monophasic truncated waveforms for defibrillation [9, 10]. Another defibrillation waveform used in AED is the pulsed biphasic waveform (PBW) [11]. As BTE waveform, the PBW consists of two phases of current flowing in opposite directions. However, each of the two phases in PBW includes a set of alternating active and inactive phases.

The defibrillation efficacy may differ when different biphasic waveforms are used. However, the efficacy of different biphasic waveforms has not been compared in human studies. The Guidelines 2010 [6], therefore state that "*For biphasic defibrillators, providers should use the manufacturer's recommended energy dose. If the manufacturer's recommended dose is not known, defibrillation at the maximal dose may be considered.*"

7.2.2 Energy, Current, Waveform Duration

Energy is still the most common parameter used to indicate the strength of the shock. However, there is growing evidence that energy is not the best indicator as the current flowing through the myocites defibrillates the heart[12, 13]. Recent investigations by our own group highlighted large differences in the current delivered by the different AEDs [14, 15]. Although there were several reports on the importance of the current as the leading parameter, there is as yet no evidence on the proper amount of current needed to successfully defibrillate a fibrillating heart nor is there a precise quantity of current above which the damage to the cells occurred [12].

Besides the current, the other variable of paramount importance is the shock duration. Although the data on this issue are quite scarce, there is some evidence that the first phase shock duration should be around 5 ms (msec), whereas the total waveform duration should be no longer than 20 ms [16]. Above this value, refibrillation might occur.

7.2.3 Monitoring the Quality of CPR

Large observational clinical studies have provided important information about the positive impact of bystander CPR on survival after out-of-hospital CA [17, 18]. Quality of CPR, including adequate compression rate and depth, complete chest recoil after each compression, and voiding excessive ventilation, is likely to be one of the key factors that affect resuscitation and survival. However, the quality of both in-hospital and out-of-hospital CPR is not optimal. Using a sternal pad to monitor chest compressions and ventilations, Abella et al. [19] found that the quality of multiple parameters of CPR often did not meet published guideline recommendations, even when performed by well-trained hospital staff for in-hospital cardiac arrest (CA) patients.

Wik and colleagues [20] studied the quality of CPR during out-of-hospital CA by using a monitor/defibrillator equipped with sensors that measure and record variables related to CPR performance. They concluded that chest compressions performed by ambulance personnel in their study were often too shallow and that overall CPR performance did not meet current guidelines. Their study also suggested that CPR quality and patient survival may be improved by using resuscitation aids that give rescuers feedback to deliver chest compressions of correct depth and rate with minimal interruptions.

Real-time CPR prompting and feedback technologies such as visual and auditory prompting devices can improve the quality of CPR. The application of automated computer-based audible feedback system also showed an improvement in the quality of CPR during manikin training when incorporated into an AED [21]. Using an extra chest pad mounted on the lower part of the sternum with an accelerometer and a pressure sensor, Kramer-Johansen et al. [22] demonstrated that quality of CPR was greatly improved with a real-time automatic feedback in a prospective non-randomized interventional study of out-of-hospital CA. Therefore, instructions from the AED may be highly valuable in aiding the performance of CPR.

7.2.4 Automated Pulse Detection

The use of AEDs by minimally trained individuals who lack the skills to differentiate CA from other causes of collapse may increase the probability of an incorrect diagnosis between CA, shock, breathing arrhythmia (irregular heartbeat), or asphyxia. Identification of blood circulation by detecting a pulse can help the rescuer to perform optimal intervention. However, detecting the presence of a pulse is difficult in weak patients, such as a victim in shock or CA [23]. Thus automated pulse detection is of critical importance during CA especially in out-of-hospital settings.

To examine the use of four parameters extracted from the impedance cardiogram as predictors of cardiac output, Johnston et al. [24] recorded the ECG and impedance through two defibrillation pads placed in an anterior-apical position in 107 CA victims. Their study validated that the impedance cardiogram measured from conventional defibrillation electrodes was a potential hemodynamic sensor for AED. The changes in transthoracic impedance coincident with cardiac contractions and arterial pressure pulses have been confirmed with echocardiography and blood pressure measurements. Pellis et al. [25] also expanded AEDs to include detection of cardiac, respiratory, and cardiorespiratory arrest by using the same electrodes currently applied for defibrillation in an experimental study. Losert and colleagues [26] validated that transthoracic impedance changes measured via defibrillator pads to monitor the sign of circulation in CA victims. Implementation of this technology into AEDs will allow AEDs to affirmatively recognize pulseless electrical activity and prompt chest compression without repetitive interruptions for ECG analyses. The priorities of CPR interventions therefore may be improved by the detection of the presence or absence of the pulse, including the distinction between dysrhythmic and asphyxial CA.

7.2.5 Optimizing the Time of Defibrillation

Since characteristics of VF waveform change over time and with CPR, which exhibit ability for prognostication of defibrillation success, several retrospective case series, animal studies, and theoretical models suggest that it is possible to predict the probability of shock outcome and to optimize the timing of defibrillation by analyzing the VF waveform [27]. The search for defibrillation prediction features gained from VF waveforms dates back to 20 years, and recently published review articles [28, 29] provide excellent overviews of various techniques developed for VF waveform analysis. Approaches for optimizing timing of defibrillation, including measures based on time domain methods, frequency domain methods including wavelet-based transformation, nonlinear dynamics methods, and a combination of these methods, have gained some success in clinical trials. Presently, the measurements of amplitude spectrum analysis (AMSA) parameter seem to provide reliable information on the optimal timing for defibrillation [30].

7.3   The Development of the Public Access Defibrillation: From Historical Perspective to Present

The goal of early defibrillation gave rise to the development of AEDs available to nonprofessional rescuer. In the early 1970s, Diack and colleagues described experimental and clinical experience with the first AED [31]. Subsequently, other studies provided supportive evidence for the potential role of such a device in achieving a rapid defibrillation [32, 33]. In 1984, Cummins et al. assessed the performance of AED used by paramedics to detect VF and deliver countershocks in out-of-hospital CA patients [34]. This study confirmed the sensitivity and specificity of the AED algorithms as well as the safety and efficacy of the device. In 1988, Weaver and coworkers [35] presented their data on the comparison of initial treatment with AED by firefighters who arrived first at the scene, with the results of standard defibrillation administered by paramedics who arrived slightly after the firefighters. Their findings supported the widespread use of the AED as an important part of the treatment of out-of-hospital CA, although the overall impact on community survival rates was still uncertain. These studies, together with the improved portability and ease of use of AED, have led to the expansion of defibrillation to trained first-responders who often arrive at the scene of an arrest before paramedics. Studies on the use of AED by such personnel have shown a dramatic reduction in the time before defibrillation and have thus enhanced survival.

Highly evident data on the effects of early defibrillation by lay people were documented when the AEDs were located in public places such as in the casinos in Las Vegas, in the airports, and on the airplanes. In 1991, Quantas Airlines initiated a program using AEDs on overseas flights and at major terminals with selected crew trained for CPR and use of AED [36, 37]. In 1997, a major U.S. airline began equipping its aircrafts with AEDs. Flight attendants were trained in the use of the defibrillator and applied the device when passengers had a lack of consciousness, pulse, or respiration. Page et al. [38] reported the results of AED use on 200 patients between June 1997 and July 1999 from American Airlines. Of those patients with VF, the rate of survival to discharge from the hospital after shock with the AED was 40%. Based on these experiences, several U.S. and international airlines have installed AEDs.

Valenzuela et al. [39] studied a prospective series of cases of sudden CA in casinos where *"personnel using an AED can improve survival after out-of-hospital CA due to VF. Intervals of no more than 3 min from collapse to defibrillation are necessary to achieve the highest survival rates."*

In 2002, Caffrey et al. [40] performed a 2-year prospective study at three Chicago airports to assess whether random bystander-witnessing out-of-hospital CA would retrieve and successfully use AEDs. Among the 21 CA persons, 18 had VF and 10 patients were alive and neurologically intact at 1 year.

Due to the high prevalence of CA at home accounting for more than 70% of the arrests, it was thought that placing the AEDs in families where members are at higher risk of sudden cardiac death could be associated with increased survival. Moore and his collaborators [41] assessed the ability of 34 family members of CA survivors to learn and retain defibrillation skills using an AED in 1987. McDaniel et al. [42] tested the practical aspects of home AED use in high risk patients after myocardial infarction in 1988. In the following year, Eisenberg and coworkers [43] evaluated the use of AEDs in the homes of high risk cardiac patients, but only *"a small potential for AEDs to save high risk patients"* were found. These results partly limited the enthusiasm for placement of AEDs in the home of high risk patients.

In a recent international, multicenter clinical trial, Bardy et al. [44] evaluated the benefit of the availability of AEDs in the homes of patients with a previous anterior-wall myocardial infarction who were not otherwise candidates for implantation of a cardioverter defibrillator. Their data showed that there was no significant reduction in death from any cause with a home AED. The authors concluded that *"access to a home AED did not significantly improve overall survival, as compared with reliance on conventional resuscitation methods."*

More recently, Jorgenson et al. reported the effectiveness of home AEDs on survival. Although the number of patients treated was low (25 in 7 years), they supported the use of home AEDs as 8 of 12 patients found in VF survived to hospital discharge. Nevertheless, all the 12 patients were in the group of witnessed CA [45].

The combination of ease-to-use, low cost, and negligible maintenance makes public access AED potentially attractive for the treatment of VF. Through the widespread deployment of defibrillators within a community, the "collapse-to-shock" time can decrease and survival rates may increase. According to a 2003 nationwide survey of workplaces by the American College of Environmental and Occupational Medicine (ACOEM), 34% of those who have implemented an AED program have used their AED at least once in order to help save a life with an overall primary success rate of 71% [46].

7.4   Legislation

There is a large variety of regulations around the world as per the PAD projects. Overall, most of the countries in Europe do not have a specific law. The use of AED is based on individual decision and/or on the training of lay people. In 2010, Bahr and coworkers reported a survey on 36 European countries on the existence of specific legislation for the use of AEDs. Among the 36 countries only 7 have a law establishing the rules for the use of AEDs, 27 do not have any legislation at all, whereas 2 reported not to know if there is a legislation [47]. Table 7.1 summarizes the overall situation.

Italy is one of the few countries in which specific laws on AEDs were promulgated in the last decade. The first national decree, presented in 2000, allowed the use of AEDs to stewards and flight attendants following a successful course on BLSD [48]. In the following year, the first law stated that non-doctors were allowed to use an AED in the out-of-hospital setting provided an adequate training course and a successful attendance to a course [49].

In 2004, this law was amended with the extension to the in-hospital setting, thus allowing nurses and other personnel to use the AED following a course successfully passed [50].

The major implementation under the legislative point of view, however, occurred in 2011 in which a large and overall well-detailed decree focused on many items such as the responsibility of the projects, the figures or associations in charge of training, the validity of a certificate, and the goals of the entire projects [51]. This decree demanded of the Regional governments the whole organization and the responsibility which, in turn, were left to the local (provincial) 118 Emergency Services. On one hand this led to a certain level of rules by defining

Table 7.1 Legislation on AED use in European countries. Bahr et al., Resuscitation, [47]

Presence of legislation	No legislation			Data not available
Austria	Bulgaria	Ireland	Russian Federation	Albania
Belgium	Croatia	Lithuania	Serbia	Bosnia and Herzegowina
Cyprus	Czech Republic	Luxemburg	Slovenia	
France	Denmark	Macedonia	Sweden	
Greece	Estonia	Malta	Switzerland	
Italy	Finland	Netherlands	Turkey	
Spain	Germany	Norvay	UK	
	Hungary	Poland	Ukraine	
	Iceland	Portugal		

not only the responsibility but also the practical aspects of training. Overall an improved homogeneity emerged. On the other hand, however, other discrepancies arose among the Italian Regions with contrasting rules such as the validity of a certificate not recognized in Regions different from where the course was held. Another paradox was the requirement of some local 118 EMS which made mandatory the attendance (and the successful overcoming) of a course for a specific AED model, thus obliging people to attend different courses according to the AED models employed.

Lombardia Region made a step forward in the attempt to overcome many of the controversial aspects that emerged in the national and regional legislations [52]. In our document, indeed, we first recognized the validity of a certificate for every kind of AED. Secondly, those who passed a course in another region were fully recognized by our Regional EMS without the need to attend another course if held within 2 years. Thirdly, we defined those persons whose AED use is mandatory (all personnel working in the emergency setting and those who work on every ambulance service even if not dedicated to the emergency interventions). A list of other people to whom the use of AED was either recommended or advised was then presented. Concurrently, we also listed the places where the AEDs should be located. The document ends up with the modality to prepare a PAD project and the information to be provided to our Regional EMS staff.

Particular attention was paid to sport societies and to sport facilities according to a more recent national law which established the need that every amateur and professional sport society must have an AED. This law was recently approved with detailed recommendation on AED location and adequate trained personnel.

Some considerations can emerge regarding the opportunity of having a specific legislation on AEDs. On one hand one may raise questions about the uselessness of specific laws stating that any law could be too restrictive and that the laws would impede a proper diffusion and use of AED. In other nations anyone who witnesses a person with a loss of consciousness (potentially a CA patient) may use an AED without any restriction since the AEDs are safe and avoid misuse by simply following their vocal prompts. The Good Samaritan Laws applied in the USA indeed follows this rule. This is true in Italy as well. Our legislation indeed does not impede the use of AED by those who are not certified or by those who did not attend a course. There are no penalties for those who apply an AED without training. The main reason for having established national (and consequently regional) statements is to emphasize the importance of being trained not only in AED use (which is the easiest part) but also in CPR and how to combine both maneuvers. Based on the current epidemiological data, VF accounts for about 20–40 % of the presenting CA rhythms [53–55]. Yet, early and uninterrupted chest compression is by far more important than a delayed application of an AED. Accordingly, the use alone of an AED without at least some chest compression would limit the potential benefits of a rescue by lay people.

Although not all would agree with the national and regional legislation, it is our personal belief that our country has made important steps forward with the introduction of these laws.

7.5   Implementation of the PAD Programs

Although there is no formula for determining the optimal number of defibrillators and their appropriate placement, deployment should be based on shortened response time (an ideal collapse to shock goal $\leq$3–5 min) and on CA risk factors that exist within the population. Usually, number and location are based on local strategies and resources. Nielsen and coworkers in Denmark reported more than 5,000 AEDs registered in their nation but estimates suggest that more than 15,000 AEDs were sold for a population of 5.5 million inhabitants [56]. To be most effective, Atkins suggested that the PAD projects (and therefore the location of the AEDs) should be acknowledged by the local EMS. In the absence of proper check of the equipment, batteries and pads have progressively expired thus making the AED ineffective [57].

Based on these recommendations, our group began the strategy of precisely mapping almost every AED on our regional territory (Lombardia Region). This led to the identification of more than 600 AEDs for a population of 10 million inhabitants, which were categorized and precisely located. For each AED, a person responsible for the project and for the maintenance was identified. Every AED was mapped according to its geographical coordinates and was inserted into a dynamic software that highlights the position on a satellite map.

Another point of improvement is the placement of the AEDs within boxes or cabinets electronically connected to the 118 dispatch centers and therefore alarmed. Any device removal will trigger an immediate alarm at the Operative Center. This project, however, is still in progress and data will be needed for an adequate assessment of this strategy.

7.6   Impact of PAD Projects on Survival

The real impact of the PAD projects or the public AEDs by laypeople has only been recently documented. Overall, interventions on CA patients by laypeople account for only 2 % of the total treatments, with most of them being carried out by the EMS personnel. In a study by Weisfeldt and coworkers on public AEDs, only 289 of 13,769 CA patients were initially treated by laypeople but only 170 were shocked before EMS arrival [58]. Comparable proportions were also reported by Rea [59], though showing a gradual increase from 0.6 to 2.4 % in 2006 in the proportion of patients rescued by laypeople. Kitamura in his nationwide study reported a progressive rise in the proportion of patients saved by public AEDs which increased from 1.2 to 6.2 % [60]. Our unpublished results in the province of Bergamo (Lombardia Region) highlighted comparable proportions (Table 7.2).

Table 7.2 Data from out-of-hospital cardiac arrest in Bergamo province (Lombardia Region, North Italy)

	2003	2004	2005	2006	2007	2008	2009	2010	2011	2012
Cardiac arrest initially treated by EMS	14	111	204	191	163	177	195	239	231	268
Cardiac arrest initially treated by PAD			1	6	3		1	1	5	4
Total	14	111	205	197	166	177	196	240	236	272

Despite the low proportion of patients shocked by laypeople, survival among these patients is very high ranging from 55 to 65 % [39, 40, 45, 56]. More so, Nielsen and coworkers observed in their population of VF patients that more than 70 % were in VF [56]. This result is indeed challenging as in the last decade a progressive decline in the proportion of patients in VF was widely documented. If Nielsen's results are confirmed in other studies, the epidemiology of CA and the presenting rhythm will have to be further re-evaluated.

7.7 Conclusions

PAD projects have been introduced to strength the chain of survival by reducing the time window from cardiac arrest to the onset of CPR. Also, a prompt defibrillation by laypeople is desirable. The evidence suggests that the results are more effective when the PAD projects are strongly linked to the local EMS. This will further prompt a close connection with the dispatch centers able to locate the closest AED. Besides the use of AEDs, however, it must be remembered that early chest compression represents the most importance initial treatment when an AED is not immediately available.

References

1. Go AS, Mozaffarian D, Roger VL et al (2013) Heart disease and stroke statistics–2013 update: a report from the American Heart Association. Circulation 127(1):e6–e245
2. http://www.laerdal.com/au/docid/36016554/The-Importance-of-Early-Defibrillation
3. Valenzuela TD, Roe DJ, Cretin S et al (1997) Estimating effectiveness of cardiac arrest interventions: a logistic regression survival model. Circulation 96:3308–3313
4. Nolan JP, Hazinski MF, Billi JE, Boettiger BW, Bossaert LB et al (2010) International consensus on cardiopulmonary resuscitation and emergency cardiovascular care science with treatment recommendations. Resuscitation 81S:e1–e330
5. Field JM, Hazinski MF, Sayre MR, Chameides L, Schexnayder SM, Hemphill R, Samson RA (2010) American heart association guidelines for cardiopulmonary resuscitation and emergency cardiovascular care. Circulation 122:s640–s933
6. Nolan JP, Soar J, Zideman DA, Biarent D, Bossaert LL, Deakin C, Koster RW, Wyllie J, Böttiger B (2010) On behalf of the ERC guidelines writing group. European resuscitation council guidelines for resuscitation. Resuscitation 81:1219–1451

7. Chen B, Wang K, Wang J et al (2012) Novel Ventricular Fibrillation/Tachycardia Detection Algorithms Used for Automated External Defibrillators. Recent Pat Eng 6:217–225

8. Li Y, Bisera J, Weil MH et al (2012) An algorithm used for ventricular fibrillation detection without interrupting chest compression. IEEE Trans Biomed Eng Jan 59:78–86

9. Morrison LJ, Dorian P, Long J et al (2005) Out-of-hospital cardiac arrest rectilinear biphasic to monophasic damped sine defibrillation waveforms with advanced life support intervention trial (ORBIT). Resuscitation 66:149–157

10. Stothert JC, Hatcher TS, Gupton CL et al (2004) Rectilinear biphasic waveform defibrillation of out-of-hospital cardiac arrest. Prehosp Emerg Care 8:388–392

11. Didon JP, Fontaine G, White RD et al (2008) Clinical experience with a low-energy pulsed biphasic waveform in out-of-hospital cardiac arrest. Resuscitation 76:350–353

12. Kerber RE, Kouba C, Martins J, Kelly K, Low R, Hoyt R, Ferguson D, Bailey L, Bennett P, Charbonnier F (1984) Advance prediction of transthoracic impedance in human defibrillation and cardioversion: importance of impedance in determining the success of low-energy shock. Circulation 70:303–308

13. Dalzell GWN, Cunnigham SR, Anderson J, Adgey AAJ (1989) Initial experience with a microprocessor controlled current based defibrillator. Br Heart J 61:502–505

14. Kette F, Locatelli L, Bozzola M, Zoli A, Li Y, Salmoiraghi M, Ristagno G, Andreassi A (2013) Electrical features of eighteen automated external defibrillators: a systematic evaluation. Resuscitation. doi:pii: S0300-9572(13)00298-0. 10.1016/j.resuscitation.2013.05.017

15. Bozzola M (2012) Automated external defibrillators: comparison of different waveforms. Resuscitation 83:e56

16. Shan Y, Ristagno G, Fuller M, Sun S, Li Y, Weil MH, Russell J, Tang W (2010) The effects of phase duration on defibrillation success of dual time constant biphasic waveforms. Resuscitation 81:236–241

17. SOS-KANTO Study Group (2007) Cardiopulmonary resuscitation by bystanders with chest compression only (SOS-KANTO): an observational study. Lancet 369:920–926

18. Kitamura T, Iwami T, Kawamura T et al (2010) Conventional and chest-compression-only cardiopulmonary resuscitation by bystanders for children who have out-of-hospital cardiac arrests: a prospective, nationwide, population-based cohort study. Lancet 375:1347–1354

19. Abella BS, Alvarado JP, Myklebust H et al (2005) Quality of cardiopulmonary resuscitation during in-hospital cardiac arrest. JAMA 293:305–310

20. Wik L, Kramer-Johansen J, Myklebust H et al (2005) Quality of cardiopulmonary resuscitation during out-of-hospital cardiac arrest. JAMA 293:299–304

21. Handley AJ, Handley SA (2003) Improving CPR performance using an audible feedback system suitable for incorporation into an automated external defibrillator. Resuscitation 57:57–62

22. Kramer-Johansen J, Myklebust H, Wik L et al (2006) Quality of out-of-hospital cardiopulmonary resuscitation with real time automated feedback: a prospective interventional study. Resuscitation 71:283–292

23. Dick WF, Eberle B, Wisser G et al (2000) The carotid pulse check revisited: what if there is no pulse? Crit Care Med 28:N183–N185

24. Johnston PW, Imam Z, Dempsey G et al (1998) The trans-thoracic impedance cardiogram is a potential haemodynamic sensor for an automated external defibrillator. Eur Heart J 19:1879–1888

25. Pellis T, Bisera J, Tang W et al (2002) Expanding automatic external defibrillators to include automated detection of cardiac respiratory, and cardio-respiratory arrest. Crit Care Med 30:S176–S178

26. Losert H, Risdal M, Sterz F et al (2007) Thoracic-impedance changes measured via defibrillator pads can monitor signs of circulation. Resuscitation 73:221–228

27. Reed MJ, Clegg GR, Robertson CE (2003) Analysing the ventricular fibrillation waveform. Resuscitation 57:11–20

28. Callaway CW, Menegazzi JJ (2005) Waveform analysis of ventricular fibrillation to predict defibrillation. Curr Opin Crit Care 11:192–199
29. Li Y, Tang W (2012) Optimizing the timing of defibrillation: the role of ventricular fibrillation waveform analysis during cardiopulmonary resuscitation. Crit Care Clin 28:199–210
30. Ristagno G, Gullo A, Berlot G, Lucangelo U, Geheb E, Bisera J (2008) Prediction of successful defibrillation in human victims of out-of-hospital cardiac arrest: a retrospective electrocardiographic analysis. Anaesth Intensive Care 36:46–50
31. Diack AW, Welborn WS, Rullman RG et al (1979) An automatic cardiac resuscitator for emergency treatment of cardiac arrest. Med Instrum 13:78–83
32. Jaggarao NS, Heber M, Grainger R et al (1982) Use of an automated external defibrillator-pacemaker by ambulance staff. Lancet 2:73–75
33. Rozkovec A, Crossley J, Walesby R et al (1983) Safety and effectiveness of a portable external automatic defibrillator-pacemaker. Clin Cardiol 6:527–533
34. Cummins RO, Eisenberg M, Bergner L (1984) Sensitivity, accuracy, and safety of an automatic external defibrillator. Lancet 2:318–320
35. Weaver WD, Hill D, Fahrenbruch CE et al (1988) Use of the automatic external defibrillator in the management of out-of-hospital cardiac arrest. N Engl J Med 319:661–666
36. O'Rourke M, Donaldson E (1995) Management of ventricular fibrillation in commercial airliners. Lancet 345:515–516
37. O'Rourke MF, Donaldson E, Geddes JS (1997) An airline cardiac arrest program. Circulation 96:2849–2853
38. Page RL, Joglar JA, Kowal RC et al (2000) Use of automated external defibrillators by a U.S. airline. N Engl J Med 343:1210–1216
39. Valenzuela TD, Roe DJ, Nichol G et al (2000) Outcomes of rapid defibrillation by security officers after cardiac arrest in casinos. N Engl J Med 343:1206–1209
40. Caffrey S, Willoughby P, Pepe P, Becker L (2002) Public use of automated external defibrillators. N Engl J Med 347:1242–1247
41. Moore JE, Eisenberg MS, Cummins RO et al (1987) Lay person use of automatic external defibrillation. Ann Emerg Med 16:669–672
42. McDaniel CM, Berry VA, Haines DE et al (1988) Automatic external defibrillation of patients after myocardial infarction by family members: practical aspects and psychological impact of training. Pacing Clin Electrophysiol 11:2029–2034
43. Eisenberg MS, Moore J, Cummins RO et al (1989) Use of the automatic external defibrillator in homes of survivors of out-of-hospital ventricular fibrillation. Am J Cardiol 63:443–446
44. Bardy GH, Lee KL, Mark DB et al (2008) Home use of automated external defibrillators for sudden cardiac arrest. N Engl J Med 358:1793–1804
45. Jorgenson DB, Yount TB, White RD, Lin PY, Esienberg MS, Becker LB (2013) Impact of sudden cardiac arrest in the home. A safety and effectiveness study on privately-owned AEDs. Resuscitation 84:149–153
46. Utilization and Impact of AEDs in the Workplace: A Survey of Occupational Health Physicians (2003) American college of occupational and environmental medicine. Available at: http://www.acoem.org/AEDSurveyResults.aspx
47. Bahr J, Bossaert L, Handley A, Koster R, Vissers B, Monsieur K (2010) AED in Europe. Report on a survey. Resuscitation 81:168–174
48. Decree (2000) September 21, 2000: use of semi-automated external defibrillators on board of aircrafts and training courses for chief stewards
49. Law 120 (2001) April 3, 2001. Use of in the out-of-hospital setting. GU 88, April 14, 2001
50. Law 69 (2004) March 16, 2004. Modification of art. 1 of the law 120 re semiautomated external defibrillators
51. Decree (2011) March 18, 2011. Criteria for diffusion of semi-automated external defibrillators

52. Lombardia Regional Government Deliberation 4717 (2013) January 23, 2013. Regional guidelines on the use of semi-automated external defibrillators and on PAD projects diffusion on the regional land
53. Cobb LA, Fahrenbruch CE, Olsufka M, Copass MK (2002) Changing incidence of out-of-hospital ventricular fibrillation, 1980–2000. JAMA 288(23):3008–3013
54. Herlitz J, Engdahl J, Svensson L, Young M, Angquist KA, Holmberg S (2004) Decrease in the occurrence of ventricular fibrillation as the initially observed arrhythmia after out-of-hospital cardiac arrest during 11 years in Sweden. Resuscitation 60(3):283–290
55. Kette F, Pellis T (2007) Pordenone cardiac arrest cooperative study group (PACS). Increased survival despite a reduction in out-of-hospital ventricular fibrillation in north-east Italy. Resuscitation 72(1):52–58
56. Nielsen AM, Folke F, Lippert FK, Rasmussen LS (2010) Use and benefits of public access defibrillation in a nation-wide network. Resuscitation 84:430–434
57. Atkins DL (2010) Realistic expectations for public access defibrillation programs. Ciurr opin Crtic Care 16:191–195
58. Weisfeldt ML, Sitlani CM, Ornato JP, Rea T, Aufderheide TP, Davis D, Dreyer J, Hess EP, Jui J, Maloney J, Sopko G, Powell J, Nichol G, Morrison LJ (2010) ROC Investigators. Survival after application of automatic external defibrillators before arrival of the emergency medical system: evaluation in the resuscitation outcomes consortium population of 21 million. J Am Coll Cardiol 55(16):1713–1720
59. Rea TD, Olsufka M, Bennis B, White L, Yin L, Becker L, Copass M, Eisenberg M, Cobb L (2010) A population-base investigation of public access defibrillation: role of emergency medical service care. Resuscitation 81:163–167
60. Kitamura T, Iwami T, Nagao K, Tanaka H, Hiraide A (2010) Nation-wide public access defibrillation in Japan. NEJM 362:994–1004

Part III
Optimization of Cardiopulmonary and Cerebral Resuscitation on Sudden Cardiac Death

Mechanical Versus Manual CPR

8

Giuseppe Ristagno

8.1 Introduction

Cardiac arrest represents a dramatic clinical event that can occur suddenly and often without premonitory signs. This condition is characterized by sudden loss of consciousness caused by the lack of cerebral blood flow, which occurs when the heart ceases to pump. Indeed, it represents a leading cause of death in the Western world, with as many as 350,000–700,000 people in the United States, Canada, and Europe sustaining cardiac arrest each year [1, 2]. Cardiopulmonary resuscitation (CPR), including chest compression, often in conjunction with electrical defibrillation, has the potential of re-establishing spontaneous circulation (ROSC). Despite major efforts to improve outcomes from cardiac arrest, average survival rate remains dismal and presents a large variation with a spread between 2 and 39 % [3, 4]. Both in heavily populated larger cities and in sparsely populated rural communities, delayed response by emergency medical services compromises outcomes such that survival is more disappointing.

During cardiac arrest, coronary blood flow ceases, accounting for a progressive and severe energy imbalance. Intramyocardial hypercarbic acidosis is associated with depletion of high energy phosphates and correspondingly severe global myocardial ischemia [5]. The ischemic left ventricle becomes contracted ushering in the stone heart [6]. After onset of contracture, the probability of ROSC becomes remote. There is now evidence that the highest priority of intervention is to re-establish systemic blood flow promptly by external chest compression, and thereby achieve and maintain threshold levels of coronary and cerebral perfusion.

G. Ristagno (✉)
Department of Cardiovascular Research, IRCCS – Istituto di Ricerche Farmacologiche
"Mario Negri", via La Masa 19, 20156 Milan, Italy
e-mail: gristag@gmail.com

A. Gullo and G. Ristagno (eds.), *Resuscitation*,
DOI: 10.1007/978-88-470-5507-0_8, © Springer-Verlag Italia 2014

Accordingly, effective, consistent, and uninterrupted chest compression is now designated as the primary intervention for management of cardiac arrest. Both survival and neurological recovery are contingent upon initiating chest compression within <5 min [7, 8]. Accordingly, bystander initiated chest compressions by minimally trained, nonprofessional rescuers subsequently supported by well-organized professional emergency medical providers have significantly increased survival from out-of-hospital cardiac arrest.

8.2   Quality of CPR

In addition to the benefits of prompt intervention, it is also the quality of chest compressions delivered in both in- and out-of-hospital settings that has proven to be a determinant of outcomes. Indeed, blood flows generated by chest compression are dependent on the pressure gradient between the aortic and the venous pressures. Coronary perfusion pressure (CPP), defined as the difference between simultaneously measured minimal aortic pressure and right atrial pressure during compression diastole, is highly correlated with coronary blood flow during cardiac resuscitation and is currently recognized as the best single indicator of the likelihood of ROSC [9]. Based on both experimental and clinical observations, ROSC can be predicted when CPP is maintained above 15 mmHg during compressions [9, 10]. Resuscitative strategies that increase CPP, including high quality chest compressions as well as the use of vasopressor, have been therefore supported and considered more effective in restore circulation. In fact, although chest compression produces less than 50 % of prearrest stroke volumes, threshold levels of myocardial and cerebral blood flows are restored such as to minimize ischemic myocardial and cerebral ischemic injury [11].

The evidence is secure that the quality of chest compression is a major determinant of successful resuscitation. A good quality CPR should be performed with: adequate chest compression depth and rate; duty cycle; minimal interruptions; and complete chest recoil [12]. Yet, there is persuasive evidence that conventional manual chest compressions are often performed ineffectively. Indeed, whereas 23 % of victims were resuscitated after what Wik et al. defined as "good CPR," only 1 % were resuscitated with "not good CPR" [13]. In both in-hospital and out-of-hospital settings, the quality of CPR, and specifically chest compressions, was also the major determinant of the ROSC. Based on 176 victims of out-of-hospital cardiac arrest, only 28 % of rescuers performed competent chest compressions in which the anterior–posterior diameter was decreased by approximately 5 cm so as to conform to the international guidelines [14]. An inadequate depth of chest compressions was also reported in 67 instances of in-hospital cardiac arrest [15]. Human observational studies also showed that interruptions of chest compressions are common, averaging 24–57 % of the total arrest time [13].

However, even well-trained professional providers cannot maintain effective chest compression for intervals that exceed 2 min [16, 17]. This limitation is in addition to the documented inconsistency of depth and rate of compressions [14–18]. The challenges are even greater during evacuation and transport of victims. Therefore, the option of using mechanical devices is attractive. Mechanical chest compression potentially overcomes operator fatigue, slow rates of compression, and inadequate depth of compression. A mechanical compressor would also allow for the delivery of an electrical shock without interruption of manual compression for the protection of the rescuer.

8.3 Mechanical Compression

Several new devices have recently been introduced to facilitate mechanical chest compression [19]. Both the AutoPulse (ZOLL Medical Corporation, USA) and the Lund University Cardiac Arrest System (LUCAS) (LUCAS, PhysioControl, Sweden) have demonstrated equivalency and potentially even greater effectiveness than manual chest compression.

8.4 AutoPulse

The AutoPulse is a battery powered load-distributing band, mechanical CPR device. Its functioning is based on the concept that distributing force over the entire chest through a band improves the effectiveness of chest compressions by delivering more total energy to the torso. The device adjusts automatically to the size and shape of each patient and is constructed around a backboard that contains a motorized rotating shaft. It utilizes a load-distributing band, which is connected to the rotating shaft to compress the chest. The band is tightened or relaxed around the chest rhythmically to provide a "squeezing" effect during the compression phase [20]. AutoPulse-CPR features are reported in Table 8.1.

Earlier animal studies of pigs and clinical studies in the setting of in-hospital cardiac arrest have reported better hemodynamics during mechanical compression with AutoPulse in comparison to standard manual CPR [21, 22]. Subsequently, nonrandomized human series have reported increased rates of sustained ROSC

Table 8.1 AutoPulse-CPR features

Compression depth: 20 % of chest anterior–posterior diameter
Rate of compression: 80/min
Duty cycle: equal compression/decompression time
Compression/ventilation ratio: 30/2 or continuous compressions
Full chest recoil allowed

[23] and increased survival to hospital discharge following out-of-hospital cardiac arrest with AutoPulse in comparison to standard CPR (9.7 versus 2.9 %) [24]. Based on these results, the ASPIRE trial (AutoPulse Assisted Prehospital International Resuscitation) was initiated [25]. It was a multicenter, randomized trial of patients experiencing out-of-hospital cardiac arrest in the United States and Canada. The trial compared mechanical cardiopulmonary resuscitation with AutoPulse device (AutoPulse-CPR) to traditional manual CPR (manual-CPR). The primary end point was survival to 4 h after the 911 call, while secondary end points were survival to hospital discharge and neurological outcome. Enrollment was suspended early due to safety concerns, after approximately 1,000 patients. No difference existed in the primary end point of survival to 4 h. However, survival to hospital discharge was 9.9 % in the manual-CPR group and 5.8 % in the Auto-Pulse-CPR. More importantly, a significantly worse neurologic outcome was observed when AutoPulse-CPR was compared with manual-CPR (3.1 versus 7.5 %, $p = 0.006$). However, a subsequently posthoc analysis of this study revealed significant heterogeneity among study sites [26]. Indeed, one site (site C) made a potentially important protocol change midtrial, and enrollment at that site was noted to be independently associated with outcome. The protocol change at site C also appeared to have resulted in a delay in application of AutoPulse-CPR. Before and after the protocol change survival in patients receiving AutoPulse-CPR decreased from 19.6 to 4 %. At the time the trial was suspended, the outcomes of patients at the other sites appeared to have been trending in favor of the intervention.

A more recent prospective cohort evaluation compared resuscitation outcomes before and after switching from manual CPR to AutoPulse-CPR in a multicenter emergency department trial, enrolling 1,011 patients (459 in the manual CPR and 552 patients in the AutoPulse-CPR) [27]. The rate of survival to hospital discharge tended to be higher in the Autopulse-CPR phase (3.3 %) versus the manual one (1.3 %). There were also more survivors in the AutoPulse group with cerebral performance category 1 compared to the manual group ($p = 0.01$).

Finally, another multicenter randomized clinical trial, the "Circulation Improving Resuscitation Care (CIRC)" trial was conducted by Dr. Wik [28] and compared AutoPulse versus "high quality" manual CPR in over 4,000 out-of-hospital cardiac arrest patients in the USA and Europe. The trial had unique features: [1] training of all EMS providers in a standardized deployment strategy and continuous monitoring for protocol compliance; [2] a pre-trial simulation study of provider compliance with the trial protocol; [3] three distinct study phases (in-field training, run-in, and statistical inclusion) to minimize the Hawthorne effect and other biases; [4] monitoring of the CPR process using either transthoracic impedance or accelerometer data; [5] randomization at the subject level after the decision to resuscitate is made to reduce selection bias; [6] use of specific statistical tests with sufficient power to determine superiority, inferiority, or equivalence. Although the full article has not been published yet, preliminary results have shown equivalence in ROSC, 24 h survival, survival to hospital discharge, and hands-off fraction between the two CPR approaches.

8.5   LUCAS

The LUCAS chest compression system is a portable piston device composed of: a back plate, which is positioned underneath the patient as a support for the external chest compressions; an upper part mounted on two arms, which contains the battery and the compression mechanism with a disposable suction cup; a stabilization strap which helps to secure the position of the device in relation to the patient. Two versions of the device have been produced. The original LUCAS 1, is a pnuematically driven device that requires no electrical supply, but is powered by compressed air from a portable compressed air cylinder or wall outlet. The LUCAS 2, instead is a battery powered device. LUCAS CPR features are reported in Table 8.2.

Currently, there are no published multicenter randomized human studies comparing LUCAS CPR with standard CPR. Nevertheless, animal studies and clinical observations have reported better hemodynamics during LUCAS CPR in comparison to manual CPR. A single study of pigs with VF showed that LUCAS CPR improved hemodynamic and short-term survival rates compared with standard CPR [29]. Indeed, after 5 min of untreated VF, animals were subjected to 20-min CPR with either LUCAS or manual CPR. Significantly higher CPP was observed during LUCAS CPR. All the pigs in the mechanical group achieved ROSC compared with only 37 % in the manual group. Another animal study randomized pigs to a 15-min CPR with either LUCAS or manual compression [30]. During CPR, the cortical cerebral blood flow was significantly higher in the group treated with LUCAS ($p = 0.041$). End-tidal CO2, an indirect measurement of the achieved cardiac output during CPR, was also significantly higher in the group treated with the LUCAS device ($p = 0.009$). Greater EtCO2 was also consistently measured over a 15-min interval of LUCAS CPR in comparison with manual CPR in a prospective clinical study including 126 out-of-hospital cardiac arrest patients [31].

Six case series involving overall approximately 200 patients have reported variable success in use of the LUCAS device when implemented after an unsuccessful period of manual CPR [32–37]. One study, in particular, was a good quality case series including 100 patients [33]. Of the 43 witnessed cases treated with LUCAS within 15 min from ambulance call: 24 had VF and 15 (63 %) of these cases achieved ROSC and 6 (25 %) of them survived with a good neurological

Table 8.2 Lucas CPR features

Compression depth: 5 cm
Rate of compression: 100/min
Duty cycle: equal compression/decompression time
Compression/ventilation ratio: 30/2 or continuous compressions
Full chest recoil allowed

recovery after 30 days; 19 patients, instead, were found in asystole at rescuers' arrival and 5 (26 %) of them achieved ROSC and 1 (5 %) survived for over 30 days. Another study using concurrent controls in witnessed out-of-hospital cardiac arrest was unable to show benefit in ROSC, survival to hospital, and survival to hospital discharge with the use of the LUCAS device over the use of manual CPR [38].

More recently, LUCAS versus manual CPR have been compared in a randomized prospective pilot study, enrolling 149 patients with out-of-hospital cardiac arrest in two Swedish cities [39]. This pilot study reported no difference in ROSC, 4 h survival, and survival to hospital discharge between the two CPR approaches. Nevertheless, this was only a pilot investigation and data were used for power calculation in one of the two currently underway randomized multicenter trials [40, 41].

Indeed, the role of LUCAS CPR will be clarified after completion and publication of the results of the following two ongoing studies: (1) The prehospital randomized assessment of a mechanical compression device in cardiac arrest (PARAMEDIC) trial, that enrolls 4,000 patients in England, Wales, and Scotland, in order to assess effects of LUCAS CPR over manual CPR on 30-day survival [40]; and (2) The LUCAS in Cardiac arrest study (LINC): a study comparing conventional adult out-of-hospital cardiopulmonary resuscitation with a concept with mechanical chest compressions and simultaneous defibrillation that enrolls 2,500 patients with the intent to compare the effects of LUCAS CPR over manual CPR on 4-h survival [41].

8.6   Conclusions

At the moment, there are insufficient data to support or refute the use of a mechanical compressor instead of manual CPR. Currently undergoing multicenter randomized clinical trials comparing mechanical versus manual CPR will clarify the role of mechanical chest compression. There is some low-quality evidence that mechanical CPR can improve consistency and reduce interruptions in chest compressions. Nevertheless, it has to be recognized that mechanical devices for CPR warrant: continuous high quality CPR; compression during transport; no interruptions in CPR; no rescuer fatigue; and more importantly hands free for other procedures. It may be reasonable therefore to consider mechanical CPR to maintain continuous chest compression while undergoing CT scan or similar diagnostic studies, or interventional procedures treatments, i.e., primary angioplasty, when provision of manual CPR would be difficult. Finally, in order to ensure the best result from the use of a mechanical CPR it is important to consider the implementation of cardiac arrest teams specially trained in applying and starting mechanical compressor, i.e., with a "pit-crew" protocol, so as to reduce the interruption in CPR [20]. Interruptions in chest compressions to apply a mechanical device, in fact, can be as low as 20 s, but are often much longer, i.e., almost 2 min [42].

References

1. Travers AH, Rea TD, Bobrow BJ et al (2010) Part 4: CPR Overview 2010 American Heart Association guidelines for cardiopulmonary resuscitation and emergency cardiovascular care. Circulation 122:S676–S684
2. Lippert FK, Raffay V, Georgiou M et al (2010) European Resuscitation Council Guidelines for resuscitation 2010 section 10. The ethics of resuscitation and end-of-life decisions. Resuscitation 81:1445–1451
3. Atwood C, Eisenberg MS, Herlitz J et al (2005) Incidence of EMS-treated out-of-hospital cardiac arrest in Europe. Resuscitation 67:75–80
4. Fredriksson M, Herlitz J, Nichol G (2003) Variation in outcome in studies of out-of-hospital cardiac arrest: A review of studies conforming to the Utstein guidelines. Am J Emerg Med 21:276–281
5. Kern KB, Garewal HS, Sanders AB et al (1990) Depletion of myocardial adenosine triphosphate during prolonged untreated ventricular fibrillation: effect on defibrillation success. Resuscitation 20:221–222
6. Klouche K, Weil MH, Sun S, Tang W et al (2002) Evolution of the Stone Heart after Prolonged cardiac arrest. Chest 122:1006–1011
7. Wik L, Hansen TB, Fylling F et al (2003) Delaying defibrillation to give basic cardiopulmonary resuscitation to patients with out-of-hospital ventricular fibrillation. JAMA 289:1389–1395
8. Cobb LA, Fahrenbruch CE, Walsh TR et al (1999) Influence of cardiopulmonary resuscitation prior to defibrillation in patients with out-of-hospital ventricular fibrillation. JAMA 281:1182–1188
9. Paradis NA, Martin GB, Rosenberg J et al (1990) Coronary perfusion pressure and the return of spontaneous circulation in human cardiopulmonary resuscitation. JAMA 263:1106–1113
10. Kern KB, Ewy GA, Voorhees WD et al (1988) Myocardial perfusion pressure: a predictor of 24-hour survival during prolonged cardiac arrest in dogs. Resuscitation 16:241–250
11. Klouche K, Weil MH, Sun S et al (2002) Stroke volumes generated by precordial compression during cardiac resuscitation. Crit Care Med 30:2626–2631
12. Koster RW, Baubin MA, Bossaert L et al (2010) European Resuscitation Council Guidelines for Reuscitation 2010 section 2. adult basic life support and use of automated external defibrillators. Resuscitation 81:1277–1292
13. Wik L, Steen PA, Bircher NG (1994) Quality of bystander cardiopulmonary resuscitation influences outcome after prehospital cardiac arrest. Resuscitation 28:195–203
14. Wik L, Kramer-Johansen J, Myklebust H et al (2005) Quality of cardiopulmonary resuscitation during out-of-hospital cardiac arrest. JAMA 293:299–304
15. Abella BS, Alvarado JP, Myklebust H et al (2005) Quality of cardiopulmonary resuscitation during in-hospital cardiac arrest. JAMA 293:305–310
16. Ashton A, McCluskey A, Gwinnutt GL et al (2002) Effect of rescuer fatigue on performance of continuous external chest compressions over 3 min. Resuscitation 55:151–155
17. Ochoa FJ, Ramalle-Gomara E, Lisa V et al (1998) The effect of rescuer fatigue on the quality of chest compressions. Resuscitation 37:149–152
18. Abella BS, Sandbo N, Vassilatos P et al (2005) Chest compression rates during cardiopulmonary resuscitation are suboptimal. Circulation 111:428–434
19. Shuster M, Lim SH, Deakin CD et al (2010) Part 7: CPR techniques and devices: 2010 international consensus on cardiopulmonary resuscitation and emergency cardiovascular care science with treatment recommendations. Circulation 122(16 Suppl 2):S338–S344
20. Ong ME, Quah JL, Annathurai A et al (2013) Improving the quality of cardiopulmonary resuscitation by training dedicated cardiac arrest teams incorporating a mechanical load-distributing device at the emergency department. Resuscitation 84:508–514

21. Halperin HR, Paradis N, Ornato JP et al (2004) Cardiopulmonary resuscitation with a novel chest compression device in a porcine model of cardiac arrest: improved hemodynamics and mechanisms. J Am Coll Cardiol 44:2214–2220

22. Timerman S, Cardoso LF, Ramires JA et al (2004) Improved hemodynamic performance with a novel chest compression device during treatment of in-hospital cardiac arrest. Resuscitation 61:273–280

23. Casner M, Andersen D, Isaacs SM (2005) The impact of a new CPR assist device on rate of return of spontaneous circulation in out-of-hospital cardiac arrest. Prehosp Emerg Care 9:61–67

24. Ong ME, Ornato JP, Edwards DP et al (2006) Use of an automated, load-distributing band chest compression device for out-of-hospital cardiac arrest resuscitation. JAMA 295:2629–2637

25. Hallstrom A, Rea TD, Sayre MR et al (2006) Manual chest compression vs use of an automated chest compression device during resuscitation following out-of-hospital cardiac arrest: a randomized trial. JAMA 295:2620–2628

26. Paradis NA, Young G, Lemeshow S et al (2010) Inhomogeneity and temporal effects in AutoPulse Assisted Prehospital international resuscitation–an exception from consent trial terminated early. Am J Emerg Med 28:391–398

27. Hock Ong ME, Fook-Chong S, Annathurai A, et al (2012) Improved neurologically intact survival with the use of an automated, load-distributing band chest compression device for cardiac arrest presenting to the emergency department. Crit Care 16(4):R144

28. Lerner EB, Persse D, Souders CM et al (2011) Design of the circulation improving resuscitation Care (CIRC) trial: a new state of the art design for out-of-hospital cardiac arrest research. Resuscitation 82:294–299

29. Liao Q, Sjöberg T, Paskevicius A et al (2010) Manual versus mechanical cardiopulmonary resuscitation. An experimental study in pigs. BMC Cardiovasc Disord 10:53

30. Rubertsson S, Karlsten R (2005) Increased cortical cerebral blood flow with LUCAS; a new device for mechanical chest compressions compared to standard external compressions during experimental cardiopulmonary resuscitation. Resuscitation 65:357–363

31. Axelsson C, Karlsson T, Axelsson AB et al (2009) Mechanical active compression-decompression cardiopulmonary resuscitation (ACD-CPR) versus manual CPR according to pressure of end tidal carbon dioxide (P(ET)CO2) during CPR in out-of-hospital cardiac arrest (OHCA). Resuscitation 80:1099–1103

32. Steen S, Liao Q, Pierre L et al (2002) Evaluation of LUCAS, a new device for automatic mechanical compression and active decompression resuscitation. Resuscitation 55:285–299

33. Steen S, Sjoberg T, Olsson P et al (2005) Treatment of out-of-hospital cardiac arrest with LUCAS, a new device for automatic mechanical compression and active decompression resuscitation. Resuscitation 67:25–30

34. Larsen AI, Hjornevik AS, Ellingsen CL et al (2007) Cardiac arrest with continuous mechanical chest compression during percutaneous coronary intervention. A report on the use of the LUCAS device. Resuscitation 75:454–459

35. Deakin CD, O'Neill JF, Tabor T (2007) Does compression-only cardiopulmonary resuscitation generate adequate passive ventilation during cardiac arrest? Resuscitation 75:53–59

36. Bonnemeier H, Olivecrona G, Simonis G et al (2009) Automated continuous chest compression for in-hospital cardiopulmonary resuscitation of patients with pulseless electrical activity: a report of five cases. Int J Cardiol 136:e39–e50

37. Wagner H, Terkelsen CJ, Friberg H et al (2010) Cardiac arrest in the catheterisation laboratory: a 5-year experience of using mechanical chest compressions to facilitate PCI during prolonged resuscitation efforts. Resuscitation 81:383–387

38. Axelsson C, Nestin J, Svensson L et al (2006) Clinical consequences of the introduction of mechanical chest compression in the EMS system for treatment of out-of-hospital cardiac arrest-a pilot study. Resuscitation 71:47–55

39. Smekal D, Johansson J, Huzevka T et al (2011) A pilot study of mechanical chest compressions with the LUCAS™ device in cardiopulmonary resuscitation. Resuscitation 82:702–706
40. Perkins GD, Woollard M, Cooke MW et al (2010) Prehospital randomised assessment of a mechanical compression device in cardiac arrest (PaRAMeDIC) trial protocol. Scand J Trauma Resusc Emerg Med 18:58
41. Rubertsson S, Silfverstolpe J, Rehn L et al (2013) The study protocol for the LINC (LUCAS in cardiac arrest) study: a study comparing conventional adult out-of-hospital cardiopulmonary resuscitation with a concept with mechanical chest compressions and simultaneous defibrillation. Scand J Trauma Resusc Emerg Med 21:5
42. Yost D, Phillips RH, Gonzales L et al (2012) Assessment of CPR interruptions from transthoracic impedance during use of the LUCAS™ mechanical chest compression system. Resuscitation 83:961–965

Improving Survival from Out-of-Hospital Cardiac Arrest with Bystander Chest Compression-Only CPR: The First Component of Cardiocerebral Resuscitation

9

Karl B. Kern

9.1   Introduction

Survival after out-of-hospital cardiac arrest is dependent upon where cardiac arrest occurs. Public locations are generally better than private ones, simply because there is a greater likelihood of being witnessed and receiving bystanders' assistance. But even more important is the community's influence on survival rates from sudden unexpected cardiac arrest. Much like the common saying in real estate interactions, surviving cardiac arrest seems to be all about "Location, location and location" [1]. Even among the United States National Institutes of Health (NIH) sponsored Resuscitation Outcomes Consortium, a group of competitively selected resuscitation centers, the variability in survival rates is surprising. Nichol et al. found a fivefold (500 %) difference in survival rates after out-of-hospital cardiac arrest among these reported centers of excellence [2]. In an accompanying editorial, it was noted that such wide variability in outcome emphasizes the need for each community to "Know its Numbers," then concentrate on improving their own results by focusing on locally identified problem areas within the Chain of Survival [1].

This is what was done in Tucson, Arizona. Data from the 1990s showed that survival from out-of-hospital cardiac arrest had not changed over the entire decade, averaging 6 ± 2 % for all rhythms and 10 ± 2 % for ventricular fibrillation [3]. In collaboration with the leadership of Tucson Fire Department, a new approach entitled *"Cardiocerebral Resuscitation"* was begun. Based on more than 20 years of translational research by the University of Arizona Sarver Heart Center Resuscitation Research Group, three new programs were suggested: (1) *chest*

K. B. Kern (✉)
Division of Cardiology, University of Arizona Sarver Heart Center, Tucson, AZ 85724, USA
e-mail: kernk@email.arizona.edu

A. Gullo and G. Ristagno (eds.), *Resuscitation*,
DOI: 10.1007/978-88-470-5507-0_9, © Springer-Verlag Italia 2014

compression-only CPR for basic life support, (2) a new algorithm for advanced life support provided by emergency medical services, and (3) a more aggressive approach to post-resuscitation care. The initial step is to train community populations in chest compression-only bystander CPR.

9.2   Chest Compression-Only CPR

It has been recognized for years that early CPR is a key for surviving out-of-hospital cardiac arrest. Early CPR is best accomplished with bystander CPR. Studies have shown up to a fourfold increase in survival rates when CPR is provided [4]. Table 9.1 lists the most common deterrents to bystander CPR [5]. Prominent in most such surveys is the fear of or unwillingness to perform mouth-to-mouth rescue breathing. One way to overcome this particular reluctance to help is to remove the requirement for mouth-to-mouth contact. Chest compression-only CPR does exactly that, eliminating any mouth-to-mouth breathing attempts. The idea to eliminate mouth-to-mouth breathing was originally based on the concept that circulating blood, with the oxygen it already contains, is more important in the initial resuscitation effort than is any attempt to replenish oxygen. However, the real advantage of chest compression-only CPR is that it eliminates frequent *interruptions of chest compressions* during attempts at mouth-to-mouth breathing. Assar et al. found that though laypersons are repeatedly taught to interrupt chest compressions for only 4 s while performing mouth-to-mouth breathing (2 s per breath for 2 breaths, then resume compressions), they routinely required 16 s [6]. Such frequent and lengthy interruptions result in suboptimal perfusion since a single rescuer cannot do compressions while attempting to perform rescue breathing. If compressions are performed at exactly 100/min as per the recommendations, but are interrupted after every 30 compressions with 16 s of no compressions while breathing is attempted, only about half of the resuscitation effort results in any systemic perfusion [7]. This degree of blood flow disruption during CPR results in compromised outcomes. *Decreasing such interruptions* with the use of *chest compression-only CPR* improves both perfusion [7] and outcome in clinically realistic experimental models of prolonged ventricular fibrillation cardiac arrest [8, 9] (Table 9.2).

Table 9.1 Common deterrents for bystander CPR

Fear or concern for:	
1.	Harming the victim ≈ 20 %
2.	Not performing CPR correctly ≈ 20 %
3.	Legal consequences ≈ 20 %
4.	Mouth-to-mouth contact ≈ 20 %
5.	Physically unable ≈ 20 %

Table 9.2 Advantages of chest compression-only CPR

1.		Easy to teach
2.		Easy to learn
3.		Simple to remember
4.		Less difficult to perform
5.		Fewer negative deterrents
	a.	No mouth-to-mouth contact required

9.3 Teaching Chest Compression-Only CPR to Communities

Chest compression-only CPR has been successfully taught in Tucson, Arizona, since 2003 and throughout the State of Arizona since 2005. A variety of public outreach programs have included free monthly training classes, public billboards, placards at bus stops and roadway flags (Fig. 9.1), simple instructions mailed with electric bills (Fig. 9.2), and media presentations, including both TV and radio public service announcements, as well as feature stories in print media. Other efforts include school classroom workshops (10,000 students trained in 1 year), basketball arena "3 Point Cards," with chest compression-only CPR's simple steps of (1) Check, (2) Call, and (3) Compress, explained on the back of the card–see Fig. 9.3), and actual chest compression-only CPR demonstrations at University of Arizona basketball halftime shows (Fig. 9.4).

9.4 Increasing Community Bystander CPR with Chest Compression-Only CPR

These efforts to train communities in chest compression-only CPR have paid dividends by increasing the number of bystanders who will assist and perform resuscitation efforts prior to the arrival of the EMS providers. In Arizona, such community training efforts increased bystander CPR from only 28 % in 2005 to 40 % in 2009, i.e., a 43 % gain. Interestingly, during that same period, the percentage of bystander CPR that was chest compression-only CPR rose from only 20 to 76 %, i.e., a 280 % increase [10]!

9.5 Improving Outcomes with Chest Compression-Only CPR

Does this increase in bystander CPR, especially bystander use of chest compression-only CPR, result in better outcomes after out-of-hospital cardiac arrest? Among patients with out-of-hospital cardiac arrest, layperson performance of compression-only CPR was associated with increased survival [10]. For all rhythms, survival was 5 % among those receiving no bystander CPR, 8 % for

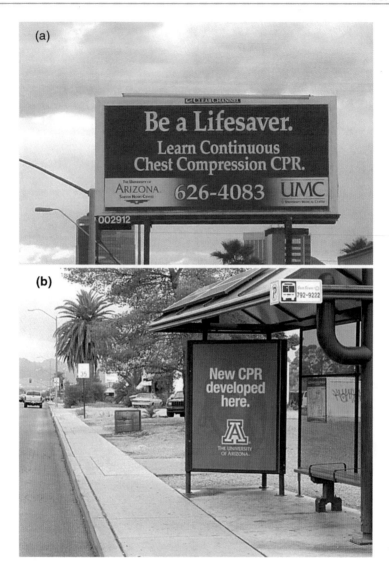

Fig. 9.1 Outdoor community announcements of a 'New' CPR (continuous chest compression CPR or chest compression-only CPR) developed at the University of Arizona. **a** Billboard. **b** Bus stop poster

those receiving bystander-attempted standard CPR (compression to ventilation ratio of 30:2), and 13 % for those receiving chest compression-only bystander CPR (OR = 1.60; CI, 1.08–2.35; $p < 0.001$). Survival with good neurological status was also better with chest compression-only CPR: 3 % with no bystander CPR, 5 % with standard CPR, and 8 % with chest compression-only CPR

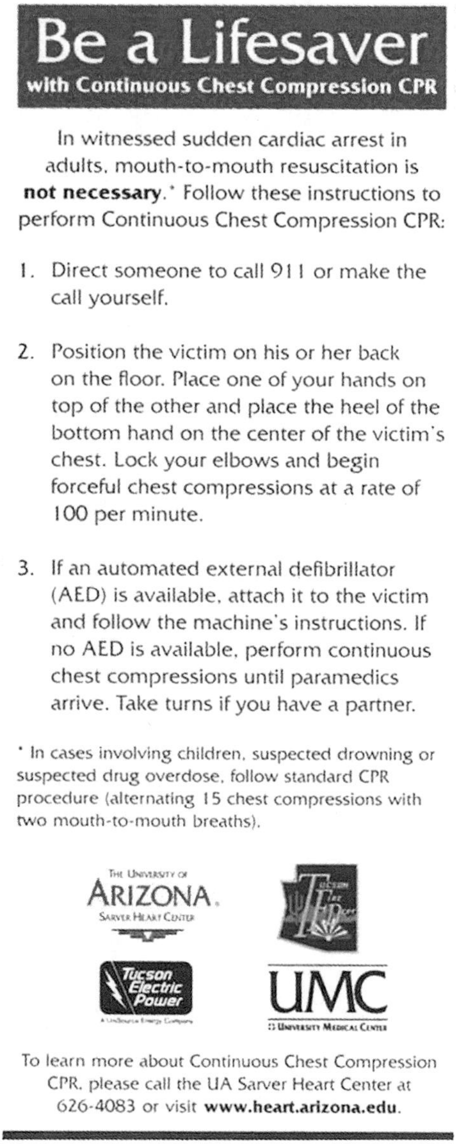

Fig. 9.2 Mail insert sent with a Tucson electric power's invoice, briefly describing chest compression-only CPR

Be a Lifesaver
with Continuous Chest Compression CPR

In witnessed sudden cardiac arrest in adults, mouth-to-mouth resuscitation is **not necessary**.* Follow these instructions to perform Continuous Chest Compression CPR:

1. Direct someone to call 911 or make the call yourself.

2. Position the victim on his or her back on the floor. Place one of your hands on top of the other and place the heel of the bottom hand on the center of the victim's chest. Lock your elbows and begin forceful chest compressions at a rate of 100 per minute.

3. If an automated external defibrillator (AED) is available, attach it to the victim and follow the machine's instructions. If no AED is available, perform continuous chest compressions until paramedics arrive. Take turns if you have a partner.

* In cases involving children, suspected drowning or suspected drug overdose, follow standard CPR procedure (alternating 15 chest compressions with two mouth-to-mouth breaths).

To learn more about Continuous Chest Compression CPR, please call the UA Sarver Heart Center at 626-4083 or visit **www.heart.arizona.edu**.

($p < 0.001$). For those with ventricular fibrillation cardiac arrest the survival rates were 18, 18, and 34 %, respectively ($p < 0.001$). Implementation of a multiyear, multifaceted, statewide public education campaign that officially endorsed and encouraged *chest compression-only CPR was associated with a significant increase in the rate of bystander CPR* for adults who experienced out-of-hospital

Fig. 9.3 "Three Point Basket" placards provided at a University of Arizona basketball game (**a**). On the backside is a description introducing chest compression-only bystander CPR (**b**)

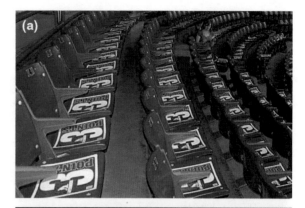

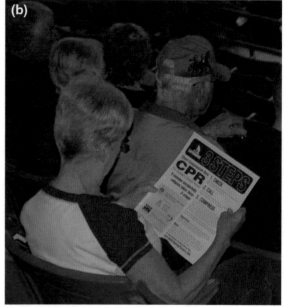

cardiac arrest. Chest compression-only CPR was independently associated with an increased rate of survival compared with no bystander CPR or conventional CPR [10].

9.6 Chest Compression-Only CPR and Cardiac Arrest Due to Noncardiac Etiologies

Resuscitation guidelines published by the American Heart Association and the European Resuscitation Council recommend standard CPR, including rescue breathing, for cardiac arrest of a noncardiac etiology such as *drowning or choking*.

Fig. 9.4 Examples of chest compression-only CPR being demonstrated for large audiences attending University of Arizona basketball games

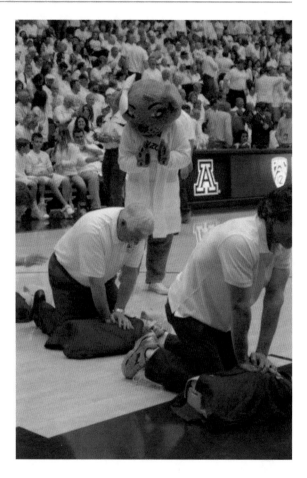

Some have been reluctant to endorse chest compression-only CPR for fear that bystanders may not be able to recognize noncardiac etiologies and may harm such victims by not attempting ventilation. Panchal et al. studied whether lay rescuers could reasonably determine which bystander CPR technique to employ, and if survival rates after arrest from noncardiac etiologies were different depending on which bystander CPR technique was provided [11]. Noncardiac etiology arrests comprised only 15 % of the total 5,793 out-of-hospital adult arrest studied. Fifty-six percent of those receiving bystander CPR for cardiac arrest of presumed cardiac etiology received chest compression-only CPR. In comparison, only 28 % of those receiving bystander CPR for noncardiac etiologies received chest compression-only CPR. Survival after arrest from noncardiac causes was only half of that seen after arrest from cardiac etiologies (3.8 vs 7.0 %; $p < 0.001$). The type of bystander CPR provided did not significantly affect survival-to-hospital discharge among those with a noncardiac etiology for their arrest; 4.0 % with no bystander CPR, 3.8 % with standard CPR, and 2.7 % with chest compression-only CPR ($p < 0.001$). In the setting of an Arizona statewide campaign endorsing chest compression-only bystander CPR for the lay public, bystanders were less likely to perform chest compression-only CPR for those with noncardiac etiologies for their arrest. *No difference in outcome* was found among such arrest victims regardless of the type of bystander CPR provided.

9.7   Conclusion

Chest compression-only bystander CPR is teachable to the lay public, who can effectively learn and perform this simple, living-saving technique. Successful community educational campaigns result in significant increases in lay public performance of bystander CPR. Most importantly, this increased incidence of willing bystanders performing chest compression-only CPR increases survival for local victims of out-of-hospital cardiac arrest.

References

1. Sanders AB, Kern KB (2008) Surviving cardiac arrest: location, location, location. JAMA 300:1462–1463
2. Nichols G, Thomas E, Callaway CW, Hedges J, Powell JL, Aufderheide TP, Rea T, Lowe R, Brown ZT, Dreyer J, Davis D, Idris A, Stiell I (2008) Regional variation in out-of-hospital cardiac arrest incidence and outcome. JAMA 300:1423–1431
3. Valenzuela TD, Kern KB, Clark LL, Berg RA, Berg M, Berg D, Otto CW, Newburn D, Ewy GA (2005) Interruptions of chest compressions during EMS resuscitation. Circulation 112:1259–1265
4. Sasson C, Rogers MAM, Dahl J, Kellerman AL (2010) Predictors of survival from out-of-hospital cardiac arrest: a systemic review and meta-analysis. Circ Cardiovasc Qual Outcomes 3:63–81
5. Coons SJ, Guy MC (2009) Performing bystander CPR for sudden cardiac arrest: behavioral intentions among the general adult population in Arizona. Resuscitation 80:334–340
6. Assar D, Chamberlain D, Colquhoun M, Donnelly P, Handley AJ, Leaves S, Kern KB (2000) Randomized controlled trials of staged teaching for basic life support: skill acquisition at Bronze level. Resuscitation 45:7–15
7. Berg RA, Sanders AB, Kern KB, Hilwig RW, Heidenreich JW, Porter ME, Ewy GA (2001) Adverse hemodynamic effects of interrupting chest compressions for rescue breathing during CPR for VF cardiac arrest. Circulation 104:2465–2470
8. Kern KB, Hilwig RW, Berg RA, Sanders AB, Ewy GA (2002) Importance of continuous chest compressions during CPR: improved outcome during a simulated single lay rescuer scenario. Circulation 105:645–649
9. Ewy GA, Zuercher M, Hilwig RW, Sanders AB, Berg RA, Otto CW, Hayes MM, Kern KB (2007) Improved neurological outcome with continuous chest compressions compared with 30:2 compressions-to-ventilations CPR in a realistic swine model of out-of-hospital cardiac arrest. Circulation 116:2525–2530
10. Bobrow BJ, Spaite D, Berg RA, Stolz U, Sanders AB, Kern KB, Vadboncoeur T, Clark LL, Gallagher J, Stapczynski JS, LoVecchio F, Mullins T, Humble W, Ewy GAE (2010) Chest

compression-only CPR by lay rescuers and survival from out-of-hospital cardiac arrest. JAMA 304:1447–1454
11. Panchal AR, Bobrow BJ, Spaite DW, Berg RA, Stolz U, Vadeboncoeur TF, Sanders AB, Kern KB, Ewy GA (2013) Chest compression-only cardiopulmonary resuscitation performed by lay rescuers for adult out-of-hospital cardiac arrest due to non-cardiac etiologies. Resuscitation 84:435–439

Reperfusion Strategies in Sudden Cardiac Arrest

10

Peter Radsel and Marko Noc

10.1 Introduction

Coronary artery disease is present in almost 80 % of patients with resuscitated sudden cardiac arrest (SCA) undergoing immediate **coronary angiography** (CAG) (1). Moreover, postmortem analyses of SCA victims indicate that unstable coronary plaque with associated thrombosis can be documented in more than 80 % (2). Accordingly, acute coronary thrombotic event leading to critical narrowing or complete coronary obstruction may be viewed as the main trigger of sudden cardiac arrest.

Feasibility and safety of "immediate invasive coronary strategy," consisting of CAG and **percutaneous coronary intervention** (CA-PCI) after resuscitated SCA, has been demonstrated already in the 1990s [1, 3]. However, since these patients have been systematically excluded from major interventional studies unequivocally demonstrating benefit in acute coronary syndromes (ACS), supporting data can be derived only from cohort studies and registries [4–6]. The data support the hypothesis that immediate CA-PCI may improve the survival of this high-risk subgroup of patients. Re-establishment of coronary perfusion may decrease myocardial ischemia and reduce infarct size which is expected to result in better hemodynamic and electrical stability in the post-resuscitation phase.

P. Radsel · M. Noc (✉)
Department of intensive internal medicine, University Medical Center Ljubljana, Zaloska 7, 1000 Ljubljana, Slovenia
e-mail: marko.noc@mf.uni-lj.si

P. Radsel
e-mail: peter.radsel@mf.uni-lj.si

A. Gullo and G. Ristagno (eds.), *Resuscitation*,
DOI: 10.1007/978-88-470-5507-0_10, © Springer-Verlag Italia 2014

10.2 Selection of Patients for Immediate Coronary Angiography

There is general agreement that immediate CAG should be performed in conscious patients after ROSC if no obvious non-coronary cause is documented [7–10]. Such decision is more complex in patients with SCA who remained comatose despite ROSC. Their hospital mortality is much higher and related also to post-resuscitation brain injury in at least 30–40 %. Since we cannot accurately predict neurological recovery on admission when immediate CAG is decided, there has always been debate if such approach is reasonable. Indeed, it was introduction of hypothermia after 2002 with a much greater proportion of patients waking up from coma that returned our focus to the fact that obstructive coronary artery disease is the background in majority of these patients. There is currently general consensus that comatose patients with **STEMI** in post-resuscitation ECG should be immediately brought to the catheterization laboratory. The strong rationale behind this that acute coronary thrombotic lesion ("ACS" lesion) suitable for CA-PCI is typically present in more than 90 % [11]. Based on these findings, immediate CAG was gradually expanded also to other patients with resuscitated SCA but without STEMI in post-resuscitation ECG [10, 12–14]. Indeed, despite absence of STEMI, "ACS" lesion suitable for CA-PCI was documented in 25–40 % [10, 11]. In this context, it is important to emphasize that also normal coronary angiogram or presence of non-obstructive coronary artery disease is a very useful diagnostic finding because it triggers the search for alternative cause of SCA. Decision for immediate CAG after SCA should therefore not be based on post-resuscitation **12-lead ECG** [11]. In comatose patients after CA without STEMI, it is reasonable to decide for immediate CAG if non-coronary cause was not confirmed at emergency department (Fig. 10.1).

Fig. 10.1 Selection of patients with resuscitated sudden cardiac arrest for immediate coronary angiography

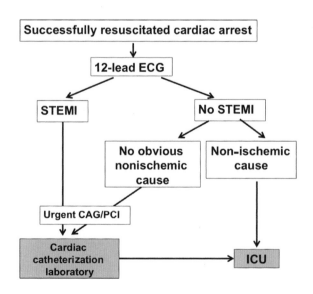

Fig. 10.2 Our exclusion criteria for urgent invasive strategy in patients with resuscitated sudden cardiac arrest

> **Exclusion criteria for urgent CAG/PCI**
>
> • **Clear noncoronary cause for cardiac arrest**
> • **Termial illness**
> • **Poor general condition (dementia, immobility, etc)**
> • **No realistic hope for neurological recovery**
>   (unwitnessed CA, no BLS, long delay to ALS, asistoly/PEA as the first rhythm, long ALS)

Rather than lack of STEMI in ECG, unfavorable features related to the setting of cardiac arrest and initial resuscitation which make neurological recovery unlikely, should argue against immediate CAG (Fig. 10.2).

10.3   Revascularization Strategy

Once coronary anatomy is defined, **revascularization** strategy should be decided. According to revascularization guidelines for STEMI and high risk non-ST elevation ACS [15, 16], CA-PCI should be primary directed toward "ACS" lesions (Picture 1) for which we can assume direct cause–effect relationship with SCA. If angiographic substrate of stable obstructive coronary artery disease is documented (Picture 2), such cause–effect relationship is possible (coronary spasm, thrombosis/spontaneous reperfusion, transient hypotension with decrease in coronary flow…)

Picture 10.1 Acute thrombotic occlusion of proximal LAD (ACS lesion) in a patient with STEMI in 12-lead post-resuscitation ECG

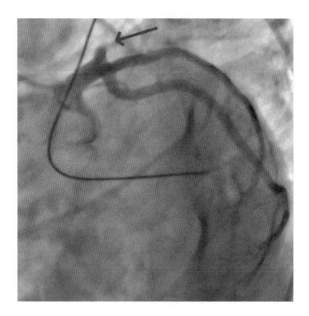

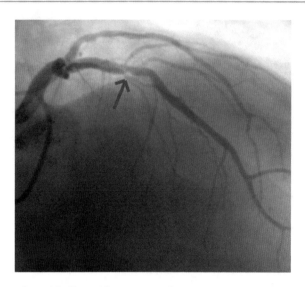

Picture 10.2 Angiographically stable coronary disease in the mid-LAD with intermediate stenosis and normal epicardial coronary flow (TIMI 3) in a patient with resuscitated SCA and no STEMI in post-resuscitation ECG

Fig. 10.3 Proposed revascularization strategy in patients with resuscitated sudden cardiac arrest

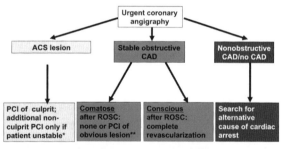

* If ischemia or hemodynamic instability after successful culprit PCI
** If considered responsible for cardiac arrest or beneficial for hemodynamic stability

but not obvious. In conscious patients who obviously have no neurological sequel, complete percutaneous or surgical revascularization should be performed according to the revascularization guidelines for stable disease [17]. In hemodynamically stable comatose patients with preserved myocardial perfusion (TIMI 3 epicardial flow, good collaterals to occluded vessels…), we usually have time to postpone percutaneous or surgical revascularization and wait for possible neurological recovery (Fig. 10.3). CA-PCI of severe obstructive non-thrombotic lesions may be beneficial in hemodynamically unstable patients if one extrapolates SHOCK trial [18]. It is important to emphasize that a combination of CA-PCI with hypothermia to improve neurological outcome is feasible, safe, and is likely to increase survival with good neurological outcome as compared to historical controls without hypothermia [13, 14, 19].

10.4   Conclusion

Despite the lack of randomized trials, immediate invasive coronary strategy in patients with resuscitated SCA has a strong pathophysiological background. Based on cohort reports and registries, immediate CAG and CA-PCI may significantly improve the outcome of survivors of SCA. Interventional cardiologist should therefore become an essential member of post-resuscitation team.

References

1. Spaulding CM, Joly LM, Rosenberg A et al (1997) Immediate coronary angiography in survivors of out-of hospital cardiac arrest. N Engl J Med 336:1629–1633
2. Davies MJ (1992) Anatomic features in victims of sudden coronary death: coronary artery pathology. Circulation 85(Suppl I):I-19–I-24
3. Kahn JK, Glazier S, Swar R et al (1995) Primary coronary angioplasty for acute myocardial infarction complicated by out-of-hospital cardiac arrest. Am J Cardiol 75:1069–1070
4. Eagle KA, Goodman SG, Avezum A et al (2002) For the GRACE investigators. Practice variation and missed opportunities for reperfusion in ST-segment-elevation myocardial infarction: findings from the Global Registry of Acute Coronary Events (GRACE). Lancet 359:373–377
5. Andersen HR, Nielsen TT, Rasmussen K, Thuesen L, Kelbaek H, Thayssen P, Abildgaard U, Pedersen F, Madsen JK, Grande P, Villadsen AB, Krusell LR, Haghfelt T, Lomholt P, Husted SE, Vigholt E, Kjaergard HK, Mortensen LS (2003) DANAMI-2 investigators. A comparison of coronary angioplasty with fibrinolytic therapy in acute myocardial infarction. N Engl J Med 349(8):733–742
6. Keeley EC, Boura JA, Grines CL (2003) Primary angioplasty versus intravenous thrombolytic therapy for acute myocardial infarction: a quantitative review of 23 randomized trials. Lancet 361:13–20
7. Gorjup V, Radsel P, Kocjancic ST, Ersen D, Noc M (2007) Acute ST-elevation myocardial infarction after successful cardiopulmonary resuscitation. Resuscitation 72:379–385
8. Sunde K, Pytte M, Jacobsen D, Mangschau A, Jensen LP, Smedsrud C, Draegni T, Steen PA (2007) Implementation of a standardised treatment protocol for post resuscitation care after out-of-hospital cardiac arrest. Resuscitation 73(1):29–39
9. Garot P, Lefevre T, Eltchaninoff H et al (2007) Six-month outcome of emergency percutaneous coronary intervention in resuscitated patients after cardiac arrest complicating ST-elevation myocardial infarction. Circulation 115:1354–1362
10. Cronier P, Vignon P, Bouferranche K et al (2011) Impact of routine percutaneous coronary intervention after out-of-hospital cardiac arrest due to ventricular fibrillation. Crit Care 15:R122
11. Radsel P, Knafelj R, Kocjancic S, Noc M (2011) Angiographic characteristics of coronary disease and postresuscitation electrocardiograms in patients with aborted cardiac arrest outside a hospital. Am J Cardiol 108:634–638
12. Werling M, Thoren AB, Axelsson C, Herlitz J (2007) Treatment and outcome in post-resuscitation care after out-of-hospital cardiac arrest when a modern therapeutic approach was introduced. Resuscitation 73:40–45
13. Batista LM, Lima FO, Januzzi JL Jr, Donahue V, Snydeman C, Greer DM (2010) Feasibility and safety of combined percutaneous coronary intervention and therapeutic hypothermia following cardiac arrest. Resuscitation 81:398–403
14. Stub D, Hengel C, Chan W et al (2011) Usefulness of cooling and coronary catheterization to improve survival in out-of-hospital cardiac arrest. Am J Cardiol 107:522–527

15. Taylor J (2012) 2012 ESC guidelines on acute myocardial infarction (STEMI). Eur Heart J 33(20):2501–2502
16. Updated ESC guidelines for managing patients with suspected non-ST-elevation acute coronary syndromes (2011) Eur Heart J 32(23):2909–2910
17. Task Force on Myocardial Revascularization of the European Society of Cardiology (ESC) and the European Association for Cardio-Thoracic Surgery (EACTS); European Association for Percutaneous Cardiovascular Interventions (EAPCI), Kolh P, Wijns W, Danchin N, Di Mario C, Falk V, Folliguet T, Garg S, Huber K, James S, Knuuti J, Lopez-Sendon J, Marco J, Menicanti L, Ostojic M, Piepoli MF, Pirlet C, Pomar JL, Reifart N, Ribichini FL, Schalij MJ, Sergeant P, Serruys PW, Silber S, Sousa Uva M, Taggart D (2010) Guidelines on myocardial revascularization. Eur J Cardiothorac Surg. Sep;38 Suppl:S1–S52
18. Hochman JS, Sleeper LA, Webb JG et al (1999) Early revascularization in acute myocardial infarction complicated with cardiogenic shock. Shock investigators. should we emergently revascularize occluded coronaries for cardiogenic shock. N Eng J Med 341:625–634
19. Knafelj R, Radsel P, Ploj T, Noc M (2007) Primary percutaneous coronary intervention and mild induced hypothermia in comatose survivors of ventricular fibrillation with ST-elevation acute myocardial infarction. Resuscitation 74:227–234

Extracorporeal Membrane Oxygenation Strategy in Cardiac Arrest

11

Margherita Scanziani, Leonello Avalli and Roberto Fumagalli

11.1 Why extracorporeal membrane 59 oxygenation (ECMO): The Last Link in the Chain of Survival?

Since the term *life support* was introduced by Peter Safar [1], it became clear that improvement of survival after cardiac arrest (CA) was not easy nor a single-step process [2]. Despite introduction of cardiopulmonary resuscitation (CPR), survival rate remains quite low and this represents a challenge to be faced, encouraging clinicians and researchers to find new solutions that would preserve and enhance previous treatments.

Although the correlation between CA mortality and its predictors is difficult to evaluate because of the complexity of the variables involved [3], survival of both in-hospital CA (IHCA) and out-hospital CA (OHCA) remains very low and it decreases by about 10 % with each minute of defibrillation delay [4], dropping dramatically if CPR lasts longer than 30 min [3, 5].

Data from the National Registry of Cardiopulmonary Resuscitation were analyzed in a large prospective observational study on in-hospital resuscitation [3]. In that study, 14,720 CAs were considered and, overall, 44 % of patients had return of spontaneous circulation (ROSC), but only 17 % survived to hospital discharge [3]. Highest ROSC and survival rate were reported for ventricular fibrillation as

M. Scanziani · L. Avalli
Department of Emergency Medicine, San Gerardo Hospital, Monza, Italy

R. Fumagalli (✉)
Department of Health Science, University of Milan-Bicocca, Monza, Italy
e-mail: roberto.fumagalli@ospedaleniguarda.it

R. Fumagalli
Ospedale Niguarda Ca' Granda, Milan, Italy

A. Gullo and G. Ristagno (eds.), *Resuscitation*,
DOI: 10.1007/978-88-470-5507-0_11, © Springer-Verlag Italia 2014

first recorded CA rhythm. Such discouraging results have been largely confirmed, with an in-hospital survival rate ranging between 10 and 22 % [5–11]. Proposed explanations for poor outcome were: comorbidities affecting hospitalized population hit by CA and lack of formal life support training of healthcare providers working in non-emergency wards [11]. To complete the picture, differences in survival rate might reflect logistic and staffing organization, as better outcome could be observed in CA events during daytime in comparison to nights or weekends [11–15].

Over the past decades, more attention has been paid to improvement of pre-hospital resuscitation practices, supporting spreading of the AHA Guidelines, implementation of Chain of Survival, and granting the possibility of early defibrillation with automated external defibrillators by lay bystander [3]. However, OHCA survival improved only slightly and, although it varies widely among studies and regions [13], it remained very low and worse than IHCA [3, 14–17].

In a systematic review and meta-analysis involving about 140,000 patients over a period of about 30 years, Sasson et al. [14] confirmed that survival of OHCA is below 10 %. Proposed explanations were: lower incidence of ventricular fibrillation as presenting rhythm in comparison to IHCA, older population, and longer delay of emergency medical service response because of urbanization and population growth. Moreover, the authors showed that, in the prehospital setting, CA survival and hospital discharge were associated with specific clinical features: witnessed CA, type of professional involved (medical or paramedical personnel or lay bystander), quality of CPR, presenting rhythm, and ROSC. When CA was witnessed and/or expert personnel performed CPR and/or initial rhythm was shockable, outcome was more favorable [14, 15]. Early defibrillation [16, 17] and also CPR quality positively affected survival [18]; on the contrary, ventricular fibrillation duration was associated with worse prognosis [19].

Lately, lack of improvement over recent years in outcome of in-hospital and out-hospital refractory CA prompted to consider new solutions. In the early 1960s, Kennedy [20] treated eight patients with refractory CA by the heart–lung machine at Cleveland Metropolitan General Hospital; all but one survived. Despite the disappointing results of first studies [21, 22], recent advances in technology with miniaturized portable device and heparin-coated circuits enabled a wider application of the technique and promoted the use of extracorporeal membrane oxygenation (ECMO) or extracorporeal life support (ECLS) in refractory CA, yielding more encouraging outcome results [11, 21, 23–26]. Massetti et al. [11] analyzed the impact of ECLS on survival in patients with in-hospital refractory CA at the University Hospital of Caen between 1997 and 2003. Among 40 patients treated with ECLS, 22 were disconnected from the device because of brain death or multiorgan failure, 18 survived after 24 h, and 8 were alive after 18 months with no neurologic abnormalities. Another 3-year long prospective observational study [25] reported the use of ECLS versus conventional CPR in patients suffering IHCA of cardiac origin and disclosed even better results. The analysis was performed on 92 patients matched by propensity score analysis to equalize potential confounding factors for prognosis. ECLS group survival rate was significantly higher compared to conventionally treated group at discharge, after 30 days and at 1 year. Later, these results were confirmed by Shin et al. [23] in a retrospective study based on similar propensity score matching and that reviewed data on 120 patients collected between 2003 and 2009. ECLS group showed significantly higher survival rate with minimal neurologic impairment in comparison to conventional CPR group at discharge and after 6 months. This was confirmed in the subgroup of patients with a cardiac etiology of CA.

Taken together, these studies might suggest that extracorporeal cardiopulmonary resuscitation is a feasible and safe therapeutic option in patients with refractory CA, even if it remains a low-level recommendation by American Guidelines (IIb) [27] in the absence of randomized trials. In this promising context, an unsolved question is whether patients who show signs of spontaneous circulation return after prolonged CPR could further benefit from ECMO [25]. In a propensity analysis on 3-year data performed by Lin et al. [28], patients who had return to spontaneous beating (ROSB) after ECLS institution, had survival rate similar to patients who had ROSC after conventional CPR at hospital discharge, after 30 days, at 6 months, and 1 year. However, as authors pointed out, patients with ROSC had a myocardium able to provide an adequate cardiac output, although supported by catecholamine, while in patients with ECLS, ROSB was achieved during ventricular unloading and adequate blood flow to peripheral organs was granted by extracorporeal support. Thus, ROSC and ROSB appear as different and not comparable physiological endpoints. As a matter of fact, ECLS could be indicated in patients with ROSC and persisting shock to sustain circulation [23] avoiding, at the same time, additional myocardial stress due to high inotropic support.

Besides the benefits on survival rate of refractory CA and on circulation support during persistent post-CA shock, ECLS claims other advantages. First, in patients with refractory CA of unknown origin, ECLS allows to perform advanced radiologic and other diagnostic examinations [29] to identify definitive treatment such as surgical or percutaneous revascularization [23, 30]. Second, ECMO provides rapid cooling and rewarming when hypothermic strategy has to be applied for neuroprotection [28]. In particular, ECLS is recommended by most recent guidelines to get fast rewarming and circulatory support in patients with CA due to accidental hypothermia [31]. Moreover, ECLS protective effects on cardiac arrhythmias were recently described by Morita et al. [32] in severe hypothermic patients with or without CA. Finally, ECLS could also be applied in cardiogenic shock caused by drugs intoxication [33, 34].

ECMO is actually used in special clinical situations to support circulation, i.e., ECMO could "buy time" in patients with terminal heart failure waiting for heart transplant [35] and, when cerebral death occurs after post-CA anoxic damage, ECMO could provide peripheral perfusion and preserve organs for donation [22]. However, a detailed description of these indications is beyond the scope of this chapter.

11.2 When ECMO: A Special Therapy for Highly Selected Patients

Kennedy et al. [20] already considered ECMO in selected patients with refractory CA and no signs of cerebral damage. For the sake of clarity, it is worthwhile to define "no-flow time" as the duration of CA before start of CPR (i.e., without any cardiac output): this time represents a key point for the success of ECMO [22]. In fact, in the clinical setting it has been reported longer no-flow time in OHCA compared to IHCA [36]. For this reason the evaluation of the no-flow time appears to be essential. In the clinical setting, another indirect index of the perfusion deficit to heart is the end tidal carbon dioxide (E_TCO_2) tension: an E_TCO_2 level lower than 10 mmHg measured 20 min after ACLS initiation seems to accurately predict death in CA with pulseless electrical activity [37]. Thus, we suggest that E_TCO_2 could drive ECMO use. The same consideration, obviously, can be applied to low-flow time. "Low-flow time" is the duration of CA with low cardiac output (i.e., during CPR). Kagawa et al. [30] showed more favorable outcome in patients treated with ECLS after IHCA compared to those after OHCA, with longer delay between circulatory collapse and ECMO in the latter [12, 36]. Actually there is no agreement on the cutoff low-flow time as it varies between authors and it also depends on the quality of CPR. Thus, in general, the shorter the low-flow time, the better the outcome expected. Although 30 min as low-flow cutoff to start ECMO has been suggested [38], evidence that ECMO allows for longer CPR duration has been reported [11, 24, 30, 36, 39]. Massetti et al. [11] reported an average of 72 min of low-flow CPR before the institution of ECMO in surviving patients; Chen et al. [38] further extended this time having a probability of survival of approximately 10 % in patients in whom CPR lasted up to 90 min. Recently, ECMO beneficial effects were also reported in patients receiving about 180 min of CPR before [37]. The explanation of the ECLS benefit on survival despite long CPR before ECMO is difficult to establish. Chen et al. [39] suggested that prompt institution of assisted perfusion with extracorporeal support could reverse evolution to multiorgan failure and reduce progressive acidosis and post-CPR myocardial stunning, providing the so-called "back from irreversibility" [11].

CPR quality is also critical for neurologic outcome. Abella et al. [40] analyzed 67 patients undergoing CPR after CA and showed that in-hospital CPR was highly variable and not consistent with current guideline recommendations, even if performed by well-trained medical personnel. Similar results were found by a study aimed at verifying quality of CPR in 167 patients with OHCA treated by paramedics and nurse anesthetists: chest compressions were too shallow and not delivered for half of the time [18]. Higher variability in chest compressions delivered in the prehospital setting compared to the emergency department was also found [41]. Other factors that could affect CPR quality and impact survival are the need for transport, and the introduction of automated band chest compression device instead of manual chest compression. Despite first discouraging results [42], recently promising data have been reported. Duchateau et al. [43] showed that in patients with OHCA treated with automated chest compression device blood pressure increased. In a prospective cohort [44] study, 1,011 patients suffering from prolonged CA in emergency department were treated with low distributing band (LBD) CPR or manual CPR. A higher rate of survival and improved neurological performance on discharge were observed in LBD CPR treated group compared to manual CPR.

Laboratory parameters have also been studied to find early predictive criteria of outcome persistent CA patients treated by cardiopulmonary bypass. Megarbane et al. [37] found that low peripheral venous oxygen saturation (SpvO$_2$ <8 %) obtained before cardiopulmonary bypass start predicted early evolution toward multiorgan failure in patients with refractory CA. Low fibrinogen, prolonged prothrombin time, and elevated lactate concentration could also suggest ECLS futility. Development of multiorgan failure was described when lactate concentration was higher than 21 mmol/L [37] as longer the duration of CA until ECLS, the greater the level lactates will reach [22]. An exception is the poisoning-related CA, where complete recovery was previously reported in patients with lactate levels up to 39 mmol/L [26]. However, a cutoff lactate level, which exactly suggests ECLS futility, has not been established yet. Interest in measuring lactate clearance during ECLS has recently grown, as ECLS was shown to significantly decrease lactate levels in 1 h [22]; moreover, a rapid decrease in lactate concentrations after 48 h on ECLS has been reported in survivors following refractory CA [26]. These data could suggest reasonable criteria for early ECLS discontinuation when futile but further studies are required. Up to now, no definitive data exist to suggest the criteria for early discontinuation of extracorporeal support for futility.

11.3 How ECMO: Advance in Technology for Extended Use

Basically, ECLS circuit consists of a portable centrifugal blood pump, a hollow fiber oxygenator with an integral heat exchanger, and bypass cannulae. Recent advances in technology allowed a wider use of ECMO: from central double-lumen cannulation to peripheral cannulation coupled with miniaturized, portable extracorporeal devices, to heparin-coated and more biocompatible circuits.

Usually, femoral vessels are percutaneously cannulated with a modified Seldinger technique [30, 36, 37, 45] or surgically [11, 22]; then, according to the patient's size, arterial (15 or 17 Fr) and venous cannulae (21 up to 29 Fr) are selected. Arterial cannula is positioned up to aortic–iliac junction, while the tip of the venous cannula is pushed into the right atrium and its correct position confirmed by radiologic examination or by echocardiography.

ECLS is in general handled by perfusionists or trained ICU personnel: blood flow is adjusted to maintain a cardiac index of 2.6 L/min or higher (we suggest an inlet venous saturation above 70 %); echocardiography is performed to verify cardiac contractility, ventricular distension, and valve opening: if necessary, low dose of dobutamine is infused to maintain pulsatile flow, to decompress left heart and minimize the risk of intracardiac clot.

Mild hypothermia [36, 46] is implemented during the first 24 h post-CA for neuroprotection; controlled or spontaneous ventilation is set to maintain an E_TCO_2 level of at least 20 mmHg and dead space is increased if necessary. Positive end-expiratory pressure is usually set at 10 cmH_2O to avoid alveolar derecruitment. After initial unfractionated heparin bolus given during the placement of arterial cannula, continuous intravenous infusion is performed to keep an activated clotting time between 160 and 180 [36] or 160 and 200 s [30, 38] or even higher when extracorporeal blood flow is reduced [11, 30, 39].

Weaning is attempted only when cardiac function improves. Weaning test is carried out by reducing ECMO blood flow, while monitoring cardiac contractility by echocardiography and by hemodynamic parameters. Sometimes, inotropic support is required to wean-off ECMO. If cardiac output increases while heart diameters remain stable under echocardiographic view, withdrawal of ECMO is conceivable [47].

Hemorrhage is one of the most serious complications and frequently requires transfusions [11, 48, 49]. In case of cannulation of femoral vessels, the following complications are reported: vena cava tears with subsequent retroperitoneal bleeding; retrograde aortic dissection [49]. Subsequent early surgical revisions were reported [11, 21].

Another complication is lower limb ischemia requiring urgent revascularization [33]. Huang et al. [50] conducted a prospective study to identify patients at risk to develop leg hypoperfusion, by measuring blood pressure in the superficial femoral artery. They proposed a mean perfusion pressure below 50 mmHg as criteria to provide distal leg reperfusion and avoid leg ischemia but also futile distal cannula insertion. Major thromboembolic events can also occur [30, 33]; finally infective complications such as pneumonia and sepsis are reported [30] mainly related to heavy sedation and multiple intravascular catheters.

11.4 Conclusion

IHCA and OHCA remain characterized by elevated mortality. The introduction of the life-support chain concept into practice improved survival rate but it appears inadequate in patients with refractory CA. With recent advances in technology, ECMO had been introduced as therapeutic option in refractory CA, and it showed beneficial effects in patients after conventional approach failure. We believe that ECMO is a special therapy that could represent a further effective link in the Chain of Survival in highly selected patients not responding to first treatment and if provided by an experienced ECMO team.

IHCA appears the most promising setting for successful ECMO application; in order to extend its use in other settings it is essential to identify criteria able to limit futility.

References

1. Safar P, Bircher N (1988) History and phases and stages of cardiopulmonary cerebral resuscitation. In: Safar P, Bircher N (eds): Cardiopulmonary Cerebral Resuscitation, 3rd edn. Philadelphia, WB Saunders Co
2. Cummins RO, Ornato JP, Thies WH, Pepe PE (1991) Improving survival from sudden cardiac arrest: the "chain of survival" concept. A statement for health professionals from the advance cardiac life support. Subcommittee and the emergency cardiac care committee. Am Heart Assoc Circ 83:1832–1847
3. Peberdy MA, Kaye W, Ornato JP et al. for the NRCPR Investigators (2003) Cardiopulmonary resuscitation of adults in the hospital: A report of 14720 cardiac arrests from the national registry of cardiopulmonary resuscitation. *Resuscitation* 58:297–308
4. Cummins RO (1989) From concept to standard-of-care? Review of the clinical experience with automated external defibrillators. Ann Emerg Med 18(12):1269–1275
5. Hajbaghery MA, Mousavi G, Akbari H (2005) Factors influencing survival after in-hospital cardiopulmonary resuscitation. Resuscitation 66:317–322
6. Tunstall-Pedoe H, Bailey L, Chamberlain DA et al (1992) Survey of 3765 cardiopulmonary resuscitation in British hospitals (the BREUS study): methods and overall results. BMJ 304:1347–1351
7. Sandroni C, Nolan J, Cavallaro F et al (2007) In-hospital cardiac arrest: Incidence, prognosis and possible measures to improve survival. Intensive Care Med 33:237–245
8. Bloom HL, Shukrullah I, Cuellar JR et al (2007) Long term survival after successful in hospital cardiac arrest resuscitation. Am Heart J 153(5):831–836
9. Chan PS, Nallamothu BK (2012) Life after death: improving outcomes following in-hospital cardiac arrest. JAMA 307(18):1917–1918
10. Girotra S, Nallamothu BK, Spertus JA et al (2012) Trends in survival after in-hospital cardiac arrest. N Engl J Med 367:1912–1920
11. Massetti M, Tasle M, Le Page O et al (2005) Back from irreversibility:extracorporeal life support for prolonged cadiac arrest. Ann Thorac Surg 79:178–184
12. Fredriksson M, Aune S, Bang A et al (2010) Cardiac arrest outside and inside hospital in a community: mechanims behind the differences in outcome and outcome in relation to time of arrest. Am Heart J 159:749–756
13. Berdowski J, Berg RA, Tijssen JGP et al (2010) Global incidences of out-of-hospital cardiac arrest and survival rates: systematic review of 67 prospective studies. Resuscitation 81:1479–1487
14. Sasson C, Roger MAM, Dahl J et al (2010) Predictors of survival from out-of-hospital cardiac arrest. A systematic review and meta-analysis. Circ Cardiovasc Qual Outcomes 3:63–81
15. Adielsson A, Holleneberg J, Karlsson T et al (2011) Increase in survival and bystander CPR in out-of-hospital shockable arrhythmia: bystander CPR and female gender are predictors of improved outcome. Experiences from Sweden in a 18 years perspective. Heart 97:1391–1396
16. Valenzuela TD, Roe DJ, Nichol G et al (2000) Outcomes of rapid defibrillation of security officers after cardiac arrest in casinos. N Engl J Med 343:1206–1209
17. Simpson PM, Goodger MS, Bendall JC (2010) Delayed versus immediate defibrillation in out-of-hospital cardiac arrest due to ventricular fibrillation: A systematic review and meta-analysis of randomized controlled trials. Resuscitation 81:925–931
18. Wik L, Kramer-Johansen J, Myklebust H et al (2005) Quality of cardiopulmonary resuscitation during in-hospital cardiac arrest. JAMA 293:299–304
19. Berdowski J, ten Haaf M, Tijssen JGP et al (2010) Time in recurrent ventricular fibrillation and survival of out-of-hospital cardiac arrest. Circ 122:1101–1108
20. Kennedy JH (1966) The role of assisted circulation in cardiac resuscitation. JAMA 197:97–100

21. Nichol G, Karmy-Jones R, Salerno C et al (2006) Systematic review of percutaneous cardiopulmonary bypass for cardiac arrest or cardiogenic shock states. Resuscitation 70:381–394
22. Le Guen M, Nicolas-Robin A, Carreira S et al (2011) Extracorporeal life support following out-of-hospital refractory cardiac arrest. Crit Care 15:R29
23. Shin TG, Choi J-H, Jo IJ et al (2011) Extracorporeal cardiopulmonary resuscitation in patients with inhospital cardiac arrest: A comparison with conventional cardiopulmonary resuscitation. Crit Care Med 39:1–7
24. Chen Y-S, Chao A, Yu H-Y et al (2003) Analysis and results of prolonged resuscitation in cardiac arrest patients reacued by extracorporeal membrane oxygenation. J Am Coll Cardiol 41:197–203
25. Chen Y-S, Lin J-W, Yu H-Y et al (2008) Cardiopulmonary resuscitation with assisted extracorporeal life-support versus conventional cardiopulmonary resuscitation in adults with in-hospital cardiac arrest: an observational study and propensity analysis. Lancet 372:554–561
26. Mégarbane B, Leprince P, Deye N et al (2007) Emergency feasibility in medical intensive care unit of extracorporeal life support for refractory cardiac arrest. Intensive Care Med 33:758–764
27. Cave DM, Gazmuri RJ, Otto CW et al (2010) Part 7: CPR techniques and devices: 2010 American heart association guidelines for cardiopulmonary resuscitation and emergency cardiovascular care. Circ 122:S720–S728
28. Lin J-W, Wang M-J, Yu H-Y et al (2010) Comparing the survival between extracorporeal rescue and conventional resuscitation in adult in-hospital cardiac arrest: propensity analysis of three-years data. Resuscitation 81:796–803
29. Kjaergaard B, Frost A, Rasmussen BS et al (2011) Extracorporeal life support makes advance radiologic examinations and cardiac interventions possible in patients with cardiac arrest. Resuscitation 82:623–626
30. Kagawa E, Inoue I, Kawagoe T et al (2010) Assessment of outcomes and differences between in- and out-of-hospital cardiac arrest treated with cardiopulmonary resuscitation with extracorporeal life support. Resuscitation 81:968–973
31. Soar J, Perkins GD, Abbas G et al (2010) European resuscitation council guidelines for resuscitation 2010 section 8. Resuscitation 81:1400–1433
32. Morita S, Inokuchi S, Yamagiwa T et al (2011) Efficacy of portable and percutaneous cardiopulmonary bypass rewarming versus that of conventional internal rewarming for patients with accidental deep hypothermia. Crit Care Med 39:1064–1068
33. Daubin C, Lehoux P, Ivascau C et al (2009) Extracorporeal life support in severe drug intoxication: a retrospective cohort study of seventeen cases. Crit Care 13:R138
34. Rona R, Cortinovis B, Marcolin R et al (2011) Extra-corporeal life support for near-fatalmulti-drug intoxication: a case report. J Med Case R 5:231
35. Fumagalli R, Bombino M, Borelli M et al (2004) Percutaneous bridge to heart transplantation by venoarterial ECMO and transaortic left ventricular venting. Int J Artif Organs 27:410–413
36. Avalli L, Maggioni E, Formica F et al (2012) Favourable survival of in-hospital compared to out-of-hospital refractory cardiac arrest patients treated with extracorporeal membrane oxygenation: an Italian tertiary care centre experience. Resuscitation 83:579–583
37. Mégarbane B, Deye N, Aout M (2011) Uselfulness of routine laboratory parameters in the decision to treat refractory cardiac arrest with extracorporeal life support. Resuscitation 82:1154–1161
38. Hartz R, LoCicero J 3rd, Sanders JH Jr et al (1990) Clinical experience with portable cardiopulmonary bypass in cardiac patients. Ann Thorac Surg 50:437–441
39. Chen Y-S, Yu H-Y, Huang S-C et al (2008) Extracorporeal membrane oxygenation support can extend the duration of cardiopulmonary resuscitation. Crit Care Med 36:2529–2535

40. Abella BS, Alvarado JP, Myklebust H, Edelson DP, Barry A, O'Hearn N, VandenHoek TL, Becker LB (2005) Quality of cardiopulmonary resuscitation during in-hospital cardiac arrest. JAMA 293:305–310
41. Roosa JR, Vadeboncoeur TF, Dommer PB et al (2012) CPR variability during ground ambulance transport of patients in cardiac arrest. Resuscitation. doi: 10.1016/j.resuscitation.2012.07.042
42. Hallstrom A, Rea TD, Sayre MR et al (2006) Manual chest compression versus use of an automated chest compression devise during resuscitation following out-of-hospital cardiac arrest. JAMA 295:2620–2628
43. Duchateau FX, Gueye P, Curac S et al (2010) Effect of the AutoPulse^{TM} automated band chest compression device on hemodynamics in out-of-hospital cardiac arrest resuscitation. Intensive Care Med 36:1256–1260
44. Hock Ong ME, Fook-Chong S, Annathurai A et al (2012) Improved neurologically intact survival with the use of an automated, load-distributing band chest compression device for cardiac arrest presenting to the emergency department. Crit Care 16:R144
45. Grasselli G, Pesenti A, Marcolin R et al (2010) Percutaneous vascular cannulation for extracorporeal life support (ECLS): a modified technique. Int J Artif Organs 33:553–557
46. Nagao K, Kikushima K, Watanabe K et al (2010) Early induction of hypothermia during cardiac arrest improves neurological outcomes in patients with out-of-hospital cardiac arrest who undergo emergency cardiopulmonary bypass and percutaneous coronary intervention. Circ J 74:77–85
47. Aissaoui N, Luyt CE, Leprince P et al (2011) Predictors of successful extracorporeal membrane oxygenation (ECMO) weaning after assistance for refractory cardiogenic shock. Intensive Care Med 37(11):1738–1745
48. Morimura N, Sakamoto T, Nagao K (2011) Extracorporeal cardiopulmonary resuscitation for out-of-hospital cardiac arrest: a review of the Japanese literature. Resuscitation 82:10–14
49. Schwarz B, Mair P, Margreiter J et al (2003) Experience with percutaneous venoarterial cardiopulmonary bypass for emergency circulatory support. Crit Care Med 31:758–764
50. Huang S-C, Yu H-Y, Ko W-J et al (2004) Pressure criterion for placement of distalperfusion catheter to prevent limb ischemia during adult extracorporeal life support. J Thorac Cardiovasc Surg 128:776–777

Part IV
Pharmacological Approach During CPR

Vasopressors During CPR

12

Antonio Maria Dell'Anna, Claudio Sandroni and Anselmo Caricato

12.1   Introduction

Cardiac arrest (CA) is the most severe medical emergency and it is often the common end of different and sometimes untreated diseases. Epidemiological data report 165,000–450,000 cases of CA each year in the United States [1, 2]. Despite recent advances in resuscitation medicine, survival rate at hospital discharge is 5–8 % for out-of-hospital CA (OHCA) and 10–15 % for in-hospital CA (IHCA) [3]. While early provision of basic life-support measures, such as good quality cardiopulmonary resuscitation (CPR), together with early automated external defibrillation may significantly increase survival after CA [4], the benefit of advanced strategies like advanced airway management or drug administration has not been clearly demonstrated [5].

Vasopressors, in particular epinephrine (adrenaline), represent the mainstay of drug therapy during resuscitation, especially after CA due to non-shockable rhythms [6]. In this chapter we will examine the rationale for their use and how they affect patients' survival.

A. M. Dell'Anna · C. Sandroni (✉) · A. Caricato
Department of Anaesthesiology and Intensive Care, Catholic University School of Medicine, Largo Gemelli 8, 00168, Rome, Italy
e-mail: sandroni@rm.unicatt.it

A. M. Dell'Anna
e-mail: anthosdel@yahoo.it

A. Caricato
e-mail: anselmo.caricato@fastwebnet.it

A. Gullo and G. Ristagno (eds.), *Resuscitation*,
DOI: 10.1007/978-88-470-5507-0_12, © Springer-Verlag Italia 2014

12.2   Rationale for Vasopressors in Cardiac Arrest

The occurrence of CA determines a sudden stop of delivery of blood flow to vital organs like heart and brain. CPR partially restores this blood flow, but the cardiac output produced is low, about 20–30 % of its normal value. The amount of blood flow to the heart depends on the coronary perfusion pressure (CPP) defined as aortic diastolic pressure minus right atrial pressure. Both experimental and human data prove that CPP lower than 15–20 mmHg during CPR is associated with poor survival and low rates of successful defibrillation [7].

Vasopressor drugs increase CPP by increasing aortic diastolic pressure and systemic vascular resistance, diverting blood flow from peripheral to vital organs. Animal studies [7, 8] demonstrated that epinephrine increases both myocardial and cerebral blood flow during CPR, and facilitates recovery of spontaneous circulation (ROSC).

12.2.1 Epinephrine

Epinephrine is an endogenous catecholamine produced by adrenal medulla, with a short (3–5 min) half-life. It acts on adrenergic receptors, especially on $\alpha 1$, $\beta 1$, and $\beta 2$. The vasoconstrictor ($\alpha 1$) effect of epinephrine increases diastolic arterial pressure [9] during CPR.

Conversely, cardiac stimulation from $\beta 1$ effect is not beneficial during CPR, since the heart is not contracting and cardiac output depends essentially on chest compression [10]. Moreover, $\beta 1$ stimulation may potentially increase myocardial oxygen consumption and worsen the imbalance between oxygen demand and supply. This possible detrimental effect has been suggested by animal studies showing an increase in cardiac lactate after epinephrine administration during CPR [11]. There is evidence that the $\beta 1$ effects of epinephrine may worsen post-resuscitation myocardial dysfunction. This consists of a transient reduction of myocardial performance from pre-arrest levels which is commonly observed after ROSC [12] and which may potentially lead to multiorgan failure and death. In an experimental model of cardiac arrest and resuscitation, Tang et al. [13] demonstrated that post-resuscitation myocardial dysfunction was more severe in animals treated with epinephrine than in those treated with α-agonist phenilephrine or with a combination of epinephrine and the $\beta 1$-blocker esmolol. Laboratory studies have shown that administration of β-blockers during CPR could reduce detrimental effects of epinephrine on the heart, at least in VF/VT arrest [14, 15]. Clinical studies are needed to assess whether this protection may be effective in human subjects as well [16].

An elegant laboratory study by Ristagno et al. [17] questioned the beneficial impact of epinephrine during CPR also on the neurological side. The study showed that despite an increase in cerebral perfusion pressure, epinephrine actually reduced microcirculatory cerebral blood flow. This effect disappeared when epinephrine was associated to α1-receptor blockade. The authors concluded that epinephrine could activate the α1-receptor subtype on cerebral and pial arterioles, inducing small-vessel constriction.

12.2.2 Vasopressin

Vasopressin is an endogenous nonapeptide, synthesized by neurons of the supra-optic and paraventricular nuclei of hypothalamus, and released in the posterior part of the pituitary gland. Vasopressin release occurs mostly during dehydration, severe hypotension, or hypovolemia [18].

Three types of vasopressin receptors have been identified: V1, V2, and V3. While the V2 receptors mediate water reabsorption and V3 mediate the effects of vasopressin on central nervous system, the V1 receptors mediate cardiovascular effects, consisting in skin, skeletal muscle, and splanchnic blood vessel vasoconstriction.

The rationale for vasopressin use during CPR derives from its capability to increase blood pressure without causing direct myocardial stimulation. In addition, there is the observation that vasopressin levels are higher in patients successfully resuscitated than in nonsurvivors after CA [19]. Animal investigations have demonstrated that vasopressin doses between 0.4 and 0.8 U/kg led to a signifi-cantly higher coronary perfusion pressure and myocardial blood flow than epi-nephrine and were associated with a higher percentage of successfully resuscitated animals [20, 21]. Moreover, vasopressin has a longer half-life (15–20 min) than epinephrine, making vasopressin apparently more resistant to increasing acidosis that arises while duration of cardiac arrest and CPR increases [22].

However, adverse cardiovascular effects of vasopressin have been described as well. They are related to the persistent vasoconstriction and increased myocardial afterload induced by this drug, as shown in laboratory model of CA [23] and in humans affected by cirrhosis [24].

12.2.3 Epinephrine Versus Vasopressin: Results of Clinical Trials

Given the potentially detrimental effects of epinephrine, an increasing interest has been directed toward vasopressin and many studies tried to define any possible beneficial and/or less detrimental effect of this vasopressor compared to epinephrine.

A first randomized trial from Lindner et al. [25] compared administration of 40 IU of vasopressin versus 1 mg of epinephrine in 40 OHCA patients who did not respond to three consecutive defibrillation shocks. Results showed that patients treated with vasopressin had a 50 % increase in survival to hospital admission and a 66 % increase of survival at 24 h. However, a subsequent randomized placebo-controlled trial from Stiell et al. [26] on 200 adult in-hospital patients comparing the same doses of the previous study did not confirm those results. Another study by Wenzel et al. [27] on 1,186 OHCA compared 40 IU of vasopressin or 1 mg of epinephrine during two consecutive ALS cycles, followed by additional boluses of epinephrine if needed. Outcomes were comparable between groups, except for a very small subgroup of asystole cardiac arrests which showed an increased survival to hospital discharge in patients treated with vasopressin compared to those who received epinephrine (12/257 [4.7 %] vs. 4/262 [1.5 %] $p = 0.04$). A meta-analysis [28] of these three studies found no differences in major outcome measures, including ROSC failure (risk ratio [RR] for vasopressin 0.81, 95 % CI: 0.58–1.12), death before hospital admission (RR 0.72, 95 % CI: 0.38–1.39), death within 24 h after hospital admission (RR 0.74, 95 % CI: 0.38–1.43), and death before hospital discharge (RR 0.96, 95 % CI: 0.87–1.05). No differences were found in subgroup analysis based on the presenting rhythms of cardiac arrest, as well.

To investigate the potential synergistic effects of vasopressin plus epinephrine, a larger multicenter placebo-controlled study was carried out on 2,894 out-of-hospital cardiac arrest patients who were randomized to receive either 1 mg of epinephrine plus 40 IU of vasopressin or epinephrine alone. In both groups, additional epinephrine was given if needed [29]. Unfortunately, the study did not show any differences between the two interventions in terms of ROSC (28.6 vs. 29.5 %; relative risk, 1.01; 95 % CI: 0.97–1.06), survival to hospital admission (20.7 vs. 21.3 %; relative risk of death, 1.01; 95 % CI: 0.97–1.05), and survival to hospital discharge (1.7 vs. 2.3 %; relative risk, 1.01; 95 % CI: 1.00–1.02). The rates of good neurological recovery were also similar in the two groups. The study included a high percentage of patients with asystole (82.4 %), which made it very suitable for investigating the possible benefit of vasopressin in that specific group suggested by the previous study.

A recent meta-analysis [30] summarized the results of clinical trials on vasopressin for cardiac arrest and it included 4,475 patients from six randomized controlled trials published from 1997 to 2009. The authors carried out a subgroup analysis according to initial cardiac rhythm and time from collapse to drug administration. Results showed that vasopressin did not improve overall rates of recovery of spontaneous circulation, long-term survival, or favorable neurological outcome. In the subgroup of patients with asystole in whom the time to drug administration was <20 min, vasopressin was associated with a significantly higher rate of both ROSC and long-term survival rates (OR 1.70 [95 % CI: 1.17–2.47] $p = 0.005$, and OR 2.84 [95 % CI: 1.19–6.79] $p = 0.02$, respectively). However, this subgroup included only 27 patients (20 in the vasopressin group and 7 in the control group) from three different trials and no data on neurological outcome were available.

Based on the results shown above, the ERC 2010 Guidelines [6] refer uniquely to epinephrine as standard vasopressor during CPR, while the AHA 2010 Guidelines [31] consider vasopressin as an alternative to the first or the second dose of epinephrine, at a dose of 40 IU.

12.3   Are Vasopressors During CPR Really Needed?

Recently, the limited evidence in favor of advanced life-support measures and the evidence of possible harm from epinephrine in the post-resuscitation phase raised the question of whether drugs should be used at all during cardiac arrest. To address this point, Olasveengen et al. designed an RCT where 851 OHCA patients were randomized to receive advanced life support (ALS) with or without intravenous drug administration [32]. To assess a possible interference from venous cannulation on CPR in the no-drug group, venous access and drugs were allowed only 5 min after ROSC. CPR quality was monitored by transthoracic impedance. Results of this trial showed that patients treated with epinephrine had significantly higher ROSC rates (40 vs. 25 %, OR 1.99 [95 % CI: 1.48–2.67] $p = 0.001$), and longer duration of CPR attempts, during which a higher number of defibrillation shocks were given. Survival to hospital discharge, however, was not significantly different between the two groups, despite a minimal trend in favor of the drug group (10.5 vs. 9.2 %, OR 1.16 [95 % CI: 0.74–1.82] $p = 0.61$).

Results of the Olasveengen study suggest that in OHCA adults the administration of drugs does not improve any relevant outcome, except short-term survival. However, the study was not specifically focused on vasopressors. Epinephrine was administered in 79 % of patients in the drug group but its specific clinical effect could not be assessed separately. Moreover, the intervention could not be blinded.

A double-blind, controlled RCT specifically designed to assess the effects of administration of epinephrine on survival from cardiac arrest was later conducted by Jacobs et al. [33]. The study was unfortunately underpowered because of ethical concerns, so that only 534 out of 4,426 previewed patients were enrolled. Results showed that the epinephrine group had a significantly higher likelihood of achieving ROSC (23.5 vs. 8.4 %; OR 3.5; [95 % CI: 2.1–6.0]) and more than twice the odds of surviving to hospital discharge, although this difference was not significant (4.0 vs. 1.9 %; OR 2.1 [0.7–6.3]).

In 2012, in a very large prospective observational study on 417,188 OHCA patients in Japan, Hagihara et al. [34] compared the outcomes of patients treated by prehospital personnel that were allowed to administer epinephrine during out-of-hospital CPR with that of patients resuscitated from prehospital personnel that were not allowed to administer epinephrine. Results confirmed that in propensity-matched patients prehospital administration of epinephrine was associated with significantly higher ROSC rates before hospital arrival (adjusted OR, 2.51 [95 % CI: 2.24–2.80] $p < 0.001$) but worse long-term outcome measures (adjusted OR for 1-month survival, 0.54 [95 % CI: 0.43–0.68] for survival with CPC 1–2: 0.21 [95 % CI: 0.10–0.44]).

Another observational study conducted in Japan [35] in 3,161 OHCA patients, of whom 1,013 (32.0 %) received epinephrine showed that patients receiving epinephrine had a significantly lower rate of neurologically intact 1-month survival as compared with the non-epinephrine group (4.1 vs. 6.1 %, $p = 0.028$).

12.4   Vasopressors for CA: Should We Keep Using Them?

Evidence presented so far suggests that vasopressors have a positive effect on immediate survival [36] after cardiac arrest but they do not improve patient-important outcomes, such as long-term survival and may possibly be detrimental on neurological outcome. There are three possible explanations for this. A first explanation could be that vasopressors often restore spontaneous circulation in patients who are simply "too ill to survive" and who will die shortly after ROSC from irreversible organ damage. However, it is also possible that the additional quota of patients who have ROSC due to the effect of vasopressors are potentially salvageable with the improvement or a better implementation of post-resuscitation care; it should be noted that in particular, implementation of therapeutic hypothermia is still incomplete in Western countries [37, 38]. A third explanation could be that vasopressors from one side increase the success rate of cardiac resuscitation because they improve coronary perfusion but on the other side also reduce the chances of survival for many resuscitated patients because of their side effects, such as increased post-resuscitation myocardial dysfunction or decreased cerebral microcirculation.

The pivotal role of microcirculation in resuscitation is also confirmed from the results of recent experimental studies showing that administering sodium nitroprusside during resuscitation increases both survival and neurological outcomes. The rationale of nitroprusside administration during CPR would consist in its vasodilator effects which could improve both cerebral blood flow and tissue perfusion [39, 40].

12.5   Conclusion

The role of vasopressors during resuscitation should be completely reassessed, based on recent evidence suggesting that they increase ROSC rates but are not associated to an increase in survival to hospital discharge. The potential harmful effects of epinephrine on post-resuscitation myocardial dysfunction, cerebral perfusion, and organ microcirculation also represent a concern. The forthcoming 2015 guidelines on resuscitation will need to provide a clear recommendation on whether administration of vasopressors during advanced life support is still indicated.

References

1. McNally B, Robb R et al (2011) Out-of-hospital cardiac arrest surveillance—Cardiac Arrest Registry to Enhance Survival (CARES), United States, 1 Oct 2005–31 Dec 2010. MMWR Surveill Summ 60:1–19
2. Mehra R (2007) Global public health problem of sudden cardiac death. J Electrocardiol 40:S118–S122

3. Sandroni C, Nolan J et al (2007) In-hospital cardiac arrest: incidence, prognosis and possible measures to improve survival. Intensive Care Med 33:237–245

4. Sasson C, Rogers MA et al (2010) Predictors of survival from out-of-hospital cardiac arrest: a systematic review and meta-analysis. Circ Cardiovasc Qual Outcomes 3:63–81

5. Stiell IG, Wells GA et al (2004) Advanced cardiac life support in out-of-hospital cardiac arrest. N Engl J Med 351:647–656

6. Deakin CD, Nolan JP et al (2010) European Resuscitation Council guidelines for resuscitation 2010 section 4 adult advanced life support. Resuscitation 81:1305–1352

7. Brown CG, Katz SE et al (1987) The effect of epinephrine versus methoxamine on regional myocardial blood flow and defibrillation rates following a prolonged cardiorespiratory arrest in a swine model. Am J Emerg Med 5:362–369

8. Kern KB, Ewy GA et al (1988) Myocardial perfusion pressure: a predictor of 24-hour survival during prolonged cardiac arrest in dogs. Resuscitation 16:241–250

9. Schumann HJ (1983) What role do alpha- and beta-adrenoceptors play in the regulation of the heart? Eur Heart J 4 (Suppl A):55–60

10. Deshmukh HG, Weil MH et al (1989) Mechanism of blood flow generated by precordial compression during CPR: I. Studies on closed chest precordial compression. Chest 95:1092–1099

11. Ditchey RV, Lindenfeld J (1988) Failure of epinephrine to improve the balance between myocardial oxygen supply and demand during closed-chest resuscitation in dogs. Circulation 78:382–389

12. Laurent I, Monchi M et al (2002) Reversible myocardial dysfunction in survivors of out-of-hospital cardiac arrest. J Am Coll Cardiol 40:2110–2116

13. Tang W, Weil MH et al (1995) Epinephrine increases the severity of post resuscitation myocardial dysfunction. Circulation 92:3089–3093

14. Bassiakou E, Xanthos T et al (2008) Atenolol in combination with epinephrine improves the initial outcome of cardiopulmonary resuscitation in a swine model of ventricular fibrillation. Am J Emer Med 26:578–584

15. Jingjun L, Yan Z et al (2009) Effect and mechanism of esmolol given during cardiopulmonary resuscitation in a porcine ventricular fibrillation model. Resuscitation 80:1052–1059

16. de Oliveira FC, Feitosa-Filho GS et al (2012) Use of beta-blockers for the treatment of cardiac arrest due to ventricular fibrillation/pulseless ventricular tachycardia: a systematic review. Resuscitation 83:674–683

17. Ristagno G, Tang W et al (2009) Epinephrine reduces cerebral perfusion during cardiopulmonary resuscitation. Crit Care Med 37:1408–1415

18. Vincent JL, Su F (2008) Physiology and pathophysiology of the vasopressinergic system: best practice & research. Clin Anaesthesiol 22:243–252

19. Lindner KH, Strohmenger HU et al (1992) Stress hormone response during and after cardiopulmonary resuscitation. Anesthesiology 77:662–668

20. Krismer AC, Lindner KH et al (2001) The effects of endogenous and exogenous vasopressin during experimental cardiopulmonary resuscitation. Anesth Analg 92:1499–1504

21. Wenzel V, Lindner KH et al (1999) Repeated administration of vasopressin but not epinephrine maintains coronary perfusion pressure after early and late administration during prolonged cardiopulmonary resuscitation in pigs. Circulation 99:1379–1384

22. Zhong JQ, Dorian P (2005) Epinephrine and vasopressin during cardiopulmonary resuscitation. Resuscitation 66:263–269

23. Prengel AW, Lindner KH et al (1996) Cardiovascular function during the postresuscitation phase after cardiac arrest in pigs: a comparison of epinephrine versus vasopressin. Crit Care Med 24:2014–2019

24. Sirinek KR, Adcock DK et al (1989) Simultaneous infusion of nitroglycerin and nitroprusside to offset adverse effects of vasopressin during portosystemic shunting. Am J Surg 157:33–37

25. Lindner KH, Dirks B et al (1997) Randomised comparison of epinephrine and vasopressin in patients with out-of-hospital ventricular fibrillation. Lancet 349:535–537
26. Stiell IG, Hebert PC et al (2001) Vasopressin versus epinephrine for inhospital cardiac arrest: a randomised controlled trial. Lancet 358:105–109
27. Wenzel V, Krismer AC et al (2004) A comparison of vasopressin and epinephrine for out-of-hospital cardiopulmonary resuscitation. N Engl J Med 350:105–113
28. Aung K, Htay T (2005) Vasopressin for cardiac arrest: a systematic review and meta-analysis. Arch Intern Med 165:17–24
29. Gueugniaud PY, David JS et al (2008) Vasopressin and epinephrine vs. epinephrine alone in cardiopulmonary resuscitation. N Engl J Med 359:21–30
30. Mentzelopoulos SD, Zakynthinos SG et al (2011) Vasopressin for cardiac arrest: meta-analysis of randomized controlled trials. Resuscitation. doi:10.1016/j.resuscitation.2011.07.015
31. Neumar RW, Otto CW et al (2010) Part 8: Adult advanced cardiovascular life support: 2010 American Heart Association guidelines for cardiopulmonary resuscitation and emergency cardiovascular care. Circulation 122:S729–S767
32. Olasveengen TM, Sunde K et al (2009) Intravenous drug administration during out-of-hospital cardiac arrest: a randomized trial. JAMA 302:2222–2229
33. Jacobs IG, Finn JC et al (2011) Effect of adrenaline on survival in out-of-hospital cardiac arrest: a randomised double-blind placebo-controlled trial. Resuscitation 82:1138–1143
34. Hagihara A, Hasegawa M et al (2012) Prehospital epinephrine use and survival among patients with out-of-hospital cardiac arrest. JAMA 307:1161–1168
35. Hayashi Y, Iwami T et al (2012) Impact of early intravenous epinephrine administration on outcomes following out-of-hospital cardiac arrest. Circ J 76:1639–1645
36. Koscik C, Pinawin A et al (2013) Rapid epinephrine administration improves early outcomes in out-of-hospital cardiac arrest. Resuscitation 84(7):915–920
37. Binks AC, Murphy RE et al (2010) Therapeutic hypothermia after cardiac arrest—Implementation in UK intensive care units. Anaesthesia 65:260–265
38. Soar J, Packham S (2010) Cardiac arrest centres make sense. Resuscitation 81:507–508
39. Schultz JC, Segal N et al (2011) Sodium nitroprusside-enhanced cardiopulmonary resuscitation improves resuscitation rates after prolonged untreated cardiac arrest in two porcine models. Crit Care Med 39:2705–2710
40. Yannopoulos D, Matsuura T et al (2011) Sodium nitroprusside enhanced cardiopulmonary resuscitation improves survival with good neurological function in a porcine model of prolonged cardiac arrest. Crit Care Med 39:1269–1274

Targeting Mitochondria During CPR

13

Raúl J. Gazmuri

13.1 Mitochondria and Cardiac Resuscitation

Sudden cardiac arrest is a major public health problem with $\sim 360,000$ cases assessed every year by Emergency Medical Services in the United States yielding a survival rate to hospital discharge that averages only 9.5 % [1]; a percentage that has improved very little over the past decade. Restoration of cardiac activity requires reperfusion by external means (i.e., CPR) of a myocardium that has been ischemic for a variable period of time. Reperfusion is obligatory to deliver the oxygen required for mitochondria to restore capability to regenerate ATP (i.e., bioenergetic function) and thus create the conditions required for resumption of an electrically organized and mechanically competent cardiac activity. Yet, reperfusion also triggers injury that largely involves generation of reactive oxygen species [2] and mitochondrial calcium overload [3, 4]. This injury further compromises mitochondrial bioenergetic function and thus the conditions required for successful cardiac resuscitation [5].

Current resuscitation methods focus almost exclusively on means to generate blood flow and terminate ventricular fibrillation (VF) but lack therapies directed at protecting mitochondria. In this chapter, basic concepts of mitochondrial function are discussed along with experimental evidence pointing to mitochondrial involvement and interventions to protect their function in helping to restore cardiac activity and lessen post-resuscitation myocardial dysfunction.

R. J. Gazmuri (✉)
Resuscitation Institute at Rosalind Franklin University of Medicine and Science,
3333 Green Bay Road, North Chicago, IL 60064, USA
e-mail: raul.gazmuri@rosalindfranklin.edu

A. Gullo and G. Ristagno (eds.), *Resuscitation*,
DOI: 10.1007/978-88-470-5507-0_13, © Springer-Verlag Italia 2014

13.2   Mitochondrial Function and Dysfunction

13.2.1 Bioenergetic Function

Mitochondria are highly abundant in myocardial tissue encompassing ∼35 % of the cardiomyocyte volume, and are "strategically" located to power contractile activity adopting a "crystal-like" structure with one mitochondrion per sarcomere [6]. Transfer of energy contained in nutrients to molecules of ATP starts with the reduction of nicotinamide adenine dinucleotide (NAD^+) to NADH and flavin adenine dinucleotide (FAD) to $FADH_2$ in the mitochondrial matrix. NADH and $FADH_2$ transfer their electrons down a redox potential through complexes I, II, III, and IV of the electron transport chain to oxygen; the final electron acceptor. Complexes I, III, and IV are also proton pumps and translocate H^+ against their electrochemical gradient from the mitochondrial matrix to the inter-mitochondrial membrane space creating a proton motive force that powers the enzyme F_oF_1 ATPsynthase to regenerate ATP from ADP and inorganic phosphate (Fig. 13.1). The newly synthesized ATP is then exchanged for ADP across the inner-mito-chondrial membrane by the adenine nucleotide translocator (ANT). The newly synthesized and translocated ATP is used to phosphorylate creatine which is then

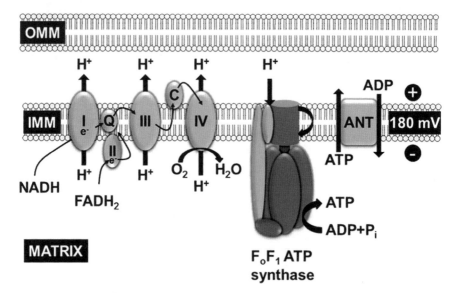

Fig. 13.1 Schematic rendition of key mitochondrial components involved in ATP synthesis via oxidative phosphorylation. *OMM*, outer mitochondrial membrane; *IMM*, inner-mitochondrial membrane; *I, II, III*, and *IV*, electron transport complexes of the respiratory chain; e⁻, electrons; Q, coenzyme Q; C, cytochrome *c*; *ANT*, adenine nucleotide translocator; *NADH*, reduced nicotinamide adenine dinucleotide; *FADH₂*, reduced flavin adenine dinucleotide

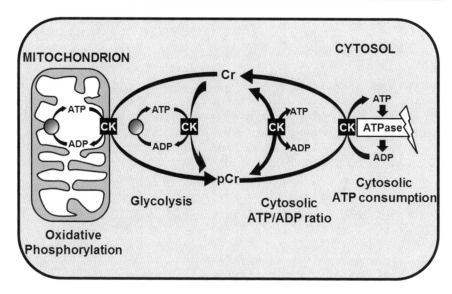

Fig. 13.2 Schematic rendition of mitochondrial *ATP* synthesis and translocation to the cytosol through the creatine phosphate shuttle. *CK*, creatine kinase; *pCr*, phosphocreatine; *Cr*, creatine

exported outside mitochondria to regenerate ATP being used in various energy requiring processes (Fig. 13.2). Measuring the amount of creatine phosphate relative to total creatine is indeed a useful indirect measurement of mitochondrial function.

13.2.2 Cell Death Signaling and Cytochrome *c* Release as Marker of Mitochondrial Injury

In addition to its bioenergetic function, mitochondria also participate in processes leading to cell death via necrosis or apoptosis. Various distinctive mechanisms have been identified including opening of the so-called mitochondrial permeability transition pore (leading to collapse of the proton motive force and uncoupling of respiration) [7] and release of various pro-apoptotic proteins, including cytochrome *c*, apoptosis-inducing factor, Smac/DIABLO, endonuclease G, and a serine protease Omi/HtrA2 [8, 9]. Of these proteins, cytochrome *c* has been the most widely studied, including work in our laboratory [10, 11].

Cytochrome *c* is a 14-kDa hemoprotein that normally resides in the outer surface of the inner-mitochondrial membrane bound to cardiolipin [12]. Cytochrome *c* plays a crucial role in oxidative phosphorylation enabling transfer of electrons from complex III to complex IV (Fig. 13.1). However, cytochrome *c* can also translocate to the cytosol under various pathological conditions including (among others) oxidative stress [13], calcium overload [14], and injury by hypoxia and reoxygenation [15, 16]. In the cytosol, cytochrome *c* forms an oligomeric complex with 2-deoxy-ATP and the apoptotic protease activating factor-1 [17]. This complex recruits procaspase-9 forming what is known as the apoptosome leading to cleavage and release of active caspase-9, which in turn cleaves and activates caspases-3, -6, and -7 [18–20]; the effectors of apoptosis.

Cytochrome c can also leave the cell and reach the bloodstream through mechanisms apparently unrelated to cell necrosis [21, 22]. In patients, elevated levels of circulating cytochrome c have been reported associated with conditions able to injure mitochondria such as cancer [23, 24], chemotherapy [21, 25], acute myocardial infarction [26], reperfusion after coronary intervention [27], possibly cardiomyopathies [28], fulminant hepatitis [29], the systemic inflammatory response syndrome [30], and influenza-associated encephalopathy [31, 32].

In a rat model of VF and CPR, we reported the release of cytochrome c to the cytosol in left ventricular tissue with activation of the mitochondrial apoptotic pathway through formation of the apoptosome as described earlier [10, 11]. However, in this model, activation of the mitochondrial apoptotic pathway did not cause cell death or was responsible for the severe myocardial dysfunction that characteristically occurs post-resuscitation [11]. In the same rat model, cytochrome c reached the bloodstream and progressively increased during CPR and the post-resuscitation period attaining levels that were inversely related to survival [10]. Thus, in rats that survived, plasma cytochrome c increased modestly to levels <2 μg/ml returning to baseline within 48–96 h. In rats that did not survive, plasma cytochrome c increased at a much faster rate and attained levels substantially higher than 2 μg/ml before demise, which was characteristically the consequence of hemodynamic deterioration.

Based on these findings, we have postulated that plasma cytochrome c could serve as biomarker of mitochondrial injury severity and be useful not only to prognosticate outcome but also to assess therapies designed to attenuate or reverse mitochondrial injury.

13.3 Mitochondrial Protection by Inhibition of the Sodium-Hydrogen Exchanger Isoform-1

Our laboratory had investigated for more than a decade the potential beneficial effects of inhibiting the sodium-hydrogen exchanger isoform-1 (NHE-1) during cardiac resuscitation, showing protective mitochondrial effects leading to functional myocardial effects that would be clinically relevant [5, 33–43].

13.3.1 Underlying Pathophysiology

The benefit associated with NHE-1 inhibition is linked to the pathophysiological process of cell injury triggered by the intense and sustained intracellular myocardial acidosis that develops during cardiac arrest after cessation of coronary blood flow

[44–46]. Intracellular acidosis activates the sarcolemmal NHE-1 bringing Na^+ into the cell in exchange for H^+ [47]. During the ensuing resuscitation effort, reperfusion of the ischemic myocardium washes-out H^+ that have accumulated in the extra-cellular space during no-flow ischemia intensifying the sarcolemmal Na^+–H^+ exchange [33, 47, 48]. Na^+ may also enter the cell through Na^+ channels and the Na^+–HCO_3^- co-transporter. The Na^+ entering the cell is not extruded as it normally would because of concomitant reduction of the Na^+–K^+ ATPase activity [49], such that progressive and prominent increases in cytosolic Na^+ occur.

The cytosolic Na^+ excess drives sarcolemmal Ca^{2+} influx through reverse mode operation of the sarcolemmal Na^+–Ca^{2+} exchanger leading to cytosolic Ca^{2+} overload [50] and subsequent mitochondrial Ca^{2+} entry; a process which is reg-ulated by the Ca^{2+} uniporter for influx and the Na^+–Ca^{2+} exchanger for efflux [51]. Mitochondria can buffer large amounts of Ca^{2+} in its matrix up to a limit when free mitochondrial Ca^{2+} rises, the mitochondrial Na^+–Ca^{2+} exchanger becomes satu-rated, and mitochondrial Ca^{2+} overload ensues [51] worsening cell injury in part by compromising its capability to sustain oxidative phosphorylation [52] and by promoting the release of pro-apoptotic factors [53].

13.3.2 Relevance to Cardiac Resuscitation

The relevance of this mechanism of injury and potential therapeutic target is highlighted by preclinical work at the Resuscitation Institute using various animal models and other capabilities at the cellular and subcellular levels over more than a decade, strongly supporting a role of NHE-1 inhibition for resuscitation from cardiac arrest [5, 33–43].

Effects during VF: Initial observations were made in an isolated rat model of VF and simulated resuscitation using the NHE-1 inhibitor cariporide [33, 34]. In these studies, infusion of the NHE-1 inhibitor cariporide during simulated resuscitation markedly attenuated left ventricular pressure increases suggesting that NHE-1 inhibition could help preserve left ventricular distensibility during cardiac resus-citation. Post-resuscitation, hearts treated with cariporide had their end-diastolic pressure–volume curves preserved suggesting a beneficial effect preventing post-resuscitation diastolic dysfunction. These observations were followed by work in a clinically more relevant swine model of VF and CPR, showing that cariporide given as bolus dose immediately before starting chest compression could also preserve left ventricular distensibility during CPR in the intact animal, evidenced by preservation of wall thickness and cavity size. Preservation of left ventricular distensibility enabled chest compression to sustain the generation of coronary perfusion pressures at stable levels in contrast to controls animals in which the coronary perfusion pressure progressively declined. As a result, higher resuscit-ability was observed in animals treated with cariporide (2/8 vs. 8/8; $p < 0.05$) [36].

We hypothesized that the observed hemodynamic benefits in the swine model could reflect the ability of chest compression to generate a greater cardiac output for a given compression depth as a result of preservation of left ventricular distensibility. In other words, a more distensible left ventricle would allow a larger volume of blood to fill the cavity before compression resulting in more blood ejected by the ensuing compression. To test this hypothesis, we conducted studies on an intact rat model of VF and CPR and measured cardiac output and regional organ blood flow using fluorescent microspheres while varying the depth of compression [38].

Two series of 14 experiments each were conducted in which rats were subjected to 10 min of untreated VF followed by 8 min of chest compression before attempting defibrillation. Compression depth was adjusted to maintain an aortic diastolic pressure between 26 and 28 mmHg in the first series and between 36 and 38 mmHg in the second series. Within each series, rats were randomized to receive cariporide (3 mg/kg) or NaCl 0.9 % (control) before starting chest compression. In rats that received cariporide, higher cardiac output and higher regional organ blood flow (including heart and brain) were generated for a given compression depth. In other words, cariporide causes a very favorable leftward shift of the flow-depth relationship as a result of maintaining left ventricular distensibility.

Because pressure is a function of flow and resistance, we further reasoned that administration of a vasopressor agent could potentiate the hemodynamic effect of shifting the flow-depth relationship to the left resulting in an even higher systemic and coronary perfusion pressure. This was indeed the case as we demonstrated in the same rat model of VF and closed-chest resuscitation [37]. These studies involved two series of 16 experiments each using epinephrine in one series and vasopressin in the other. Within each series, rats were randomized to receive cariporide or NaCl control immediately before starting chest compression with the vasopressor agents given during chest compression. A significantly higher coronary perfusion pressure was generated when either vasopressor agent was given in rats that had received cariporide. The effect was not mediated through a vascular effect as the vasoconstrictive effects of epinephrine or vasopressin were not enhanced by cariporide [37]. A similar effect was subsequently demonstrated associated with the administration of epinephrine in our pig model of VF and closed-chest resuscitation [39]. These effects on coronary perfusion pressure are important; if translated clinically they could be highly relevant because only a small increase in coronary perfusion pressure is required to have a dramatic effect on resuscitability [54].

Effects on post-resuscitation arrhythmias and refibrillation: Another prominent effect elicited by cariporide was the suppression of ventricular ectopic activity and refibrillation that typically occurs early after return of cardiac activity [34, 36, 39, 55]. This effect was associated with preservation of the action potential duration [36]; an effect that would facilitate preservation of the impulse wavelength and thus reducing the risk of reentry [55]. This is also an important effect, which if translated clinically could help stabilize initially resuscitated victim of out-of-hospital cardiac arrest and avert re-arrest episodes during initial post-resuscitation period while enroute to a hospital.

Effects on post-resuscitation myocardial function: Variable degrees of systolic dysfunction occur after resuscitation from cardiac arrest despite full restoration of coronary blood flow. This phenomenon, known as myocardial stunning, is reversible but reversibility may take hours or days and contingent on severity compromise hemodynamic function and survival. Myocardial stunning is amenable to inotropic stimulation [56, 57] and use of dobutamine has been shown to facilitate hemodynamic stabilization post-resuscitation [58]. Diastolic dysfunction also occurs in the post-resuscitation period and is linked to the same pathophysiological abnormalities responsible for decreases in distensibility; namely increases in diastolic Ca^{2+} overload and energy deficit precluding full relaxation of cardiomyocytes. Administration of NHE-1 inhibitors during CPR in our animal models also attenuated post-resuscitation left ventricular systolic and diastolic dysfunction [41, 55].

13.3.3 Mechanism of the Resuscitation Effects

We also investigated the underlying mechanism of the benefit associated with use of NHE-1 inhibitors. In a rat model of VF and closed-chest resuscitation, we examined the effects of NHE-1 inhibition and of Na^+ channel blockade (interventions collectively referred to as "Na^+-limiting interventions") on intracellular Na^+, mitochondrial Ca^{2+}, cardiac function, and plasma levels of cardiac troponin I (cTnI) [40]. For these studies, hearts were removed at specific time events; namely (i) at baseline, (ii) at 15 min of untreated VF, (iii) at 15 min of VF with chest compression provided during the last 5 min of VF, and (iv) at 60-min post-resuscitation. Rats from the last two time events were randomized to receive an Na^+-limiting intervention immediately before starting chest compression or vehicle control. The Na^+-limiting interventions included a newly developed NHE-1 inhibitor AVE4454 (1 mg/kg), lidocaine (5 mg/kg), and the combination of AVE4454 and lidocaine.

Limiting sarcolemmal Na^+ entry attenuated increases in cytosolic Na^+ and mitochondrial Ca^{2+} overload during chest compression and the post-resuscitation phase. Attenuation of cytosolic Na^+ and mitochondrial Ca^{2+} increases was accompanied by preservation of left ventricular distensibility during chest compression, less post-resuscitation myocardial dysfunction, and lower levels of cTnI. In similar studies, attenuation of post-resuscitation myocardial dysfunction by NHE-1 inhibitors was associated with lesser increases in plasma cytochrome *c* in inverse relationship with left ventricular function [43].

We also used an open-chest pig model of electrically induced VF and extracorporeal circulation to study the myocardial energy effects of inhibiting NHE-1 under conditions of controlled coronary perfusion pressure [41]. For this study, VF was induced by epicardial delivery of an alternating current and left untreated for 8 min. After this interval, extracorporeal circulation was started and the systemic (extracorporeal) blood flow adjusted to maintain a coronary perfusion pressure at

10 mmHg for 10 min before attempting defibrillation. The target coronary perfusion pressure was chosen to mimic the low coronary perfusion pressure generated by closed-chest resuscitation. Two groups of eight pigs each were randomized to receive the NHE-1 inhibitor zoniporide (3 mg/kg) or vehicle control as a right atrial bolus immediately before starting extracorporeal circulation. Like in previous studies using the NHE-1 inhibitor cariporide [36], zoniporide also prevented reductions in left ventricular distensibility during the interval of VF and extracorporeal circulation, which in control pigs was characterized by progressive reductions in cavity size and progressive thickening of the left ventricular wall. Importantly, these effects occurred without changes in coronary blood flow or coronary vascular resistance indicating that the favorable myocardial effects of NHE-1 inhibition during resuscitation are not likely to be mediated through increases in blood flow and oxygen availability.

Myocardial tissue measurements indicated that administration of zoniporide prevented progressive loss of oxidative phosphorylation during the interval of simulated resuscitation. This effect was supported by a higher creatine phosphate-to-creatine (pCr/Cr) ratio, higher ATP/ADP ratio, and lesser increases in adenosine in animals treated with zoniporide. These measurements are consistent with regeneration of ADP into ATP by mitochondria instead of downstream degradation to adenosine, with the newly formed ATP being used to regenerate creatinine phosphate; all indicative of preserved mitochondrial bioenergetic function.

These changes were accompanied with prominent amelioration of myocardial lactate increases, attaining levels which were inversely proportional to the pCr/Cr ratio at 8 min of VF and extracorporeal circulation, suggesting a shift away from anaerobic metabolism consequent to preservation of mitochondrial bioenergetic function in pigs treated with zoniporide.

These energy effects are consistent with NHE-1 inhibition protecting mitochondrial bioenergetic function—probably as a result of limiting mitochondrial Ca^{2+} overload—and supportive of the concept that left ventricular distensibility during resuscitation is likely to be preserved by activating mitochondrial mechanisms capable of maintaining bioenergetic function.

13.3.4 Barriers to Clinical Translation

Unfortunately, efforts by pharmaceutical companies to develop NHE-1 inhibitors for clinical use have been modest at best and targeted only myocardial infarction [59–61] and myocardial protection during coronary artery bypass surgery (CABG) [60, 62]. Although the studies in acute myocardial infarction were inconclusive—with only one of three studies showing myocardial benefits [59]—studies in patients undergoing CABG—best represented by the EXPEDITION trial [62]—demonstrated a prominent myocardial protective effect providing proof-of-concept and lending support for NHE-1 inhibition in this clinical setting. The EXPEDITION trial compared cariporide with placebo in 5,761 high risk patients undergoing CABG. Cariporide—given intravenously before surgery and after surgery for 48 h—reduced the incidence of postoperative myocardial infarction from 18.9 % in the placebo group to 14.4 % in the treatment group ($p < 0.001$). Unfortunately and unexpectedly, patients who received cariporide had higher incidence of occlusive strokes. In subsequent analysis, the risk of stroke was linked to an enhanced platelet aggregation effect related to a very high dose of cariporide used in the study. However, the effect was unrelated to the mode of action and was not observed with other NHE-1 inhibitors.

Experts in the field have attributed the inconclusive findings of NHE-1 inhibition for acute myocardial infarction to the diminishing efficacy of NHE-1 inhibition when given only at the time of reperfusion after an extended period of coronary occlusion [63, 64]; a concept that is also supported by studies in a porcine model of coronary occlusion and reperfusion [65]. Likewise, the benefit observed in the CABG population can be explained by the administration of NHE-1 inhibitors before the anticipated episodes of myocardial ischemia [62]. In contrast to acute myocardial infarction and CABG, cardiac arrest is characterized by rapid development of intense myocardial ischemia (and other organs including the brain) but without infarction thus enabling to intervene on tissues suffering potentially reversible injury.

13.3.5 Alternative Strategies

Pending clinical development of NHE-1 inhibitors, we examined alternative mitochondrial protective strategies using compounds that are clinically available for other uses hypothesizing that mitochondrial protection through non-genomic activation of protective pathways such as Akt or the use of antioxidants could be beneficial. Applying this paradigm with first examined whether erythropoietin administered at the start of CPR could be as effective as an NHE-1 inhibitor. Studies in rat models of VF and CPR demonstrated a similar effect on left ventricular distensibility and an effect favoring reversal of post-resuscitation myocardial dysfunction in the presence of dobutamine [58, 66]. In these studies, use of erythropoietin was associated with activation of Akt and PKCε in myocardial tissue and preservation of activity of complex IV of the electron transport chain. These effects, consistent with activation of mitochondrial protective mechanisms, were also associated with an inverse relationship between plasma cytochrome c and left ventricular function. However, in a more recent study using a swine model of VF and resuscitation by ECC, we could not reproduce the beneficial effects on myocardial distensibility observed in rats. Moreover, no effects on myocardial energy metabolism or mitochondrial protective pathways could be demonstrated despite a modest favorable effect on post-resuscitation left ventricular systolic function [67].

Examination of other potential interventions in our rat model, including vitamin C [68] and estrogens (Unpublished) was not only ineffective but also associated with decreased resuscitability and survival.

13.4 Conclusions

Our experience using various animal models of VF and resuscitation over the last 15 years indicates that mitochondria play a key role in resuscitation from cardiac arrest and that therapies aimed at protecting mitochondrial bioenergetic function have the potential for facilitating initial resuscitation and subsequent survival. Based on our work we continue to look forward to the clinical development of NHE-1 inhibitors for reducing mitochondrial Ca^{2+} overload as the most promising experimental pharmacological intervention for cardiac resuscitation.

References

1. Go AS, Mozaffarian D, Roger VL, Benjamin EJ, Berry JD, Borden WB, Bravata DM, Dai S, Ford ES, Fox CS, Franco S, Fullerton HJ, Gillespie C, Hailpern SM, Heit JA, Howard VJ, Huffman MD, Kissela BM, Kittner SJ, Lackland DT, Lichtman JH, Lisabeth LD, Magid D, Marcus GM, Marelli A et al (2013) Heart disease and stroke statistics–2013 update: a report from the American Heart Association. Circulation 127(1):e6–e245
2. Weisfeldt ML, Zweier J, Ambrosio G, Becker LC, Flaherty JT (1988) Evidence that free radicals result in reperfusion injury in heart muscle. Basic Life Sci 49:911–919
3. Dong Z, Saikumar P, Weinberg JM, Venkatachalam MA (2006) Calcium in cell injury and death. Annu Rev Pathol 1:405–434
4. Halestrap AP (2006) Calcium, mitochondria and reperfusion injury: a pore way to die. Biochem Soc Trans 34(Pt 2):232–237
5. Gazmuri RJ, Radhakrishnan J (2012) Protecting mitochondrial bioenergetic function during resuscitation from cardiac arrest. Crit Care Clin 28(2):245–270
6. Vendelin M, Beraud N, Guerrero K, Andrienko T, Kuznetsov AV, Olivares J, Kay L, Saks VA (2005) Mitochondrial regular arrangement in muscle cells: a "crystal-like" pattern. Am J Physiol Cell Physiol 288(3):C757–C767
7. Halestrap AP, Clarke SJ, Javadov SA (2004) Mitochondrial permeability transition pore opening during myocardial reperfusion–a target for cardioprotection. Cardiovasc Res 61(3):372–385
8. Cai J, Yang J, Jones DP (1998) Mitochondrial control of apoptosis: the role of cytochrome c. Biochim Biophys Acta 1366(1–2):139–149
9. Green DR, Reed JC (1998) Mitochondria and apoptosis. Science 281(5381):1309–1312
10. Radhakrishnan J, Wang S, Ayoub IM, Kolarova JD, Levine RF, Gazmuri RJ (2007) Circulating levels of cytochrome c after resuscitation from cardiac arrest: a marker of mitochondrial injury and predictor of survival. Am J Physiol Heart Circ Physiol 292:H767–H775
11. Radhakrishnan J, Ayoub IM, Gazmuri RJ (2009) Activation of caspase-3 may not contribute to postresuscitation myocardial dysfunction. Am J Physiol Heart Circ Physiol 296(4):H1164–H1174
12. Ott M, Robertson JD, Gogvadze V, Zhivotovsky B, Orrenius S (2002) Cytochrome c release from mitochondria proceeds by a two-step process. Proc Natl Acad Sci USA 99(3):1259–1263

13. von Harsdorf R, Li PF, Dietz R (1999) Signaling pathways in reactive oxygen species-induced cardiomyocyte apoptosis. Circulation 99(22):2934–2941
14. Petrosillo G, Ruggiero FM, Pistolese M, Paradies G (2004) Ca2+-induced reactive oxygen species production promotes cytochrome c release from rat liver mitochondria via mitochondrial permeability transition (MPT)-dependent and MPT-independent mechanisms: role of cardiolipin. J Biol Chem 279(51):53103–53108
15. de Moissac D, Gurevich RM, Zheng H, Singal PK, Kirshenbaum LA (2000) Caspase activation and mitochondrial cytochrome C release during hypoxia-mediated apoptosis of adult ventricular myocytes. J Mol Cell Cardiol 32(1):53–63
16. Loor G, Kondapalli J, Iwase H, Chandel NS, Waypa GB, Guzy RD Vanden Hoek TL, Schumacker PT (2011) Mitochondrial oxidant stress triggers cell death in simulated ischemia-reperfusion. Biochim Biophys Acta 1813(7):1382–1394
17. Li P, Nijhawan D, Budihardjo I, Srinivasula SM, Ahmad M, Alnemri ES, Wang X (1997) Cytochrome c and dATP-dependent formation of Apaf-1/caspase-9 complex initiates an apoptotic protease cascade. Cell 91(4):479–489
18. Budihardjo I, Oliver H, Lutter M, Luo X, Wang X (1999) Biochemical pathways of caspase activation during apoptosis. Annu Rev Cell Dev Biol 15:269–290
19. Saleh A, Srinivasula SM, Acharya S, Fishel R, Alnemri ES (1999) Cytochrome c and dATP-mediated oligomerization of Apaf-1 is a prerequisite for procaspase-9 activation. J Biol Chem 274(25):17941–17945
20. Zou H, Li Y, Liu X, Wang X (1999) An APAF-1.cytochrome c multimeric complex is a functional apoptosome that activates procaspase-9. J Biol Chem 274(17):11549–11556
21. Renz A, Burek C, Mier W, Mozoluk M, Schulze-Osthoff K, Los M (2001) Cytochrome c is rapidly extruded from apoptotic cells and detectable in serum of anticancer-drug treated tumor patients. Adv Exp Med Biol 495:331–334
22. Zager RA, Johnson AC, Hanson SY (2004) Proximal tubular cytochrome c efflux: determinant, and potential marker, of mitochondrial injury. Kidney Int 65(6):2123–2134
23. Osaka A, Hasegawa H, Tsuruda K, Inokuchi N, Yanagihara K, Yamada Y, Aoyama M, Sawada T, Kamihira S (2009) Serum cytochrome c to indicate the extent of ongoing tumor cell death. Int J Lab Hematol 31(3):307–314
24. Liu X, Xie W, Liu P, Duan M, Jia Z, Li W, Xu J (2006) Mechanism of the cardioprotection of rhEPO pretreatment on suppressing the inflammatory response in ischemia-reperfusion. Life Sci 78(19):2255–2264
25. Barczyk K, Kreuter M, Pryjma J, Booy EP, Maddika S, Ghavami S, Berdel WE, Roth J, Los M (2005) Serum cytochrome c indicates in vivo apoptosis and can serve as a prognostic marker during cancer therapy. Int J Cancer 116(2):167–173
26. Alleyne T, Joseph J, Sampson V (2001) Cytochrome-c detection: a diagnostic marker for myocardial infarction. Appl Biochem Biotechnol 90(2):97–105
27. Marenzi G, Giorgio M, Trinei M, Moltrasio M, Ravagnani P, Cardinale D, Ciceri F, Cavallero A, Veglia F, Fiorentini C, Cipolla CM, Bartorelli AL, Pelicci P (2010) Circulating cytochrome c as potential biomarker of impaired reperfusion in ST-segment elevation acute myocardial infarction. Am J Cardiol 106(10):1443–1449
28. Narula J, Pandey P, Arbustini E, Haider N, Narula N, Kolodgie FD, Dal Bello B, Semigran MJ, Bielsa-Masdeu A, Dec GW, Israels S, Ballester M, Virmani R, Saxena S, Kharbanda S (1999) Apoptosis in heart failure: release of cytochrome c from mitochondria and activation of caspase-3 in human cardiomyopathy. Proc Natl Acad Sci USA 96(14):8144–8149
29. Sakaida I, Kimura T, Yamasaki T, Fukumoto Y, Watanabe K, Aoyama M, Okita K (2005) Cytochrome c is a possible new marker for fulminant hepatitis in humans. J Gastroenterol 40(2):179–185
30. Adachi N, Hirota M, Hamaguchi M, Okamoto K, Watanabe K, Endo F (2004) Serum cytochrome c level as a prognostic indicator in patients with systemic inflammatory response syndrome. Clin Chim Acta 342(1–2):127–136

31. Hosoya M, Nunoi H, Aoyama M, Kawasaki Y, Suzuki H (2005) Cytochrome c and tumor necrosis factor-alpha values in serum and cerebrospinal fluid of patients with influenza-associated encephalopathy. Pediatr Infect Dis J 24(5):467–470

32. Hosoya M, Kawasaki Y, Katayose M, Sakuma H, Watanabe M, Igarashi E, Aoyama M, Nunoi H, Suzuki H (2006) Prognostic predictive values of serum cytochrome c, cytokines, and other laboratory measurements in acute encephalopathy with multiple organ failure. Arch Dis Child 91:469–472

33. Gazmuri RJ, Hoffner E, Kalcheim J, Ho H, Patel M, Ayoub IM, Epstein M, Kingston S, Han Y (2001) Myocardial protection during ventricular fibrillation by reduction of proton-driven sarcolemmal sodium influx. J Lab Clin Med 137(1):43–55

34. Gazmuri RJ, Ayoub IM, Hoffner E, Kolarova JD (2001) Successful ventricular defibrillation by the selective sodium-hydrogen exchanger isoform-1 inhibitor cariporide. Circulation 104:234–239

35. Gazmuri RJ, Ayoub IM, Kolarova JD, Karmazyn M (2002) Myocardial protection during ventricular fibrillation by inhibition of the sodium-hydrogen exchanger isoform-1. Crit Care Med 30(4 Suppl):S166–S171

36. Ayoub IM, Kolarova JD, Yi Z, Trevedi A, Deshmukh H, Lubell DL, Franz MR, Maldonado FA, Gazmuri RJ (2003) Sodium-hydrogen exchange inhibition during ventricular fibrillation: Beneficial effects on ischemic contracture, action potential duration, reperfusion arrhythmias, myocardial function, and resuscitability. Circulation 107:1804–1809

37. Kolarova J, Yi Z, Ayoub IM, Gazmuri RJ (2005) Cariporide potentiates the effects of epinephrine and vasopressin by nonvascular mechanisms during closed-chest resuscitation. Chest 127(4):1327–1334

38. Kolarova JD, Ayoub IM, Gazmuri RJ (2005) Cariporide enables hemodynamically more effective chest compression by leftward shift of its flow-depth relationship. Am J Physiol Heart Circulatory Physiol 288:H2904–H2911

39. Ayoub IM, Kolarova J, Kantola RL, Sanders R, Gazmuri RJ (2005) Cariporide minimizes adverse myocardial effects of epinephrine during resuscitation from ventricular fibrillation. Crit Care Med 33(11):2599–2605

40. Wang S, Radhakrishnan J, Ayoub IM, Kolarova JD, Taglieri DM, Gazmuri RJ (2007) Limiting sarcolemmal Na+ entry during resuscitation from VF prevents excess mitochondrial Ca2+ accumulation and attenuates myocardial injury. J Appl Physiol 103:55–65

41. Ayoub IM, Kolarova J, Kantola R, Radhakrishnan J, Gazmuri RJ (2007) Zoniporide preserves left ventricular compliance during ventricular fibrillation and minimizes post-resuscitation myocardial dysfunction through benefits on energy metabolism. Crit Care Med 35:2329–2336

42. Ayoub IM, Kolarova J, Gazmuri RJ (2010) Cariporide given during resuscitation promotes return of electrically stable and mechanically competent cardiac activity. Resuscitation 81(1):106–110

43. Radhakrishnan J, Kolarova JD, Ayoub IM, Gazmuri RJ (2011) AVE4454B—a novel sodium-hydrogen exchanger isoform-1 inhibitor—compared less effective than cariporide for resuscitation from cardiac arrest. Transl Res 157(2):71–80

44. von Planta M, Weil MH, Gazmuri RJ, Bisera J, Rackow EC (1989) Myocardial acidosis associated with CO2 production during cardiac arrest and resuscitation. Circulation 80:684–692

45. Kette F, Weil MH, Gazmuri RJ, Bisera J, Rackow EC (1993) Intramyocardial hypercarbic acidosis during cardiac arrest and resuscitation. Crit Care Med 21(6):901–906

46. Noc M, Weil MH, Gazmuri RJ, Sun S, Bisera J, Tang W (1994) Ventricular fibrillation voltage as a monitor of the effectiveness of cardiopulmonary resuscitation. J Lab Clin Med 124:421–426

47. Karmazyn M, Sawyer M, Fliegel L (2005) The na(+)/h(+) exchanger: a target for cardiac therapeutic intervention. Curr Drug Targets Cardiovasc Haematol Disord 5(4):323–335

48. Imahashi K, Kusuoka H, Hashimoto K, Yoshioka J, Yamaguchi H, Nishimura T (1999) Intracellular sodium accumulation during ischemia as the substrate for reperfusion injury. Circ Res 84(12):1401–1406

49. Avkiran M, Ibuki C, Shimada Y, Haddock PS (1996) Effects of acidic reperfusion on arrhythmias and Na(+)-K(+)-ATPase activity in regionally ischemic rat hearts. Am J Physiol 270(3 Pt 2):H957–H964

50. An J, Varadarajan SG, Camara A, Chen Q, Novalija E, Gross GJ, Stowe DF (2001) Blocking Na(+)/H(+) exchange reduces [Na(+)](i) and [Ca(2+)](i) load after ischemia and improves function in intact hearts. Am J Physiol 281(6):H2398–H2409

51. Gunter TE, Buntinas L, Sparagna G, Eliseev R, Gunter K (2000) Mitochondrial calcium transport: mechanisms and functions. Cell Calcium 28(5–6):285–296

52. Yamamoto S, Matsui K, Ohashi N (2002) Protective effect of Na+/H+ exchange inhibitor, SM-20550, on impaired mitochondrial respiratory function and mitochondrial Ca2+ overload in ischemic/reperfused rat hearts. J Cardiovasc Pharmacol 39(4):569–575

53. Borutaite V, Brown GC (2003) Mitochondria in apoptosis of ischemic heart. FEBS Lett 541(1–3):1–5

54. Paradis NA, Martin GB, Rivers EP, Goetting MG, Appleton TJ, Feingold M, Nowak RM (1990) Coronary perfusion pressure and the return of spontaneous circulation in human cardiopulmonary resuscitation. JAMA 263:1106–1113

55. Ayoub IM, Kolarova J, Gazmuri RJ (2009) Cariporide given during resuscitation promotes return of electrically stable and mechanically competent cardiac activity. Resuscitation 81:106–110

56. Ellis SG, Wynne J, Braunwald E, Henschke CI, Sandor T, Kloner RA (1984) Response of reperfusion-salvaged, stunned myocardium to inotropic stimulation. Am Heart J 107(1):13–19

57. Meyer RJ, Kern KB, Berg RA, Hilwig RW, Ewy GA (2002) Post-resuscitation right ventricular dysfunction: delineation and treatment with dobutamine. Resuscitation 55(2):187–191

58. Radhakrishnan J, Upadhyaya MP, Ng M, Edelheit A, Moy HM, Ayoub IM, Gazmuri RJ (2013) Erythropoietin facilitates resuscitation from ventricular fibrillation by signaling protection of mitochondrial bioenergetic function in rats. Am J Transl Res 5(3):316–326

59. Rupprecht HJ, vom DJ, Terres W, Seyfarth KM, Richardt G, Schultheibeta HP, Buerke M, Sheehan FH, Drexler H (2000) Cardioprotective effects of the Na(+)/H(+) exchange inhibitor cariporide in patients with acute anterior myocardial infarction undergoing direct PTCA. Circulation 101(25):2902–2908

60. Boyce SW, Bartels C, Bolli R, Chaitman B, Chen JC, Chi E, Jessel A, Kereiakes D, Knight J, Thulin L, Theroux P (2003) Impact of sodium-hydrogen exchange inhibition by cariporide on death or myocardial infarction in high-risk CABG surgery patients: results of the CABG surgery cohort of the GUARDIAN study. J Thorac Cardiovasc Surg 126(2):420–427

61. Zeymer U, Suryapranata H, Monassier JP, Opolski G, Davies J, Rasmanis G, Linssen G, Tebbe U, Schroder R, Tiemann R, Machnig T, Neuhaus KL (2001) The Na(+)/H(+) exchange inhibitor eniporide as an adjunct to early reperfusion therapy for acute myocardial infarction. Results of the evaluation of the safety and cardioprotective effects of eniporide in acute myocardial infarction (ESCAMI) trial. J Am Coll Cardiol 38(6):1644–1650

62. Mentzer RM Jr, Bartels C, Bolli R, Boyce S, Buckberg GD, Chaitman B, Haverich A, Knight J, Menasche P, Myers ML, Nicolau J, Simoons M, Thulin L, Weisel RD (2008) Sodium-hydrogen exchange inhibition by cariporide to reduce the risk of ischemic cardiac events in patients undergoing coronary artery bypass grafting: results of the EXPEDITION study. Ann Thorac Surg 85(4):1261–1270

63. Murphy E, Allen DG (2009) Why did the NHE inhibitor clinical trials fail? J Mol Cell Cardiol 46(2):137–141

64. Karmazyn M (2013) NHE-1: still a viable therapeutic target. J Mol Cell Cardiol. 61:77–82

65. Klein HH, Pich S, Bohle RM, Lindert-Heimberg S, Nebendahl K (2000) Na(+)/H(+) exchange inhibitor cariporide attenuates cell injury predominantly during ischemia and not at onset of reperfusion in porcine hearts with low residual blood flow. Circulation 102(16):1977–1982
66. Singh D, Kolarova JD, Wang S, Ayoub IM, Gazmuri RJ (2007) Myocardial protection by erythropoietin during resuscitation from ventricular fibrillation. Am J Ther 14:361–368
67. Borovnik-Lesja V, Whitehouse K, Baetiong A, Artin B, Radhakrishnan J, Gazmuri RJ (2013) High-dose erythropoietin during cardiac resuscitation lessens post-resuscitation myocardial stunning in swine. Transl Res 162(2):110–121
68. Motl J, Radhakrishnan J, Ayoub IM, Grmec S, Gazmuri RJ (2012) Vitamin C compromises cardiac resuscitability in a rat model of ventricular fibrillation. Am J Ther. Jun 16 [Epub]

The Potential Contribution of Corticosteroids to Positive Cardiac Arrest Outcomes

14

Iosifina Koliantzaki, Spyros G. Zakynthinos and Spyros D. Mentzelopoulos

14.1 Introduction

Over the past 50 years, the majority of research on cardiac arrest has focused on improving the rate of return of spontaneous circulation (ROSC); however, many interventions improved ROSC without improving long-term survival. The translation of optimized basic life support and advanced life support interventions into the best possible outcomes is sine qua non in optimal post-arrest care. There is a scarcity of data reported from the post-arrest in-hospital phase, and no generally accepted, evidence-based protocol exists, other than brain protection-oriented intensive care. For any further improvement in post-arrest care, we first have to determine the relative contribution of potential, outcome-determining factors [1].

The importance of these factors leads to the addition of a fifth ring, post-resuscitation care (Fig. 14.1), to the "Chain of Survival." The idea is not new; the hospital ring was included by Niemann [2] in 1982, and more recently, by Engdahl et al. [3].

I. Koliantzaki · S. G. Zakynthinos · S. D. Mentzelopoulos (✉)
Department of Intensive Care Medicine, University of Athens Medical School,
Evaggelismos Hospital, 45–47 Ipsilandou Street, GR-10675, Athens, Greece
e-mail: sdmentzelopoulos@yahoo.com

I. Koliantzaki
e-mail: josephine.koliantzaki@hotmail.com

S. G. Zakynthinos
e-mail: szakynthinos@yahoo.com

A. Gullo and G. Ristagno (eds.), *Resuscitation*,
DOI: 10.1007/978-88-470-5507-0_14, © Springer-Verlag Italia 2014

143

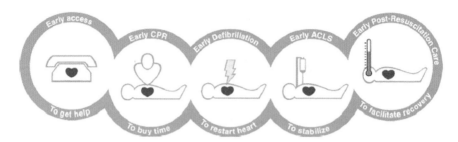

Fig. 14.1 The chain of Survival. Reproduced with permission from Ref. [1]. *CPR* Cardiopulmonary resuscitation; *ACLS* Advanced cardiac life support

14.2 Pharmacological Effects of Corticosteroids

Corticosteroids are a class of chemicals involved in a wide range of physiological processes, including stress response, immune response, and regulation of inflammation, carbohydrate metabolism, protein catabolism, blood electrolyte levels, and behavior. The possible effect of exogenously administered steroids on cardiac arrest outcomes was already hypothesized in 1988. Still, there is no definitive evidence on their efficacy when given to cardiac arrest patients after ROSC.

The physiological effects of glucocorticoids can be summarized as follows:

1. Anti-inflammatory effects: Glucocorticoids inhibit inflammatory and allergic reactions by decreasing the production of interleukin (IL)-2 as well as the proliferation of T-lymphocytes, histamine, and serotonin release, and prostaglandin and leukotriene synthesis.
2. Renal effects: Glucocorticoids restore glomerular filtration rate and renal blood flow to normal following adrenalectomy; in addition, they facilitate free water excretion (clearance) and uric acid secretion.
3. Vascular effects: In pharmacological doses, cortisol enhances the vasopressor effect of norepinephrine. In the absence of cortisol, the vasopressor action of catecholamines is diminished, and hypotension ensues.
4. Stress adaptation: Corticosteroids allow mammals to adapt to various stresses in order to maintain homeostasis. Stress is associated with the activation of the hypothalamic–pituitary–adrenal axis.
5. Corticosteroids also have gastric, psychoneural, and antigrowth effects.
6. Metabolic effects: Glucocorticoids stimulate gluconeogenesis through: (a) increase in protein catabolism and decrease in protein synthesis, resulting in more amino acids being available to the liver for glyconeogenesis; (b) decrease in insulin sensitivity and glucose utilization in adipose tissue; and (c) increase in lipolysis, so as to offer more substrate for gluconeogenesis.

14.3 Retrospective Data on Steroids in Cardiac Arrest

The potential usefulness of steroids in cardiac arrest has been previously assessed in two retrospective studies. Grafton et al. [4] examined the effect of steroid treatment on the early neurological outcome and in-hospital survival of 458 consecutive patients admitted after out-of-hospital cardiac arrest. Two hundred and thirteen patients (47 %) received median doses of 24, 16, and 16 mg of dexamethasone or its equivalent on days 1, 2, and 3 post-ROSC, respectively; the reported median duration of treatment was 3.4 days, and 87 % of these patients received steroid treatment for one week or less. Of those receiving steroids, 128/213 (60 %) regained consciousness, and of those not receiving steroids, 150/245 (61 %) regained consciousness. There was no reported comparison of patient baseline characteristics, despite the fact that the use of steroids was nonrandomized. However, findings remained unchanged after using logistic regression to adjust for differences in potential effect modifiers between the two treatment groups. These factors were: witnessed or not witnessed cardiac arrest, use of epinephrine or norepinephrine during resuscitation, and motor examination findings, response of the pupils to light, presence of spontaneous eye movements, and blood glucose level on hospital admission. According to the authors, these results could not support any role of steroids in the treatment of global brain ischemia due to cardiac arrest.

One year later, an article published in JAMA [5], concluded that "The routine clinical practice of administering glucocorticoids after global brain ischemia is not justified." This was a retrospective analysis of prospectively collected data aimed at evaluating the efficacy of thiopental in global cerebral ischemia. The study included 262 initially comatose, cardiac arrest survivors, who made no purposeful response to pain after ROSC. These patients were divided into four groups which received either no glucocorticoids, or glucocorticoids at low doses (i.e., equivalent to 1–20 mg of dexamethasone), or glucocorticoids at medium doses (i.e., equivalent to 20–50 mg of dexamethasone), or glucocorticoids at high doses (i.e., equivalent to >70 mg of dexamethasone) within the first 8 h following ROSC. The paper did not report a comparison of the baseline characteristics of the four patient groups. Also, the glucocorticoid doses administered within 8–24 h post-ROSC were unknown. Furthermore, the extent of the protocolized use of post-ROSC hyperventilation (titrated to a $PaCO_2$ of 25–35 mmHg) was not compared among the four groups; hyperventilation may adversely affect cerebral blood flow and neurological outcome [6]. Finally, cardiac arrest due to noncardiac causes (an independent predictor of poor outcome [7]) was more frequent in the steroid-treated patients. In that study, neurological outcome was scored using a modification of the Glasgow–Pittsburgh Cerebral Performance Category Scale. Steroid-treated groups versus the "no steroid" group had no significant improvement in overall survival or neurological recovery [5].

14.4 Defining the Postcardiac Arrest Syndrome

ROSC after prolonged, complete, whole-body ischemia is an unnatural pathophysiological state created by successful cardiopulmonary resuscitation (CPR). In the early 1970s, Negovsky recognized that the pathology caused by complete, whole-body ischemia and reperfusion was unique in that it had a clearly definable cause, time course, and constellation of pathophysiological processes [8–10]. Negovsky named this state "post-resuscitation disease." Although appropriate at the time, the term "resuscitation" is now used more broadly to include treatment of various shock states in which circulation has not ceased. Moreover, the term "post-resuscitation" implies that the act of resuscitation has ended. Negovsky stated that "a second, more complex phase of resuscitation begins when patients regain spontaneous circulation after cardiac arrest (Fig. 14.2) [8]." Therefore, the term "postcardiac arrest syndrome" seems more appropriate.

The high mortality rate of patients who initially achieve ROSC after cardiac arrest can be attributed to a unique pathophysiological process that involves multiple organs. Although prolonged, whole-body ischemia initially causes global tissue and organ injury, additional damage occurs during and after reperfusion [11, 12]. The unique features of postcardiac arrest pathophysiology are often superimposed on the disease or injury that caused the cardiac arrest, as well as underlying comorbidities. Therapies that focus on individual organs may compromise other injured organ systems. The four key components of postcardiac arrest syndrome are (1) postcardiac arrest brain injury, (2) postcardiac arrest myocardial dysfunction, (3) ischemia/reperfusion-triggered, systemic inflammatory response, and (4) persistent underlying pathology [13].

Fig. 14.2 The phases of the postcardiac arrest syndrome. Reproduced with permission from Ref. [13]

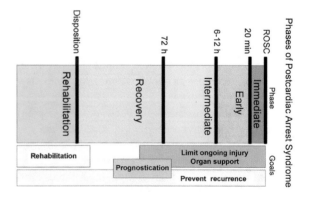

14.5   Postischemic Myocardial Dysfunction and Corticosteroids

Postcardiac arrest myocardial dysfunction contributes to the low survival rate after in-hospital and out-of-hospital cardiac arrest [14–16]. Laboratory and clinical evidence, however, indicates that this phenomenon is both responsive to therapy and reversible [16–21]. Immediately after ROSC, heart rate and blood pressure are extremely variable. It is important to recognize that normal or elevated heart rate and blood pressure immediately after ROSC can be caused by a transient increase in local myocardial and circulating catecholamine concentrations [22, 23]. Using an experimental model of coronary microembolization, Hori et al. [24] demonstrated that after a rapid (i.e., 5–10 min lasting) recovery from the immediate, microembolization-induced ischemic myocardial dysfunction, a progressive and more prolonged (i.e., lasting for approximately 4 days) contractile dysfunction develops in the presence of an unchanged regional myocardial blood flow [25]. This perfusion–contraction mismatch was associated with a local inflammatory response characterized by leukocyte infiltration [25]. In subsequent studies, a causal role for tumor necrosis factor (TNF) and sphingosine in this progressive contractile dysfunction was demonstrated [26, 27]. Interestingly, high-dose (i.e., 30 mg/kg) methylprednisolone, even when given after microembolization, prevented the progressive contractile dysfunction [28].

Glucocorticoids have been used for their anti-inflammatory action in the treatment of a wide variety of diseases [29]. More specifically, glucocorticoids attenuate leukocyte/endothelium interactions [30–33], as well as the generation and release of inflammatory cytokines and mediators [34–38]. Cardioprotective effects of glucocorticoids in the acute setting of myocardial ischemia/reperfusion have been shown experimentally with regard to structural and functional myocardial damage [39–45].

The inflammation of early myocardial ischemia is characterized by leukocyte infiltration [46, 47], a process involving the expression of L-selectin, CD11/CD18-complex, and adhesion molecules [48, 49]. Glucocorticoids suppress the expression of L-selectin and CD11/CD18 on leukocytes [32, 33], and the expression of endothelial leukocyte adhesion molecule-1 and the intercellular adhesion molecule-1 [30]. Glucocorticoids have previously been shown to inhibit the expression of mRNA of TNF in immunologically activated, rat, peritoneal mast cells [37], to suppress the production of TNF in the serum and the myocardium of lipopolysaccharide-stimulated rats [38], and to abolish the release of TNF into the serum of humans during cardiac surgery [36]. Glucocorticoids also attenuate the infiltration of TNF–producing macrophages/monocytes after coronary microembolization in pigs [50].

In the past, glucocorticoids have been used clinically for the treatment of acute myocardial infarction [51–53], but such treatment was abandoned because of their potentially deleterious, long-term effects on scar stability and aneurysm formation [54, 55]. However, results from chronically instrumented dogs suggest that anti-inflammatory treatment by a single dose of glucocorticoids in the presence of small, patchy microembolization-induced infarcts exerts no adverse effects [28]. Furthermore, a more recent meta-analysis of human data from 11 controlled trials suggested a possible mortality benefit for corticosteroid treatment of myocardial infarction [56].

14.6 Postcardiac Arrest Systemic Inflammatory Response and Corticosteroids

The American Heart Association Guidelines 2010 for Cardiopulmonary Resuscitation and Emergency Cardiovascular Care state that the postcardiac arrest syndrome has similarities to septic shock [57, 58]. However, the efficacy of corticosteroids remains controversial in patients with sepsis [59–61]. The mechanisms underlying the postcardiac arrest syndrome involve a whole-body ischemia and reperfusion that triggers a systemic inflammatory response [58, 62]. Altogether, the high levels of circulating cytokines, the presence of endotoxin in plasma, and the dysregulated production of cytokines found in cardiac arrest patients resemble the immunological profile found in patients with sepsis [58].

The postcardiac arrest syndrome seems to be causally related to an early systemic inflammatory response, leading to an inflammatory imbalance [62, 63], and is also associated with an "endotoxin tolerance," as observed in severe sepsis [64]. Additional disturbances include activation of the coagulation cascade [65, 66], platelet activation with formation of thromboxane A2 [67], and an alteration of soluble E-selectin and P-selectin [63] have been described.

The postcardiac arrest syndrome can be temporally subdivided into four phases (Fig. 14.2) [62]: (1) Within the first 24-h post-arrest, a microcirculatory dysfunction from the multifocal hypoxia leads to rapid release of toxic enzymes and free radicals into the cerebrospinal fluid and blood; (2) over the next 1–3 days, cardiac and systemic functions improve, but intestinal permeability increases, predisposing the patient to sepsis and the multiple organ dysfunction syndrome; (3) during the subsequent days, a serious infection may occur causing rapid clinical deterioration; and (4) the patient either dies of a secondary complication or the primary disease that caused the cardiac arrest, or undergoes a frequently prolonged, partial or complete recovery.

The Surviving Sepsis Campaign guidelines 2012 for the management of severe sepsis and septic shock suggest stress-dose hydrocortisone therapy (daily dose: 200 mg) only for patients who are poorly responsive to fluid and vasopressor therapy [68]. However, in cardiac arrest patients, treatment-refractory shock is a common post-ROSC complication [69]. Furthermore, post-resuscitation shock is frequently partly due to a post-arrest adrenal insufficiency or dysfunction [58, 62, 70], which in turn constitutes an independent predictor of mortality at 1 week after resuscitation [71]. In light of these facts, in our recently published, single-center (sample size: 100 patients), randomized, double-blind, placebo-controlled study of vasopressor-requiring, in-hospital cardiac arrest [69], we administered 40 mg of methylprednisolone during CPR, and stress-dose hydrocortisone (300 mg/day for a maximum of 7 days followed by gradual taper) to patients fulfilling a clearly defined criterion for post-resuscitation shock. Our CPR intervention also included vasopressin (dose range: 20–100 IU) and epinephrine. The control group received standard, epinephrine-based CPR according to the contemporary guidelines for resuscitation. Intervention group results showed a combination of improved post-arrest hemodynamics and central venous oxygen saturation, post-arrest cytokine levels and organ/system function, and survival to hospital discharge (Fig. 14.3). Survival to hospital discharge was improved in the total intervention group (Fig. 14.3a) as well as in the subgroup of patients with post-resuscitation shock (Fig. 14.3b). Furthermore, multivariate Cox regression analysis showed that the assignment to the intervention group and completion of a full post-arrest course of hydrocortisone was associated with a hazard ratio of 0.15 (95 % confidence interval: 0.06–0.38, $P < 0.001$) for in-hospital death during follow-up. These results were consistent with a steroid-associated benefit in cardiac arrest. However, the combined nature of our intervention precluded a precise determination of the relative contribution of the steroids to the positive outcomes of the intervention group.

Another pilot (sample size: 100 patients), randomized, unblinded study of out-of-hospital cardiac arrest [72], showed improved rates of ROSC in its intervention group patients, who received a single dose of 100 mg of hydrocortisone during CPR. Interestingly, and consistently with prior findings [70], patients of the study's control arm with a serum cortisol level of more than 20 μg/dL had a ROSC rate of 43 %, as opposed to a ROSC rate of 25 % that was observed in controls with a serum cortisol level of less than 20 μg/dL.

14.7 Corticosteroids and Neuroprotection

To date, there is no published data showing that peri-arrest glucocorticoids are neuroptotective [73]. In the peri-arrest period, there is a multifactorial disruption of the blood–brain barrier (BBB), involving the enhanced production of nitric oxide, inflammatory cytokines, and vascular endothelial growth factor [74]. According to recent evidence, several of these mechanisms could constitute potential targets of corticosteroid treatment. Corticosteroids promote BBB integrity through their interaction with astrocytic cells, which results in upregulation of the endothelial tight junction proteins such as occludin and claudin-5 [75]. Glucocorticoids regulate the expression of leukocyte adhesion molecule genes in endothelial cells [76], and suppress the production of the pro-inflammatory cytokines [34–38, 77]. Methylprednisolone attenuates axonal changes (e.g., myelin fragmentation and presence of edematous vesicles), caused by experimental cerebral edema [78]. In addition, 17-beta estradiol suppresses the expression of inducible nitric oxide synthase and neuronal nitric oxide synthase, thus attenuating the BBB disruption after experimental, hypovolemic cardiac arrest [79]. However,

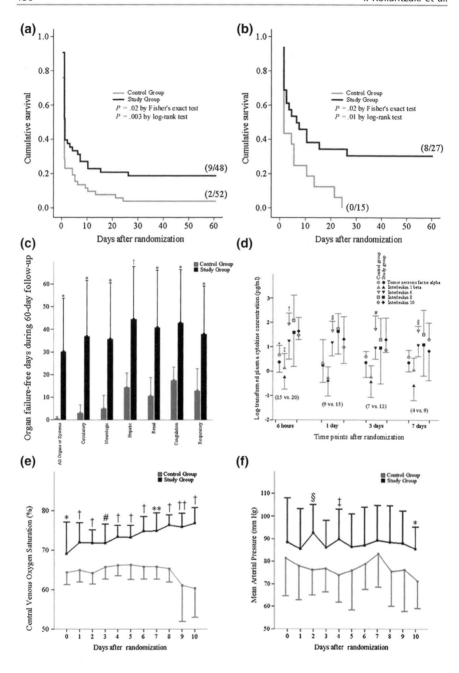

◀ **Fig. 14.3** Main results of patient follow-up. Reproduced with permission from Ref. [69]. Study group denotes intervention group. **a, b** Probability of survival to day 60 postrandomization, which was identical to survival to hospital discharge, in all 100 patients (**a**) and in the 42 patients with post-resuscitation shock (**b**). Parentheses, survivors/total number of patients. **c** Organ failure-free days in patients who completed a full course of hydrocortisone ($n = 12$) or saline-placebo ($n = 6$) according to protocol. Bars, mean; Error-bars, standard deviation; *, $P = 0.001$; †, $P < 0.001$. **d** Plasma-cytokines in post-resuscitation shock. Parentheses, number of controls versus number of study-group patients; Symbols, mean; Error-bars, standard deviation; *, $P = 0.04$; †, $P = 0.003$; §, $P = 0.02$; #, $P = 0.01$; ‡, $P = 0.06$. **e, f** Central-venous oxygen saturation (**e**) and mean arterial pressure (**f**) in post-resuscitation shock. Dots, mean; Error-bars, standard deviation. *, $P = 0.03$; †, $P < 0.001$; §, $P = 0.006$; #, $P = 0.005$; ‡, $P = 0.01$; **, $P = 0.002$; ††, $P = 0.04$

during the course of ischemic insults, insensitivity to glucocorticoids ensues, due to proteasome-induced degradation of the glucocorticoid receptor [80, 81]. This suggests that the inhibition of the proteasomal degradation pathway may constitute a prerequisite for the glucocorticoid-associated preservation of BBB integrity [80, 81]. Consequently, in cardiac arrest, it is still highly uncertain whether peri-arrest and/or post-arrest hydrocortisone can directly confer neuroprotection.

14.8   Conclusions

Preceding retrospective studies with inherent methodological limitations do not support the use of low-dose corticosteroids during and after CPR. However, more recent laboratory data and clinical results are consistent with a possible, low-dose corticosteroid-associated, benefit in cardiac arrest, especially in patients with post-resuscitation shock. Such potential benefit can be explained mainly by the hemodynamic and anti-inflammatory effects of hydrocortisone, as a direct neuroprotective effect seems rather unlikely. Controversies and unclear mechanisms of hydrocortisone action and possible efficacy should be addressed by a large, multicenter, randomized, placebo-controlled evaluation of stress-dose hydrocortisone in cardiac arrest.

14.9   Financial and Competing Interests Disclosure

The authors have no relevant affiliations or financial involvement with any organization or entity with a financial interest in or a financial conflict with the subject matter or materials discussed in the manuscript. This includes employment, consultancies, honoraria, stock ownership or options, expert testimony, grants or patents received or pending, or royalties. No writing assistance has been utilized in the production of this manuscript.

References

1. Langhelle A, Nolan J, Herlitz J et al (2005) Recommended guidelines for reviewing, reporting, and conducting research on post-resuscitation care: the Utstein style. Resuscitation 66:271–283
2. Niemann JT (1982) Perfusing during cardiopulmonary resuscitation. In: Harwood AL (ed) Cardiopulmonary resuscitation. Williams & Wilkins, Baltimore, pp 34–54
3. Engdahl J, Abrahamsson P, Bang A et al (2000) Is hospital care of major importance for outcome after out-of-hospital cardiac arrest? Experience acquired from patients with out-of-hospital cardiac arrest resuscitated by the same Emergency Medical Service and admitted to one of two hospitals over a 16-year period in the municipality of Goteborg. Resuscitation 43:201–211
4. Grafton ST, Longstreth WT Jr (1988) Steroids after cardiac arrest: a retrospective study with concurrent, nonrandomized controls. Neurology 38:1315–1316
5. Jastremski M, Sutton-Tyrrell K, Vaagenes P et al (1989) Glucocorticoid treatment does not improve neurological recovery following cardiac arrest. JAMA 262:3427–3430
6. Aufderheide TP, Lurie KG (2004) Death by hyperventilation: a common and life-threatening problem during cardiopulmonary resuscitation. Crit Care Med 32(9 Suppl):S345–S351
7. Meaney PA, Nadkarni VM, Kern KB, Indik JH, Halperin HR, Berg RA (2010) Rhythms and outcomes of adult in-hospital cardiac arrest. Crit Care Med 38:101–108
8. Negovsky VA (1972) The second step in resuscitation: the treatment of the "post-resuscitation disease". Resuscitation 1:1–7
9. Negovsky VA (1988) Postresuscitation disease. Crit Care Med 16:942–946
10. Negovsky VA, Gurvitch AM (1995) Post-resuscitation disease: a new nosological entity: its reality and significance. Resuscitation 30:23–27
11. Opie LH (1989) Reperfusion injury and its pharmacologic modification. Circulation 80:1049–1062
12. White BC, Grossman LI, Krause GS (1993) Brain injury by global ischemia and reperfusion: a theoretical perspective on membrane damage and repair. Neurology 43:1656–1665
13. Neumar RW, Nolan JP, Adrie C et al (2008) Post-cardiac arrest syndrome: epidemiology, pathophysiology, treatment, and prognostication. A consensus statement from the International Liaison Committee on Resuscitation (American Heart Association, Australian and New Zealand Council on Resuscitation, European Resuscitation Council, Heart and Stroke Foundation of Canada, InterAmerican Heart Foundation, Resuscitation Council of Asia, and the Resuscitation Council of Southern Africa); the American Heart Association Emergency Cardiovascular Care Committee; the Council on Cardiovascular Surgery and Anesthesia; the Council on Cardiopulmonary, Perioperative, and Critical Care; the Council on Clinical Cardiology; and the Stroke Council. Circulation 118:2452–2483
14. Laver S, Farrow C, Turner D, Nolan J (2004) Mode of death after admission to an intensive care unit following cardiac arrest. Intensive Care Med 30:2126–2128
15. Herlitz J, Ekström L, Wennerblom B, Axelsson A, Bång A, Holmberg S (1995) Hospital mortality after out-of-hospital cardiac arrest among patients found in ventricular fibrillation. Resuscitation 29:11–21
16. Laurent I, Monchi M, Chiche JD et al (2002) Reversible myocardial dysfunction in survivors of out-of-hospital cardiac arrest. J Am Coll Cardiol 40:2110–2116
17. Huang L, Weil MH, Tang W, Sun S, Wang J (2005) Comparison between dobutamine and levosimendan for management of postresuscitation myocardial dysfunction. Crit Care Med 33:487–491
18. Ruiz-Bailén M, Aguayo de Hoyos E, Ruiz-Navarro S et al (2005) Reversible myocardial dysfunction after cardiopulmonary resuscitation. Resuscitation 66:175–181
19. Cerchiari EL, Safar P, Klein E, Cantadore R, Pinsky M (1993) Cardiovascular function and neurologic outcome after cardiac arrest in dogs: the cardiovascular post-resuscitation syndrome. Resuscitation 25:9–33

20. Kern KB, Hilwig RW, Berg RA et al (1997) Postresuscitation left ventricular systolic and diastolic dysfunction: treatment with dobutamine. Circulation 95:2610–2613
21. Kern KB, Hilwig RW, Rhee KH, Berg RA (1996) Myocardial dysfunction after resuscitation from cardiac arrest: an example of global myocardial stunning. J Am Coll Cardiol 28:232–240
22. Rivers EP, Wortsman J, Rady MY, Blake HC, McGeorge FT, Buderer NM (1994) The effect of the total cumulative epinephrine dose administered during human CPR on hemodynamic, oxygen transport, and utilization variables in the postresuscitation period. Chest 106:1499–1507
23. Prengel AW, Lindner KH, Ensinger H, Grünert A (1992) Plasma catecholamine concentrations after successful resuscitation in patients. Crit Care Med 20:609–614
24. Hori M, Inoue M, Kitakaze M et al (1986) Role of adenosine in hyperemic response of coronary blood flow in microcirculation. Am J Physiol 250:H509–H518
25. Dörge H, Neumann T, Behrends M et al (2000) Perfusion-contraction mismatch with coronary microvascular obstruction: role of inflammation. Am J Physiol 279:H2587–H2592
26. Dörge H, Schulz R, Belosjorow S et al (2000) Coronary microembolization: the role of TNF in contractile dysfunction. J Mol Cell Cardiol 34:51–62
27. Thielmann M, Dörge H, Martin C et al (2002) Myocardial dysfunction with coronary microembolization: signal transduction through a sequence of nitric oxide, tumor necrosis factor-alpha, and sphingosine. Circ Res 90:807–813
28. Skyschally A, Haude M, Dörge H et al (2004) Glucocorticoid treatment prevents progressive myocardial dysfunction resulting from experimental coronary microembolization. Circulation 109:2337–2342
29. Falkenstein E, Tillmann H-C, Christ M et al (2000) Multiple actions of steroid hormones: a focus on rapid, nongenomic effects. Pharmacol Rev 52:513–555
30. Cronstein BN, Kimmel SC, Levin RI et al (1992) A mechanism for the anti-inflammatory effects of corticosteroids: the glucocorticoid receptor regulates leukocyte adhesion to endothelial cells and expression of endothelial-leukocyte adhesion molecule 1 and intercellular adhesion molecule 1. Proc Natl Acad Sci 89:9991–9995
31. Springer TA (1994) Traffic signals for lymphocyte recirculation and leukocyte emigration: the multistep paradigm. Cell 76:301–314
32. Filep JG, Delalandre A, Payette Y et al (1997) Glucocorticoid receptor regulates expression of L-selectin and CD11/CD18 on human neutrophils. Circulation 96:295–301
33. Nakagawa M, Bondy GP, Waisman D et al (1999) The effect of glucocorticoids on the expression of L-selectin on polymorphonuclear leukocyte. Blood 93:2730–2737
34. Radomski MW, Palmer RMJ, Moncada S (1990) Glucocorticoids inhibit the expression of an inducible, but not the constitutive, nitric oxide synthase in vascular endothelial cells. Proc Natl Acad Sci 87:10043–10047
35. Amano Y, Lee SW, Allison AC (1993) Inhibition by glucocorticoids of the formation of interleukin-1 alpha, interleukin-1 beta, and interleukin-6:mediation by decreased mRNA stability. Mol Pharmacol 43:176–182
36. Teoh KHT, Bradley CA, Gauldie J, et al (1995). Steroid inhibition of cytokine-mediated vasodilation after warm heart surgery. Circulation. 92(suppl II): 347–363
37. Williams CM, Coleman JW (1995) Induced expression of mRNA for IL-5, IL-6, TNF-alpha, MIP-2 and IFN-gamma in immunologically activated rat peritoneal mast cells: inhibition by dexamethasone and cyclosporin A. Immunology 86:244–249
38. Meng X, Ao L, Brown JM et al (1997) LPS induces late cardiac functional protection against ischemia independent of cardiac and circulating TNF-alpha. Am J Physiol 42:H1894–H1904
39. Libby P, Maroko PR, Bloor CM et al (1973) Reduction of experimental myocardial infarct size by corticosteroid administration. J Clin Invest 52:599–607
40. Spath JA Jr, Lane DL, Lefer AM (1974) Protective action of methylprednisolone on the myocardium during experimental myocardial ischemia in the cat. Circ Res 35:44–51

41. Hammerman H, Kloner RA, Hale S et al (1983) Dose-dependent effects of short-term methylprednisolone on myocardial infarct extent, scar formation, and ventricular function. Circulation 68:446–452
42. Wynsen JC, Preuss KC, Gross GJ et al (1988) Steroid-induced enhancement of functional recovery of postischemic, reperfused myocardium in conscious dogs. Am Heart J 116:915–925
43. D'Amico M, Di Filippo C, La M et al (2000) Lipocortin 1 reduces myocardial ischemia-reperfusion injury by affecting local leukocyte recruitment. FASEB J 14:1867–1869
44. Valen G, Kawakami T, Tähepold P et al (2000) Glucocorticoid pretreatment protects cardiac function and induces cardiac heat shock protein 72. Am J Physiol 279:H836–H843
45. Sun L, Chang J, Kirchhoff SR et al (2000) Activation of HSF and selective increase in heat-shock proteins by acute dexamethasone treatment. Am J Physiol 278:H1091–H1097
46. Dreyer WJ, Michael LH, West MS et al (1991) Neutrophil accumulation in ischemic canine myocardium: insights into time course, distribution, and mechanism of localization during early reperfusion. Circulation 84:400–411
47. Entman ML, Michael L, Rossen RD et al (1991) Inflammation in the course of early myocardial ischemia. FASEB J 5:2529–2537
48. Gumina RJ, Newman PJ, Kenny D et al (1997) The leukocyte cell adhesion cascade and its role in myocardial ischemia-reperfusion injury. Basic Res Cardiol 92:201–213
49. Jordan JE, Zhao Z-Q, Vinten-Johansen J (1999) The role of neutrophils in myocardial ischemia-reperfusion injury. Cardiovasc Res 43:860–878
50. Arras M, Strasser R, Mohri M et al (1998) Tumor necrosis factor-alpha is expressed by monocytes/macrophages following cardiac microembolization and is antagonized by cyclosporine. Basic Res Cardiol 93:97–107
51. Gerisch RA, Compeau L (1956) Treatment of acute myocardial infarction in man with cortisone. Am J Cardiol 1:535–536
52. Dall JLC, Peel AAF (1963) A trial of hydrocortisone in acute myocardial infarction. Lancet 2(7317):1097–1098
53. Barzilai D, Plavnick J, Hazani A et al (1972) Use of hydrocortisone in the treatment of acute myocardial infarction: a summary of a clinical trial in 446 patients. Chest 61:488–491
54. Bulkley BH, Roberts WC (1974) Steroid therapy during acute myocardial infarction: a cause of delayed healing and of ventricular aneurysm. Am J Med 56:244–250
55. Roberts R, DeMello V (1976) Deleterious effects of methylprednisolone in patients with myocardial infarction. Circulation 53(suppl I):I-204–I-206
56. Giugliano GR, Giugliano RP, Gibson CM, Kuntz RE (2003) Meta-analysis of corticosteroid treatment in acute myocardial infarction. Am J Cardiol 91:1055–1059
57. Peberdy MA, Callaway CW, Neumar RW et al (2010) Part 9: post-cardiac arrest care: 2010 American Heart Association Guidelines for cardiopulmonary resuscitation and emergency cardiovascular care. Circulation 122: S768–S786
58. Adrie C, Adib-Conquy M, Laurent I et al (2002) Successful cardiopulmonary resuscitation after cardiac arrest as a "sepsis-like" syndrome. Circulation 106:562–568
59. Minneci PC, Deans KJ, Banks SM, Eichacker PQ, Natanson C (2004) Corticosteroids for septic shock. Ann Intern Med 141:742–743
60. Sprung CL, Annane D, Keh D et al (2008) Hydrocortisone therapy for patients with septic shock. N Engl J Med 358(111–124):194
61. Annane D, Sebille V, Charpentier C et al (2002) Effect of treatment with low doses of hydrocortisone and fludrocortisone on mortality in patients with septic shock. JAMA 288:862–871
62. Adrie C, Laurent I, Monchi M, Cariou A, Dhainaou JF, Spaulding C (2004) Postresuscitation disease after cardiac arrest: a sepsis-like syndrome? Curr Opin Crit Care 10:208–212
63. Geppert A, Zorn G, Karth GD et al (2000) Soluble selectins and the systemic inflammatory response syndrome after successful cardiopulmonary resuscitation. Crit Care Med 28:2360–2365

64. Munoz C, Carlet J, Fitting C et al (1991) Dysregulation of in vitro cytokine production by monocytes during sepsis. J Clin Invest 88:1747–1754
65. Gando S, Kameue T, Nanzaki S et al (1997) Massive fibrin formation with consecutive impairment of fibrinolysis in patients with out-of-hospital cardiac arrest. Thromb Haemost 77:278–282
66. Böttinger BW, Motsch J, Böhrer H et al (1995) Activation of blood coagulation after cardiac arrest is not balanced adequately by activation of endogenous fibrinolysis. Circulation 92:2572–2578
67. Gando S, Kameue T, Nanzaki S et al (1997) Platelet activation with massive formation of thromboxane A2 during and after cardiopulmonary resuscitation. Intensive Care Med 23:71–76
68. Dellinger RP, Levy MM, Rhodes A et al (2013) Surviving sepsis campaign: international guidelines for management of severe sepsis and septic shock, 2012. Intensive Care Med 39:165–228
69. Mentzelopoulos SD, Zakynthinos SG, Tzoufi M et al (2009) Vasopressin, epinephrine, and corticosteroids for in-hospital cardiac arrest. Arch Intern Med 169:15–24
70. Hékimian G, Baugnon T, Thuong M et al (2004) Cortisol levels and adrenal reserve after successful cardiac arrest resuscitation. Shock 22:116–119
71. Kim JJ, Hyun SY, Hwang SY et al (2011) Hormonal responses upon return of spontaneous circulation after cardiac arrest: a retrospective cohort study. Crit Care 15:R53
72. Tsai MS, Huang CH, Chang WT et al (2007) The effect of hydrocortisone on the outcome of out-of-hospital cardiac arrest patients: a pilot study. Am J Emerg Med 25:318–325
73. Peberdy MA, Callaway CW, Neumar RW et al (2010) Part 9: post-cardiac arrest care: 2010 American Heart Association Guidelines for Cardiopulmonary Resuscitation and Emergency Cardiovascular Care. Circulation 122(18 Suppl 3): S768-786. Erratum in Circulation (2011) 124:e403; 123(6):e237
74. Kaur C, Ling EA (2008) Blood brain barrier in hypoxic-ischemic conditions. Curr Neurovasc Res 5(1):71–81
75. Kröll S, El-Gindi J, Thanabalasundaram G et al (2009) Control of the blood–brain barrier by glucocorticoids and the cells of the neurovascular unit. Ann N Y Acad Sci 1165:228–239
76. Dietrich JB (2004) Endothelial cells of the blood–brain barrier: a target for glucocorticoids and estrogens. Front Biosci 9:684–693
77. Almawi WY, Lipman ML, Stevens AC et al (1991) Abrogation of glucocorticoid-mediated inhibition of T cell proliferation by the synergistic action of IL-1, IL-6, and IFN-γ. J Immunol 146:3523–3527
78. Kozler P, Riljak V, Pokorný J (2011) Methylprednisolone reduces axonal impairment in the experimental model of brain edema. Neuro Endocrinol Lett 32:831–835
79. Semenas E, Sharma HS, Nozari A, Basu S, Wiklund L (2011) Neuroprotective effects of 17β-estradiol after hypovolemic cardiac arrest in immature piglets: the role of nitric oxide and peroxidation. Shock 36:30–37
80. Kleinschnitz C, Blecharz K, Kahles T et al (2011) Glucocorticoid insensitivity at the hypoxic blood–brain barrier can be reversed by inhibition of the proteasome. Stroke 42:1081–1089
81. Thal SC, Schaible EV, Neuhaus W et al (2013) Inhibition of proteasomal glucocorticoid receptor degradation restores dexamethasone-mediated stabilization of the blood–brain barrier after traumatic brain injury. Crit Care Med 41:1305–1315

Pharmacological Induction of Hypothermia

15

Yinlun Weng, Shijie Sun and Wanchun Tang

Marked protection provided by therapeutic hypothermia after traumatic ischemic-hypoxic damage has been deeply studied, contributing to satisfactory clinic effects. Several physical methods to induce therapeutic hypothermia have been established, and briefly can be divided into two categories: invasive and non invasive. Recently, pharmacological hypothermia is drawing increasing attention as a neuroprotective alternative approach worthy of further clinical development. This chapter reviews the hypothermic effect of several classes of hypothermia-inducing drugs: the cannabinoids, opioid receptor activators, transient receptor potential vanilloid, neurotensins, thyroxine derivatives, dopamine receptor agonists, and cholecystokinin. Recent findings have extended our knowledge of the thermoregulatory mechanisms of the above drugs. A better understanding of the roles of the hypothermia-inducing drugs in neuroprotection may have broad clinical implications. Till date, there is few data that uniquely elicit that pharmacologically induced hypothermia is the sole or specific mechanism on neuroprotection. However, some mechanisms underlying the protection of hypothermia are overlapped with the current evidence on the intrinsic effects of the above drugs.

Y. Weng
Sun Yat-sen Memorial Hospital, Sun Yat-sen University, Yanjiang West Road, 510120, Guangzhou, China
e-mail: yearonyung@126.com

S. Sun · W. Tang (✉)
The Institute of Critical Care Medicine, Bob Hope Drive, Rancho Mirage, CA 92270, USA
e-mail: wanchun.tang@me.com

S. Sun
e-mail: ShijieSun@aol.com

A. Gullo and G. Ristagno (eds.), *Resuscitation*,
DOI: 10.1007/978-88-470-5507-0_15, © Springer-Verlag Italia 2014

15.1 Cannabinoids

There are two main receptors within the cannabinoid system: cannabinoid receptors 1 and 2. In the brain, the cannabinoid receptor 1, one of the most abundant Gi/o-protein-coupled receptors, was found in the hypothalamus responsible for regulation of temperature [1–6]. At the cellular level, cannabinoid receptor 1 is also abundant in the plasma membranes of the axon and axonal terminals, where it typically mediates the release of neurotransmitters [5]. Numerous evidences suggest that cannabinoid 1 receptors participate in the prevention of neurodegenerative disease or protection from ischemic insults [7–10]. The neuroprotective effects of cannabinoid agonists were related either to specific mechanisms played by these agonists or by a cannabinoid-induced hypothermia [11]. Among them, however, cannabinoid-induced hypothermia was the primary mechanism which was principally triggered by activation of cannabinoid receptor 1. Several neurological neurotransmitters were demonstrated to be involved, such as the release of GABA (Gamma-amino Butyric Acid, GABA) [12, 13] and the dopamine [14]. As cannabinoid-induced regulation of body temperature is, however, dose-dependent, further evidence is necessary to establish optimal application standards for the cannabinoid-based hypothermic treatment [15].

It is well documented that cannabinoids may have therapeutic potential in disorders resulting from cerebral ischemia, including stroke, and may protect neurons from injury through a variety of mechanisms [9]. The beneficial mechanisms were related to the decrease of inflammatory factors [16], reduction of apoptotic cell death, maintenance of mitochondrial integrity and functionality [17], activation of extracellular signal-regulated kinases, increase of S-100 protein, and mitigation of glutamatergic excitotoxicity, TNF-alpha release and iNOS expression [18, 19]. These effects are achieved through two parallel CB1-dependent and -independent mechanisms [20, 21].

15.2 Opioid Receptor Agonists

The opioid system was reported to be involved in thermoregulation. Indeed, naloxone has been reported to antagonize the hypothermic effects played by morphine [22–24]. The main subtype of opioid receptors involved in thermoregulation and hypothermia induction is the kappa-receptor, while the mu-receptor is related to hyperthermia. The magnitude of hypothermic effects produced by kappa- opioid agonists is related to the degree of their selectivity for the kappa-receptor [25]. The kappa-opioid receptor is primarily located outside the brain; thus peripheral application of kappa-receptor agonists could produce dose-dependent hypothermia [26, 27].

Moreover, the existence of subtypes of the different receptors may well explain the different effects of one single drug on thermoregulation [28]. Anatomical, histochemical, and pharmacological evidence suggests that the opioid system probably interacts with the dopaminergic, adrenergic, serotonergic, cholinergic, and other transmitter systems [25–28]. Thus, it can be hypothesized that the opioid system interacts with other neurotransmitter systems known to be involved in thermoregulation. However, studies carried out so far do not present a clear picture of these interrelationships in terms of thermoregulation. In view of the recent findings that several neuropeptides play marked effects on body temperature, exploration of opioid interactions with these systems should prove to be a fruitful approach to deepen the understanding of the opioid system and its function in the thermoregulation.

Kappa-receptor agonists, have been demonstrated effective in preventing brain swelling in parallel with reducing infarction after an ischemic insult [29, 30], but the use of opioid receptor agonist is limited to the early phase of cerebral edema [31, 32]. This was related mainly to the attenuation of ischemia-evoked nitric oxide production [33], the reduction of $Na(+)-K(+)$-ATPase activity [34], and a significant prolonged neuron survival [35–37].

15.3   Transient Receptor Potential Vanilloid

Studies have demonstrated that many pathophysiological processes were mediated by transient receptor potential (TRP) channels, including pain, respiratory reflex hypersensitivity, cardiac hypertrophy, thermoregulation, and ischemic cell death. The superfamily of mammalian *TRP* channels consists of around 30 proteins which can be divided into six subfamilies: ankyrin (TRPA), canonical, melastatin (TRPM), mucolipin, polycystin, and vanilloid (TRPV). Till date, nine of the proteins are found highly sensitive to temperature and are referred to as the thermo-TRP channels, which include the heat-activated TRPV1 as well as the cold-activated TRPA1 and TRPM8 [38–41].

No consensus in the literature was achieved on the hypothermic response to systemically administered TRPV1 agonists. Most evidence is in support of the central mediation hypothesis: (1) the TRPV1 channel was demonstrated to be widely distributed in the hypothalamus; [42–44], (2) TRPV1 agonist was able to cross the blood–brain barrier; [45, 46], (3) the primary action mode after application of TRPV1 agonist lies on the glutamatergic preoptic anterior hypothalamus neurons; [43, 47], (4) a reduced or low hypothermic response to TRPV1 agonist was observed in rats with decreased hypothalamic sensitivity [48]. Moreover, several authors also suggested a contribution of a peripheral action of TRPV1 agonists to the hypothermic response.

However, there was no definite data illustrating that TRPV1-induced hypothermia could directly contribute to the beneficial neurologic outcomes in rat models of ischemia.

15.4   Neurotensin

At least three subtypes of receptors are involved in pathophysiologic processes of neurotensin: neurotensin-1 and neurotensin-2 receptor, both members of the hepta-helical transmembrane domain G protein-coupled receptor superfamily; and neurotensin-3 receptor, which is identical to gp95/sortilin, with only a single transmembrane domain [29–31].

Neurotensin is abundant in the preoptic area of the hypothalamus [49]. Early in the 1980s, neurotensin was first reported to elicit hypothermic effect by acting on the hypothamalus in rodents [50, 51]. Neurotensin-induced hypothermia is thought to be caused by a downward shift of the physiological temperature set point ("regulated hypothermia"). Previous results using neurotensin analogs or peptide nucleic acids suggested that neurotensin receptor 1 was implicated in neurotensin-induced hypothermia, but the nonspecificity of these molecules aroused some doubt. Neurotensin normally does not cross the blood–brain barrier and is quickly metabolized when administered systemically. In terms of wide clinic application, many neurotensin analogs emerge as new options with the ability to penetrate the blood–brain barrier and prolong the hypothermia duration.

Previously, several neurotensin receptor 1 agonists were demonstrated to induce hypothermia in a dose-dependent manner without causing shivering or altering physiological parameters. These analogs ultimately reduced cerebral infarct volumes and improved neurologic outcomes [52–54]. The specific mechanisms involved would be increase in bcl-2 expression, decrease in caspase-3 activation, and suppression of cell death [53, 54].

15.5   Thyroxine Derivatives

Thyroxine is the principal secretion form of thyroid hormone (TH), constituting 95 % of all TH found in human circulation. When deiodinated and decarboxylated, thyroxine is transformed into 3-iodothyonamine (T1AM) and thyronamine (T0AM). It was reported that when injected peripherally, T1AM and T0AM rapidly induced hypothermia through a mechanism independent of gene transcription. T1AM and T0AM are agonists of trace amine associated receptor 1 (TAAR1), a G-protein coupled receptor activated by phenylethylamine, tyramine, methamphetamine, and its congeners. Although T1AM and T0AM can dose-dependently couple TAAR1 to the production of cAMP, it is not yet clear whether TAAR1 is an endogenous receptor for these molecules [55].

There has been data demonstrating that T1AM and T0AM are potent neuroprotectants in neurologic ischemia disease. Hypothermia induced by T1AM and T0AM may partially underlie neuroprotection [55].

15.6 Dopamine Receptor Agonists

Dopamine (DA) is one of the major neurotransmitters in the mammalian central nervous system (CNS). The receptors for DA have been classified into three subtypes: the D1, D2, and D3 receptor subtype [56]. There were data suggesting that hypothermia in mammals are centrally mediated by D2 receptor mechanism, and this centrally mediated D2 receptor mechanism may be modulated by the D1 receptor [57]. Furthermore, the dopamine D1 receptor agonist was also reported to produce hypothermia that was antagonized by D1 receptor antagonists, but not by the dopamine D2/3 receptor antagonists. This supports the evidence that activation of dopamine D1 receptors may play a determinant role in inducing hypothermia in rats [58]. Further evidence finally demonstrated that hypothermia did not result from a selective stimulation of the D3 receptor [59].

There is lack of evidence, however, that D1 or 2 receptor agonist-induced hypothermia would provide protective effects in neurologic ischemic diseases.

15.7 Cholecystokinin

It was first reported in 1981 that centrally administrated cholecystokinin was able to produce hypothermia in rats [38, 60, 61]. Specific mechanisms of cholecystokinin-induced hypothermia after peripheral or central application, however, remain unclear [39, 40, 60]. Hypothermia may either be produced by different mechanisms, such as inhibition of central nervous system function without specific relation to central body temperature control, interruption of afferent or efferent nervous pathways, or a decrease of regulated level of body temperature. The central action of cholecystokinin was not supported by the long latency of the thermoregulatory response observed after central administration of cholecystokinin [39, 40, 60]. An alternative explanation for the cholecystokinin-induced hypothermia after peripheral injection could be a direct skin vasodilatation. Besides, a nervous afferent mechanism, such as the vagal afferentation shown to be an important way of influencing central regulation of food intake could also play relevant roles on specific thermoregulatory sites [41]. The hypothermic action of the peptide in mammals seems to depend on cholecystokinin-1 receptors, since administration of cholecystokinin-1 receptor antagonists attenuated these hypothermic effects, while the cholecystokinin-2 receptor antagonist had no effect on this response [42–45].

Although the concept of pharmacological hypothermia induced by cholecystokinin was not widely raised, there are some data revealing that cholecystokinin to some extent plays a vital role in protecting from brain ischemia disease. Yasui M et al. demonstrated that in rats subjected to stroke, cholecystokinin prevented the dysfunction of CA1 pyramidal neurons [46]. Moreover, in a rat model of global ischemia after cardiac arrest, cholecystokinin octapeptide indeed induced hypothermia, and improved post-resuscitation myocardial dysfunction and overall neurological performance after intravenous injection of CCK8 at a dose of 200 µg/kg [47].

References

1. Herkenham M, Lynn AB, Little MD, Johnson MR, Melvin LS, de Costa BR, Rice KC (1990) Cannabinoid receptor localization in brain. Proc Natl Acad Sci USA 87:1932–1936
2. Herkenham M, Lynn AB, Johnson MR, Melvin LS, de Costa BR, Rice KC (1991) Characterization and localization of cannabinoid receptors in rat brain: a quantitative in vitro autoradiographic study. J Neurosci 11:563–583 (the official journal of the Society for Neuroscience)
3. Tsou K, Brown S, Sanudo-Pena MC, Mackie K, Walker JM (1998) Immunohistochemical distribution of cannabinoid cb1 receptors in the rat central nervous system. Neuroscience 83:393–411
4. Piomelli D (2003) The molecular logic of endocannabinoid signalling. Nat Rev Neurosci 4:873–884
5. Mackie K (2006) Cannabinoid receptors as therapeutic targets. Annu Rev Pharmacol Toxicol 46:101–122
6. Di Marzo V (2008) Targeting the endocannabinoid system: to enhance or reduce? Nat Rev Drug Discov 7:438–455
7. Jin KL, Mao XO, Goldsmith PC, Greenberg DA (2000) Cb1 cannabinoid receptor induction in experimental stroke. Ann Neurol 48:257–261
8. Sinor AD, Irvin SM, Greenberg DA (2000) Endocannabinoids protect cerebral cortical neurons from in vitro ischemia in rats. Neurosci Lett 278:157–160
9. Nagayama T, Sinor AD, Simon RP, Chen J, Graham SH, Jin K, Greenberg DA (1999) Cannabinoids and neuroprotection in global and focal cerebral ischemia and in neuronal cultures. J Neurosci 19:2987–2995
10. Braida D, Pozzi M, Sala M (2000) Cp 55,940 protects against ischemia-induced electroencephalographic flattening and hyperlocomotion in mongolian gerbils. Neurosci Lett 296:69–72
11. Viscomi MT, Oddi S, Latini L, Bisicchia E, Maccarone M, Molinari M (2010) The endocannabinoid system: a new entry in remote cell death mechanisms. Exp Neurol 224:56–65
12. Rawls SM, Cabassa J, Geller EB, Adler MW (2002) Cb1 receptors in the preoptic anterior hypothalamus regulate win 55212–2 [(4,5-dihydro-2-methyl-4(4-morpholinylmethyl)-1-(1-naphthalenyl-carbonyl)-   6h-pyrrolo[3,2,1ij]quinolin-6-one]-induced   hypothermia. J Pharmacol Exp Ther 301:963–968
13. Rawls SM, Tallarida RJ, Kon DA, Geller EB, Adler MW (2004) Gabaa receptors modulate cannabinoid-evoked hypothermia. Pharmacol Biochem Behav 78:83–91
14. Gonzalez B, Paz F, Floran L, Aceves J, Erlij D, Floran B (2009) Cannabinoid agonists stimulate [3h]gaba release in the globus pallidus of the rat when g(i) protein-receptor coupling is restricted: Role of dopamine d2 receptors. J Pharmacol Exp Ther 328:822–828
15. Sulcova E, Mechoulam R, Fride E (1998) Biphasic effects of anandamide. Pharmacol Biochem Behav 59:347–352
16. Fernandez-Lopez D, Faustino J, Derugin N, Wendland M, Lizasoain I, Moro MA, Vexler ZS (2012) Reduced infarct size and accumulation of microglia in rats treated with win 55,212–2 after neonatal stroke. Neuroscience 207:307–315
17. Alonso-Alconada D, Alvarez A, Alvarez FJ, Martinez-Orgado JA, Hilario E (2012) The cannabinoid win 55212–2 mitigates apoptosis and mitochondrial dysfunction after hypoxia ischemia. Neurochem Res 37:161–170
18. Alonso-Alconada D, Alvarez FJ, Alvarez A, Mielgo VE, Goni-de-Cerio F, Rey-Santano MC, Caballero A, Martinez-Orgado J, Hilario E (2010) The cannabinoid receptor agonist win 55,212–2 reduces the initial cerebral damage after hypoxic-ischemic injury in fetal lambs. Brain Res 1362:150–159

19. Hu B, Wang Q, Chen Y, Du J, Zhu X, Lu Y, Xiong L, Chen S (2010) Neuroprotective effect of win 55,212-2 pretreatment against focal cerebral ischemia through activation of extracellular signal-regulated kinases in rats. Eur J Pharmacol 645:102–107

20. Fernandez-Lopez D, Martinez-Orgado J, Nunez E, Romero J, Lorenzo P, Moro MA, Lizasoain I (2006) Characterization of the neuroprotective effect of the cannabinoid agonist win-55212 in an in vitro model of hypoxic-ischemic brain damage in newborn rats. Pediatr Res 60:169–173

21. Martinez-Orgado J, Fernandez-Frutos B, Gonzalez R, Romero E, Uriguen L, Romero J, Viveros MP (2003) Neuroprotection by the cannabinoid agonist win-55212 in an in vivo newborn rat model of acute severe asphyxia. Brain Res Mol Brain Res 114:132–139

22. Clark WG, Cumby HR (1978) Hyperthermic responses to central and peripheral injections of morphine sulphate in the cat. Br J Pharmacol 63:65–71

23. Geller EB, Hawk C, Keinath SH, Tallarida RJ, Adler MW (1983) Subclasses of opioids based on body temperature change in rats: Acute subcutaneous administration. J Pharmacol Exp Ther 225:391–398

24. Rosow CE, Miller JM, Poulsen-Burke J, Cochin J (1982) Opiates and thermoregulation in mice. Ii. Effects of opiate antagonists. J Pharmacol Exp Ther 220:464–467

25. Hayes AG, Skingle M, Tyers MB (1985) Effect of beta-funaltrexamine on opioid side-effects produced by morphine and u-50, 488h. J Pharm Pharmacol 37:841–843

26. Geller EB, Rowan CH, Adler MW (1986) Body temperature effects of opioids in rats: intracerebroventricular administration. Pharmacol Biochem Behav 24:1761–1765

27. Maldonado R, Dauge V, Callebert J, Villette JM, Fournie-Zaluski MC, Feger J, Roques BP (1989) Comparison of selective and complete inhibitors of enkephalin-degrading enzymes on morphine withdrawal syndrome. Eur J Pharmacol 165:199–207

28. Lin MT, Uang WN, Chan HK (1984) Hypothalamic neuronal responses to iontophoretic application of morphine in rats. Neuropharmacology 23:591–594

29. Kusumoto K, Mackay KB, McCulloch J (1992) The effect of the kappa-opioid receptor agonist ci-977 in a rat model of focal cerebral ischaemia. Brain Res 576:147–151

30. Silvia RC, Slizgi GR, Ludens JH, Tang AH (1987) Protection from ischemia-induced cerebral edema in the rat by u-50488h, a kappa opioid receptor agonist. Brain Res 403:52–57

31. Yang L, Wang H, Shah K, Karamyan VT, Abbruscato TJ (2011) Opioid receptor agonists reduce brain edema in stroke. Brain Res 1383:307–316

32. Gueniau C, Oberlander C (1997) The kappa opioid agonist niravoline decreases brain edema in the mouse middle cerebral artery occlusion model of stroke. J Pharmacol Exp Ther 282:1–6

33. Goyagi T, Toung TJ, Kirsch JR, Traystman RJ, Koehler RC, Hurn PD, Bhardwaj A (2003) Neuroprotective kappa-opioid receptor agonist brl 52537 attenuates ischemia-evoked nitric oxide production in vivo in rats. Stroke 34:1533–1538 (a journal of cerebral circulation)

34. Furui T (1993) Potential protection by a specific kappa-opiate agonist u-50488h against membrane failure in acute ischemic brain. Neurol Med Chir 33:133–138

35. Charron C, Messier C, Plamondon H (2008) Neuroprotection and functional recovery conferred by administration of kappa- and delta 1-opioid agonists in a rat model of global ischemia. Physiol Behav 93:502–511

36. Zhang Z, Chen TY, Kirsch JR, Toung TJ, Traystman RJ, Koehler RC, Hurn PD, Bhardwaj A (2003) Kappa-opioid receptor selectivity for ischemic neuroprotection with brl 52537 in rats. Anesth Analg 97:1776–1783

37. Mackay KB, Kusumoto K, Graham DI, McCulloch J (1993) Focal cerebral ischemia in the cat: pretreatment with a kappa-1 opioid receptor agonist, ci-977. Brain Res 618:213–219

38. Zadina JE, Banks WA, Kastin AJ (1986) Central nervous system effects of peptides, 1980–1985: a cross-listing of peptides and their central actions from the first six years of the journal peptides. Peptides 7:497–537

39. Kapas L, Benedek G, Penke B (1989) Cholecystokinin interferes with the thermoregulatory effect of exogenous and endogenous opioids. Neuropeptides 14:85–92

40. Kapas L, Obal F Jr, Alfoldi P, Rubicsek G, Penke B, Obal F (1988) Effects of nocturnal intraperitoneal administration of cholecystokinin in rats: simultaneous increase in sleep, increase in eeg slow-wave activity, reduction of motor activity, suppression of eating, and decrease in brain temperature. Brain Res 438:155–164

41. Palkovits M, Kiss JZ, Beinfeld MC, Williams TH (1982) Cholecystokinin in the nucleus of the solitary tract of the rat: evidence for its vagal origin. Brain Res 252:386–390

42. Szelenyi Z, Bartho L, Szekely M, Romanovsky AA (1994) Cholecystokinin octapeptide (cck-8) injected into a cerebral ventricle induces a fever-like thermoregulatory response mediated by type b cck-receptors in the rat. Brain Res 638:69–77

43. Rezayat M, Ravandeh N, Zarrindast MR (1999) Cholecystokinin and morphine-induced hypothermia. Eur Neuropsychopharmacol 9:219–225 (the journal of the European College of Neuropsychopharmacology)

44. Pullen RG, Hodgson OJ (1987) Penetration of diazepam and the non-peptide cck antagonist, l-364,718, into rat brain. J Pharm Pharmacol 39:863–864

45. Woltman TA, Hulce M, Reidelberger RD (1999) Relative blood-brain barrier permeabilities of the cholecystokinin receptor antagonists devazepide and a-65186 in rats. J Pharm Pharmacol 51:917–920

46. Yasui M, Kawasaki K (1995) 1-cckb receptor activation protects ca1 neurons from ischemia-induced dysfunction in stroke-prone spontaneously hypertensive rats hippocampal slices. Neurosci Lett 191:99–102

47. Weng Y, Sun S, Song F Phil Chung S, Park J, Harry Weil M, Tang W (2011) Cholecystokinin octapeptide induces hypothermia and improves outcomes in a rat model of cardiopulmonary resuscitation. Crit Care Med 39:2407–2412

48. Jancso-Gabor A, Szolcsanyi J, Jancso N (1970) Stimulation and desensitization of the hypothalamic heat-sensitive structures by capsaicin in rats. J Physiol 208:449–459

49. Uhl GR (1982) Distribution of neurotensin and its receptor in the central nervous system. Ann N Y Acad Sci 400:132–149

50. Kalivas PW, Jennes L, Nemeroff CB, Prange AJ Jr (1982) Neurotensin: topographical distribution of brain sites involved in hypothermia and antinociception. J Comp Neurol 210:225–238

51. Martin GE, Bacino CB, Papp NL (1980) Hypothermia elicited by the intracerebral microinjection of neurotensin. Peptides 1:333–339

52. Torup L, Borsdal J, Sager T (2003) Neuroprotective effect of the neurotensin analogue jmv-449 in a mouse model of permanent middle cerebral ischaemia. Neurosci Lett 351:173–176

53. Choi KE, Hall CL, Sun JM, Wei L, Mohamad O, Dix TA, Yu SP (2012) 1-a novel stroke therapy of pharmacologically induced hypothermia after focal cerebral ischemia in mice. FASEB J 26(7):2799–2810 (official publication of the Federation of American Societies for Experimental Biology)

54. Babcock AM, Baker DA, Hallock NL, Lovec R, Lynch WC, Peccia JC (1993) Neurotensin-induced hypothermia prevents hippocampal neuronal damage and increased locomotor activity in ischemic gerbils. Brain Res Bull 32:373–378

55. Doyle KP, Suchland KL, Ciesielski TM, Lessov NS, Grandy DK, Scanlan TS, Stenzel-Poore MP (2007) Novel thyroxine derivatives, thyronamine and 3-iodothyronamine, induce transient hypothermia and marked neuroprotection against stroke injury. Stroke 38:2569–2576 (a journal of cerebral circulation)

56. Kebabian JW, Calne DB (1979) Multiple receptors for dopamine. Nature 277:93–96

57. Nunes JL, Sharif NA, Michel AD, Whiting RL (1991) Dopamine d2-receptors mediate hypothermia in mice: Icv and ip effects of agonists and antagonists. Neurochem Res 16:1167–1174

58. Salmi P, Ahlenius S (1997) Dihydrexidine produces hypothermia in rats via activation of dopamine d1 receptors. Neurosci Lett 236:57–59
59. Perachon S, Betancur C, Pilon C, Rostene W, Schwartz JC, Sokoloff P (2000) Role of dopamine d3 receptors in thermoregulation: a reappraisal. Neuroreport 11:221–225
60. Morley JE, Levine AS, Lindblad S (1981) Intraventricular cholecystokinin-octapeptide produces hypothermia in rats. Eur J Pharmacol 74:249–251
61. Clark WG, Lipton JM (1985) Changes in body temperature after administration of amino acids, peptides, dopamine, neuroleptics and related agents: Ii. Neurosci Biobehav Rev 9:299–371

Part V
Post-Resuscitation Care

Effectiveness of Hypothermia in Human Cardiac Arrest and Update on the Target Temperature Management-Trial

16

Tommaso Pellis, Filippo Sanfilippo, Andrea Roncarati and Vincenzo Mione

16.1 Effectiveness of Therapeutic Hypothermia

Over a decade has passed since the publication on the New England Journal of Medicine of the landmark studies that led to widespread clinical application of therapeutic hypothermia (TH) [1, 2]. After decades of clinical research, finally we found evidence in two randomized clinical trials (RCTs) of an intervention improving neurological outcome at hospital discharge. Indeed the largest RCT, the European study "Hypothermia After Cardiac Arrest" (HACA-Trial) unprecedentedly detected a survival benefit at 6 months after hospital discharge [1]. Both RCTs enrolled unconscious victims of cardiac arrest (CA) presenting with a shockable rhythm [1, 2].

Moreover in the same years a single center feasibility study looked at cooling patients in asystole or pulseless electrical activity (PEA) [3]. A subsequent meta-analysis was published that pooled the two RCTs and a feasibility study on cooling with a refrigerated head cap [4]. The results provided an astonishingly low number needed to treat only six patients to observe a benefit of hypothermia on both short- and long-term effects—i.e., improved neurological outcome and survival at hospital discharge and 6 months later.

T. Pellis (✉) · A. Roncarati · V. Mione
Anaesthesia Intensive Care and Emergency Medical Service, Santa Maria degli Angeli Hospital, Via Montereale 24, 33170, Pordenone, Italy
e-mail: thomas.pellis@gmail.com

F. Sanfilippo
Oxford Heart Centre, John Radcliffe Hospital, Oxford University Hospitals NHS Trust, Oxford, UK

A. Gullo and G. Ristagno (eds.), *Resuscitation*,
DOI: 10.1007/978-88-470-5507-0_16, © Springer-Verlag Italia 2014

As mentioned, these results are not trivial when considering that there are only three treatments supported by sound evidence in the field of cardiopulmonary resuscitation (CPR): (1) chest compressions and ventilation, (2) defibrillation for ventricular fibrillation (VF) or pulseless ventricular tachycardia (VT), and now (3) mild TH (range 32–34 °C) for 24 h in unconscious victims resuscitated from CA. This is unprecedented news since much effort devoted to other advanced life support (ALS) interventions over the past 50 years was unable to show any impact on CA and CPR outcome at hospital discharge. This includes widely accepted interventions such as airway management by endotracheal intubation and the use of drugs like epinephrine [5–7].

The majority of patients initially resuscitated from CA (approximately 70 %) die in hospital [8]. Hypothermia introduced a paradigm shift in the in-hospital treatment of post-CA patients. Indeed, because 75 % of in-hospital deaths are attributed to irreversible anoxic neurological injury, such a high mortality is likely to offer room for improvement, and TH challenged the previous widespread nihilistic approach that clinicians had toward resuscitated patients [9].

16.2   Post-Resuscitation Care

The success of hypothermia gave momentum to an in-hospital standardized approach, similar to the one employed in the links of the Chain of Survival in the out-of-hospital setting. The increased appreciation of the numerous opportunities of care held by the in-hospital phase ultimately led to what is currently named as post-resuscitation care (PRC). The first group to systematically apply a standardized 72 h treatment protocol, including hypothermia, was the Norwegian group in Oslo led by Sunde et al. [10]. A whole set of therapeutic options to limit ongoing injury, to sustain organ function and to normalize physiological parameters were considered. Clear procedures identified objectives, goals, and strategies to achieve them. Realizing that there is much to do in little time while inducing, maintaining, and gradually restoring normothermia, and while maintaining optimal intensive care standards at all time, the authors acknowledged the need for a clear understanding of clinical priorities. To achieve such objectives, at least at the beginning, a protocol of standardized care was necessary. Much effort was also posed to aggressive hemodynamic support (both pharmacological and mechanical) and urgent coronary angiography with percutaneous or surgical revascularization if necessary. Survival with good neurological recovery at 1 year from hospital discharge significantly improved from 26 % in historical controls to 56 % after the intervention period [10].

Association of TH concurrently with an aggressive PRC policy led to very consistent outcome improvements over different countries, suggesting a clear margin of benefit. Interestingly, numerous centers now report very similar rates of survival with good neurological outcome, all ranging between 54 and 59 % [11–14].

The optimism imposed by the results of TH led the International Liaison Committee on Resuscitation (ILCOR) to officially acknowledge the existence of a post-CA syndrome [15]. Negovsky was the first to understand the complexity of this state, named in 1972 as post-resuscitation disease [16]. The ILCOR consensus statement published in 2008 defines the epidemiology, pathophysiology, treatment, and even elements useful for prognostication of this syndrome [15]. With a bold step forward ILCOR provides physicians and nurses with clear objectives that can be summarized in the treatment of the four key components of the Post-CA syndrome: (1) post-CA brain injury, (2) post-CA myocardial dysfunction, (3) systemic response to ischemia and reperfusion, and (4) persistent precipitating pathology.

The 2005 European resuscitation council (ERC) guidelines did not devote much attention to TH [17]. On the contrary, the following guidelines issued in 2010 strongly emphasized, among the changes introduced, the need for implementing TH and comprehensive PRC [18]. For instance, the name of the fourth link of the Chain of Survival was changed from ALS to PRC; furthermore for the first time the brain was depicted in the logo, quite peculiar when considering that this is the ultimate goal of resuscitation but was never portrayed before [18]. Finally, almost half of the summary of changes in the ALS chapter was dedicated to TH and PRC.

On the other side of the Atlantic, the American Heart Association (AHA) 2010 guidelines introduced a dedicated fifth link to the Chain of Survival and a whole new chapter within the guidelines entitled "post-cardiac arrest care" [19].

16.3 New Evidence Supporting Therapeutic Hypothermia

Presently, there are over 4,400 references on PubMed when searching for TH and CA, but very little is new in terms of scientific evidence, since the only RCTs remain the landmark studies on which we still rely.

New information might be sought in registries, yet these are only hypothesis generating. The largest database—the Hypothermia Network Registry—including over 1,000 patients suggests that TH is beneficial not only for patients in VF as demonstrated by the landmark trials, but also for those presenting with the so-called agonal rhythms [20]. An astonishingly high survival rate was reported by the registry when compared to that of historical controls: 21% survival with good neurological outcome in patients with asystole as first detected rhythm, and 23 % for those presenting in PEA.

Expert consensus opinion in guidelines has filled the gap where the evidence is slim, so that we are now suggested to consider the use of TH also: in comatose survivors of CA with non-shockable rhythms; following in-hospital arrest; or for paediatric patients, even if the lower level of evidence for these categories is acknowledged [18]. There is also growing appreciation that it is rational to think beyond the sole hypothermia process of induction, maintenance, and rewarming. Active temperature management after restoration of normothermia in patients who do not regain consciousness should be a priority at least for the initial 72 h that follow restoration of spontaneous circulation (ROSC). Indeed a large number of patients tend to become febrile after restoration of normothermia. A hyperthermic rebound should not be underestimated as fever after any acute neurological insult (including CA) is detrimental; however, it is still unknown until when it should be considered a hazard [21]. For this reason, a rigid maintenance of normothermia should be considered at least for the first 3 days after ROSC and particularly in those patients not regaining consciousness after restoration of normothermia and sedation hold.

It is precisely with the aim of moving beyond the cooling process that five scientific societies agreed on replacing the term TH with the more appropriate one of *target temperature management* [22].

The Hypothermia Network Registry sheds also some light on adverse events related to TH [20]. Bradycardia was the most common arrhythmia (13 %) but very rarely requiring pacing, regardless of whether pharmacological or electrical, while pneumonia was the most frequent infection (41%) [20]. Bleeding requiring transfusion occurred in 4% of all patients and the risk was significantly higher if angiography/coronary intervention was performed (2.8 % vs. 6.2 %, respectively, $p = 0.02$). Sustained hyperglycemia [defined as >8 mmol/l (144 mg/dl) for >4 h] was observed in 37 % of patients. Electrolyte disorders were also quite common (18–19 %), specifically hypokalemia, hypomagnesemia, and hypophosphatemia [20]. The incidence of sepsis was low (4 %) but higher in patients with intra-vascular devices for temperature management (OR 2.6), intra-aortic ballon pump (IABP, OR 3.2), or undergoing coronary angiography (OR 4.4) [23]. Of note bleeding, infection, arrhythmia, and electrolyte disorders were not associated with increased mortality. Only sustained hyperglycemia and seizures (despite treatment) were associated with worse outcome [23].

Yet there are many unanswered questions, among them when to start hypothermia. Cooling should be started as early as possible, stated the 2010 ERC guidelines [18]. The cooling process can be started on the field and during transportation leading to a reduction in core temperature at hospital or intensive care unit (ICU) admission [24]. Our 7 years' experience is in keeping with such reports. The emergency medical service (EMS) of the province of Pordenone (north-east Italy) was able to start cooling in the out-of-hospital setting in 56 patients. Hypothermia was initiated with straightforward and inexpensive means without delaying hospital admission. This included ice-packs, means of inducing heat loss (i.e., turning off ambulance heating, opening the window, uncover patient as much as possible, and any other mean immediately at hand), and cold IV fluids. When comparing temperature at ICU admission with 117 patients that were not cooled (including in-hospital CA) there was a significant reduction in core temperature if cooling was started in the out-of-hospital setting (34.7 ± 2.1 °C vs. 35.4 ± 1.3 °C, $p < 0.01$).

Despite this strong logical and pathophysiological rationale, as yet there are no human data supporting that a reduced time to achieve the target temperature is associated with better outcomes. On the contrary, a recent Australian trial on early out-of-hospital cooling was stopped for futility after enrolling over 200 patients [24]. Also, an intra-arrest trial using transnasal evaporative cooling which allows for a very fast cooling rate, did not show improvements in ROSC or hospital discharge, despite the study not being really powered for such results [25]. Currently, four more trials are on the way, two in Australia, one in North America, and one in Europe.

What could the reasons be for this lack of benefit? One hypothesis is that if neuroprotection induced by hypothermia is not an on–off phenomenon but a spectrum with higher intensity at lower temperatures, then a patient who is difficult to cool or is cooled slowly would be exposed to a greater area under the curve of hypothermia—and thereby of neuroprotection—than a patient who achieves rapidly the target temperature. Another reason recently proposed by Oddo et al. [26], is that the impaired thermoregulation that follows ROSC is an indicator of the severity of injury, hence a determinant of post-resuscitation disease and CA prognosis. So future studies when assessing the benefit of early cooling on outcome should adjust for patient admission temperature and use the cooling rate rather than time to target temperature.

Another matter of debate is whether cooling should be extended to children and for how long. There are currently three trials and one Cochrane review on neonates, all indicating that hypothermia for 72 h at 33.5 °C is beneficial [27–29]. Once again it seems rational to use hypothermia after CA in children and, based on expert consensus, current guidelines recommend it although the length of treatment is not specified [18]. So, while waiting for the results of ongoing clinical trials, companies are now competing to produce devices that allow strict control by automatic temperature management in children of different sizes.

There is also a growing literature that suggests it might be worth regionalizing CA patients bypassing local hospitals in order to admit them directly to high-volume CA centers with percutaneous coronary intervention facilities "24/7" [30–33].

However, there are still many other areas of uncertainty, like: (1) the appropriate duration of hypothermia (does one size fit all?), (2) should we tailor the duration on an indicator of brain injury? (3) what is the optimal rewarming rate, and most of all, (4) what is the optimal depth of hypothermia?

16.4 The Target Temperature Management Trial

A critical review of the landmark studies easily reveals that they are not flawless and carry a potential risk of systematic error and random error design.

The Bernard trial was actually not a randomized trial but a quasi-randomized study as allocation was based according to odd and even days [2]. Of the 82 eligible patients only 77 were included, no justification for the missing 6 % was provided. Unscheduled interim analysis on 62 patients was performed, and no statistical correction was included in the final analysis. The two groups were uneven (43 vs. 34 patients). The discharge facility was used as a surrogate of neurological outcome. To make things worse the final result of the study depends on one single patient.

If we consider the largest study, the HACA trial, which enrolled 275 patients there are still areas of uncertainty: the study was prematurely stopped, there was no power calculation (a reasonable size would have probably included 600–700 patients), and the study lasted as long as 7 years [1]. Neurological status before CA was not investigated, early withdrawal of care was neither standardized nor reported; finally the study was highly selective since it included only 8 % of screened patients admitted to the emergency department following CA (275 of 3,551). Hence the results can be hardly generalized to the average CA population, and most of all, the controls were actually "not temperature-controlled," since the majority of them were febrile.

In conclusion, the overall quality of evidence is low at least in humans and the optimal target temperature is not yet defined at least based on high quality evidence. Therefore, although promising, hypothermia should be further investigated. These precise conclusions were drawn by a systematic review that assessed the evidence using the GRADE-methodology [34].

With the attempt of improving our knowledge on hypothermia, several ICU have joined in the attempt to investigate two subfebrile temperatures in a large general population by means of a randomized, parallel-group, and assessor-blinded clinical trial: the *target temperature management (TTM) trial* [35]. A core temperature of 36 °C was chosen as comparator to 33 °C since it is safely below febrile temperatures with allowance for temperature fluctuations and because, based on the Hypothermia Network Registry data, the median temperature at hospital admission is 36 °C. Active temperature management (36 vs. 33 °C) was continued in patients who did not regain consciousness. A total of 36 centers from 10 different countries in Europe and Australia joined this study led by the principal investigator Niklas Nielsen (Sweden).

The main objective was to assess the efficacy and safety of two TTM strategies after resuscitation from out-of-hospital CA. Enrolment of 950 patients was completed in January 2013. The intervention phase lasted 36 h, while 72 h later (that is 5 days after ROSC) a blinded neurological evaluation was performed. Patients were followed until the end of the trial.

Inclusion criteria were: unconscious adult patients with out-of-hospital CA of presumed cardiac cause with sustained ROSC. Patients too cold on admission (core temperature <30 °C) were not included, as well as those with known limitations in therapy, unlikely to survive at 6 months, or with severe preexisting neurological dysfunction. Patients could not be screened any longer than 4 h from ROSC, and if they remained in shock in spite of maximum therapeutic efforts. All presenting rhythms were included with the exception of unwitnessed asystole.

The primary endpoint was survival at the end of the trial, while the secondary was the post-CA neurological function—blindly and thoroughly evaluated not only cerebral performance categories but also modified Rankin Scale and Informant Questionnaire on Cognitive Decline in the Elderly—at 6 months, as well as safety issues (i.e., bleeding, pneumonia, etc.). Withdrawal of care was not allowed for the first 5 days, unless for predefined ethical reasons, and had to be always motivated [35]. Further details are available online at http://clinicaltrials.gov/show/NCT01020916. Publication of the trial results is expected by late 2013.

In conclusion the TTM-Trial holds promises to be a large clinical randomized and monitored trial evaluating two subfebrile temperatures, with a pragmatic design in accordance with clinical practice, and hopefully its results will apply to the majority of out-of-hospital CA patients admitted to the intensive care.

References

1. HACA (2002) Mild therapeutic hypothermia to improve the neurologic outcome after cardiac arrest. N Engl J Med 346(8):549–556
2. Bernard SA, Gray TW, Buist MD, Jones BM, Silvester W, Gutteridge G et al (2002) Treatment of comatose survivors of out-of-hospital cardiac arrest with induced hypothermia. N Engl J Med 346(8):557–563
3. Hachimi-Idrissi S, Corne L, Ebinger G, Michotte Y, Huyghens L (2001) Mild hypothermia induced by a helmet device: a clinical feasibility study. Resuscitation 51(3):275–281
4. Holzer M, Bernard SA, Hachimi-Idrissi S, Roine RO, Sterz F, Mullner M (2005) Hypothermia for neuroprotection after cardiac arrest: systematic review and individual patient data meta-analysis. Crit Care Med 33(2):414–418
5. Hasegawa K, Hiraide A, Chang Y, Brown DF (2013) Association of pre hospital advanced airway management with neurologic outcome and survival in patients with out-of-hospital cardiac arrest. J Am Med Assoc 309(3):257–266 (Epub 2013/01/17)
6. Jacobs IG, Finn JC, Jelinek GA, Oxer HF, Thompson PL (2011) Effect of adrenaline on survival in out-of-hospital cardiac arrest: a randomised double-blind placebo-controlled trial. Resuscitation 82(9):1138–1143 (Epub 2011/07/13)
7. Olasveengen TM, Sunde K, Brunborg C, Thowsen J, Steen PA, Wik L (2009) Intravenous drug administration during out-of-hospital cardiac arrest: a randomized trial. J Am Med Assoc 302(20):2222–2229 (Epub 2009/11/26)
8. Brain Resuscitation Clinical Trial II Study Group (1991) A randomized clinical study of a calcium-entry blocker (lidoflazine) in the treatment of comatose survivors of cardiac arrest. N Engl J Med 324(18):1225–1231
9. Dragancea I, Rundgren M, Englund E, Friberg H, Cronberg T (2012) The influence of induced hypothermia and delayed prognostication on the mode of death after cardiac arrest. Resuscitation (Epub 2012/09/25) 2013, 84(3):337–342
10. Sunde K, Pytte M, Jacobsen D, Mangschau A, Jensen LP, Smedsrud C et al (2007) Implementation of a standardised treatment protocol for post resuscitation care after out-of-hospital cardiac arrest. Resuscitation 73:29–39
11. Busch M, Soreide E, Lossius HM, Lexow K, Dickstein K (2006) Rapid implementation of therapeutic hypothermia in comatose out-of-hospital cardiac arrest survivors. Acta Anaesthesiol Scand 50(10):1277–1283
12. Oddo M, Schaller MD, Feihl F, Ribordy V, Liaudet L (2006) From evidence to clinical practice: effective implementation of therapeutic hypothermia to improve patient outcome after cardiac arrest. Crit Care Med 34(7):1865–1873
13. Knafelj R, Radsel P, Ploj T, Noc M (2007) Primary percutaneous coronary intervention and mild induced hypothermia in comatose survivors of ventricular fibrillation with ST-elevation acute myocardial infarction. Resuscitation 74(2):227–34 (Epub 2007/03/27)
14. Belliard G, Catez E, Charron C, Caille V, Aegerter P, Dubourg O et al (2007) Efficacy of therapeutic hypothermia after out-of-hospital cardiac arrest due to ventricular fibrillation. Resuscitation 75(2):252–259 (Epub 2007/06/08)

15. Nolan JP, Neumar RW, Adrie C, Aibiki M, Berg RA, Bottiger BW et al (2008) Post-cardiac arrest syndrome: epidemiology, pathophysiology, treatment, and prognostication. A Scientific Statement from the International Liaison Committee on Resuscitation; the American Heart Association Emergency Cardiovascular Care Committee; the Council on Cardiovascular Surgery and Anesthesia; the Council on Cardiopulmonary, Perioperative, and Critical Care; the Council on Clinical Cardiology; the Council on Stroke. Resuscitation 79(3):350–379 (Epub 2008/10/31)

16. Negovsky VA (1972) The second step in resuscitation—the treatment of the 'post-resuscitation disease'. Resuscitation 1(1):1–7

17. International Liaison Commitee on Resuscitation (2005) International Consensus on Cardiopulmonary Resuscitation and Emergency Cardiovascular Care Science with Treatment Recommendations. Part 4: advanced life support. Resuscitation 67(2–3):213–247

18. Deakin CD, Nolan JP, Soar J, Sunde K, Koster RW, Smith GB et al (2010) European resuscitation council guidelines for resuscitation Section 4: adult advanced life support. Resuscitation 81(10):1305–1352 (Epub 2010/10/20)

19. Peberdy MA, Callaway CW, Neumar RW, Geocadin RG, Zimmerman JL, Donnino M et al (2010) Part 9: post-cardiac arrest care: 2010 American heart association guidelines for cardiopulmonary resuscitation and emergency cardiovascular care. Circulation 122(18 Suppl 3):S768–786 (Epub 2010/10/22)

20. Nielsen N, Hovdenes J, Nilsson F, Rubertsson S, Stammet P, Sunde K et al (2009) Outcome, timing and adverse events in therapeutic hypothermia after out-of-hospital cardiac arrest. Acta Anaesthesiol Scand 53(7):926–934 (Epub 2009/06/25)

21. Zeiner A, Holzer M, Sterz F, Schorkhuber W, Eisenburger P, Havel C et al (2001) Hyperthermia after cardiac arrest is associated with an unfavorable neurologic outcome. Arch Intern Med 161(16):2007–2012 (Epub 2001/09/26)

22. Nunnally ME, Jaeschke R, Bellingan GJ, Lacroix J, Mourvillier B, Rodriguez-Vega GM et al (2011) Targeted temperature management in critical care: a report and recommendations from five professional societies. Crit Care Med 39(5):1113–1125 (Epub 2010/12/29)

23. Nielsen N, Sunde K, Hovdenes J, Riker RR, Rubertsson S, Stammet P et al (2011) Adverse events and their relation to mortality in out-of-hospital cardiac arrest patients treated with therapeutic hypothermia. Crit Care Med 39(1):57–64 (Epub 2010/10/21)

24. Bernard SA, Smith K, Cameron P, Masci K, Taylor DM, Cooper DJ et al (2010) Induction of therapeutic hypothermia by paramedics after resuscitation from out-of-hospital ventricular fibrillation cardiac arrest: a randomized controlled trial. Circulation 122(7):737–742 (Epub 2010/08/04)

25. Castren M, Nordberg P, Svensson L, Taccone F, Vincent JL, Desruelles D et al (2010) Intra-arrest transnasal evaporative cooling: a randomized, prehospital, multicenter study (PRINCE: Pre-ROSC IntraNasal Cooling Effectiveness). Circulation 122(7):729–736 (Epub 2010/08/04)

26. Benz-Woerner J, Delodder F, Benz R, Cueni-Villoz N, Feihl F, Rossetti AO et al (2012) Body temperature regulation and outcome after cardiac arrest and therapeutic hypothermia. Resuscitation 83(3):338–342 (Epub 2011/11/15)

27. Eicher DJ, Wagner CL, Katikaneni LP, Hulsey TC, Bass WT, Kaufman DA et al (2005) Moderate hypothermia in neonatal encephalopathy: efficacy outcomes. Pediatr Neurol 32(1):11–17 (Epub 2004/12/21)

28. Gluckman PD, Gunn AJ, Wyatt JS (2006) Hypothermia for neonates with hypoxic-ischemic encephalopathy. N Engl J Med 354(15):1643–1645 (Epub 2006/04/15)

29. Shankaran S, Laptook AR, Ehrenkranz RA, Tyson JE, McDonald SA, Donovan EF et al (2005) Whole-body hypothermia for neonates with hypoxic-ischemic encephalopathy. N Engl J Med 353(15):1574–1584 (Epub 2005/10/14)

30. Carr BG, Goyal M, Band RA, Gaieski DF, Abella BS, Merchant RM et al (2009) A national analysis of the relationship between hospital factors and post-cardiac arrest mortality. Intensive Care Med 35(3):505–511 (Epub 2008/10/22)

31. Davis DP, Fisher R, Aguilar S, Metz M, Ochs G, McCallum-Brown L et al (2007) The feasibility of a regional cardiac arrest receiving system. Resuscitation 74(1):44–51 (Epub 2007/03/10)
32. Spaite DW, Bobrow BJ, Vadeboncoeur TF, Chikani V, Clark L, Mullins T et al (2008) The impact of prehospital transport interval on survival in out-of-hospital cardiac arrest: implications for regionalization of post-resuscitation care. Resuscitation 79(1):61–66 (Epub 2008/07/12)
33. Spaite DW, Stiell IG, Bobrow BJ, de Boer M, Maloney J, Denninghoff K et al (2009) Effect of transport interval on out-of-hospital cardiac arrest survival in the OPALS study: implications for triaging patients to specialized cardiac arrest centers. Ann Emerg Med 54(2):248–255 (Epub 2009/01/27)
34. Nielsen N, Friberg H, Gluud C, Herlitz J, Wetterslev J (2011) Hypothermia after cardiac arrest should be further evaluated—a systematic review of randomised trials with meta-analysis and trial sequential analysis. Int J Cardiol 151(3):333–341 (Epub 2010/07/02)
35. Nielsen N, Wetterslev J, al-Subaie N, Andersson B, Bro-Jeppesen J, Bishop G et al (2012) Target temperature management after out-of-hospital cardiac arrest–a randomized, parallel-group, assessor-blinded clinical trial–rationale and design. Am Heart J 163(4):541–548 (Epub 2012/04/24)

New Strategies to Improve Outcome After Cardiac Arrest

17

Matthias Derwall, Anne Brücken and Michael Fries

17.1 Introduction

The advancement of resuscitation sciences in recent years has led to a considerable increase in primary survival due to simplified guidelines, public-access defibrillation initiatives, and improved training of both lay- and professional providers of CPR. Yet, this increase in patients presenting with a return of spontaneous circulation (ROSC) after cardiac arrest still does not translate into greater numbers of patients surviving until hospital discharge [1]. It is widely accepted that cerebral and myocardial lesions, defined as part of the "post-cardiac-arrest syndrome" (CAS), are responsible for the high mortality rate of survivors of cardiac arrest [2].

The introduction of mild therapeutic hypothermia (MTH) into international guidelines for post-arrest care resulted in measurable improvements in both neurological outcomes and survival, hence proving that modifying post-arrest treatment with novel interventions or drug candidates may harbor the promise to further improve outcomes from cardiac arrest.

M. Derwall · A. Brücken · M. Fries (✉)
Department of Anesthesiology, University Hospital RWTH Aachen,
Pauwelsstr. 30, 52074, Aachen, Germany
e-mail: mfries@ukaachen.de

M. Derwall
e-mail: mderwall@ukaachen.de

A. Brücken
e-mail: abruecken@ukaachen.de

A. Gullo and G. Ristagno (eds.), *Resuscitation*,
DOI: 10.1007/978-88-470-5507-0_17, © Springer-Verlag Italia 2014

Novel hemodynamic interventions aiming at improved cardiocirculatory support, extend these CAS-treatments into the intra-arrest period, and may help to improve both ROSC and overall outcomes. However, MTH still represents the current gold standard in post-arrest care.

17.2   Mild Therapeutic Hypothermia

Induced hypothermia has been used to preserve cerebral function in modern medicine for more than 50 years. First used during neurosurgical procedures [3], it was quickly adopted in other fields of surgery including thoracic interventions such as the upcoming CABG surgery and heart transplantations. While the first reports of therapeutic hypothermia reported target body temperatures below 30 °C, others used more moderate cooling to overcome or ameliorate adverse events associated with hypothermia such as cardiac arrhythmias, coagulopathy, and elevated infection rates. The moderate cooling to 33 ± 1 °C showed a reasonable proportion of preservation of neurologic functions to side effects. It was therefore proposed and tested in post-arrest care in 2002 [4], and is now widely referred to as "mild therapeutic hypothermia" (MTH) [4, 5]. The introduction of MTH into international resuscitation guidelines in 2005 recommended MTH only for unconscious adult patients with spontaneous circulation after out-of-hospital cardiac arrest, when the initial rhythm was VF [6]. Since then, guidelines have been modified to include the use of induced hypothermia for comatose adult patients with ROSC after in-hospital cardiac arrest of any initial rhythm, or after out-of-hospital cardiac arrest with an initial rhythm of pulseless electric activity or asystole [7]. With only six patients requiring treatment to save one additional life, MTH is the single most effective intervention and therefore the gold standard in post-resuscitation care today.

The molecular actions by which therapeutic hypothermia exerts its cytoprotective properties have long been thought to rely on unspecific inhibition of catabolic processes throughout the organism during the reperfusion period. Today, several molecular targets of MTH have been identified, which might serve as potential targets for drug candidates to augment the efficacy of MTH. For instance, MTH is known to induce a decrease in brain glycine and p53 protein levels [8, 9]. Furthermore, MTH blocks delta-protein kinase C and several other proteins that induce apoptotic cell death, including those from the Bcl-2 family [10].

17.3   Remaining Challenges in MTH

While therapeutic hypothermia has been widely adopted in post-arrest care worldwide, certain aspects of its application remain controversial. Although current guidelines do not recommend distinct techniques of cooling, many centers applying MTH rely on surface cooling and cooled infusions for the induction and invasive techniques such as intravascular catheters for maintaining MTH and rewarming. While the intravascular devices can provide very stable target temperatures and rewarming profiles [11], they still have the disadvantage of their invasive nature and higher costs. Furthermore, surface cooling techniques achieve shorter time spans until reaching target temperature than intravascular cooling catheters [11]. Until now, cooling catheters have failed to prove to translate their advantages over surface cooling into long-term outcome goals. The main advantage of cooling catheters is a reduced nursing time during induction and maintenance of MTH.

Another area of ongoing development in the field of therapeutic hypothermia is the application of targeted cooling. With this approach, it is possible to gain better access to the patient, while maintaining similar effectiveness than whole-body cooling in terms of cooling dynamics [12]. The desire to start cooling even during CPR procedures has led to the development of an intranasal cooling device that can be easily applied by non-physician emergency medical personnel during the resuscitation procedure. By taking advantage of the close proximity of the nasal cavity to cerebral structures, the device is able to effectively cool cerebral structures through direct conduction without interfering with other interventions such as securing the airway. As soon as a sufficient circulation is established, the device furthermore cools head and body by indirect convection via the bloodstream. While this approach provides a rapid onset of cooling, it has also been proven that it does not prevent other interventions such as chest compressions during CPR [12, 13]. It will be exciting to see whether this novel approach will translate into better ROSC and long-term neurological outcome parameters.

17.4   Neuroprotective Drug Candidates

17.4.1 Xenon and Other Gases

In recent years, several groups helped to understand the key mechanism in ischemic neuronal cell death and identify potential targets to interfere with neuronal excitotoxicity. One of these targets is believed to be the overactivated N-methyl-d-aspartate glutamate (NMDA) receptor in hypoxic-ischemic neuronal injury [14]. While several clinical trials failed to translate this knowledge into viable drugs, this receptor remains to be one of the most promising targets for potential drug candidates. Several gases that are believed to interfere with the receptor such as Isoflurane [15], Xenon [16], Helium [17], or Argon [18] have shown their safety and efficacy in animal studies.

With Xenon being extensively examined as a neuroprotective drug, we know that it acts in a synergistic pattern with therapeutic hypothermia [19]. Although Xenon is colorless and odorless, and considered to be chemically inert, it nevertheless does interact with various biological systems [20]. It can be safely used as an inhaled anesthetic, with concentrations of more than 40 % causing rapid onset of unconsciousness, which has been attributed to Xenon's ability to inhibit the NMDA receptor in the central nervous system [21]. Besides this modification of the NMDA-mediated calcium influx, Xenon appears to share further mechanisms involved in MTH-mediated neuroprotection [19], like inducing a decrease in cerebral glycine and p53 protein levels [8, 9] or pro-apoptotic proteins such as those from the Bcl-2 family [10]. In addition, Xenon appears to provide additional protection by activating the 2-pore domain potassium channel and by opening the ATP-dependent potassium channel [22].

Xenon's organ-protective properties are not limited to cardiac arrest, but have rather been shown in several models of neurological injury, including stroke, traumatic brain injury, and hypoxic-ischemic encephalopathy [23–25]. When given 1 h after successful resuscitation, inhaled Xenon improved functional recovery in a porcine model of cardiac arrest, and significantly reduced neuronal damage [16]. Xenon has also been shown to be effective within a prolonged time frame after ROSC, ranging from 10 min [26], up to 5 h [16]. Data from several small animal studies revealed a potential synergistic effect of Xenon and MTH, resulting in a significantly greater degree of protection than achieved with either of the two interventions alone [19]. Recently published data from a porcine model of prolonged cardiac arrest showed that combined short-term administration of Xenon in addition to MTH is superior to MTH alone in terms of a significant neurocognitive recovery [27]. This study furthermore revealed a preserved hemodynamic stability in the early post-resuscitation period when Xenon was given during the induction of therapeutic hypothermia. Other groups have shown in a pediatric model of hypoxic-ischemic encephalopathy that the combined administration of MTH and Xenon yields a greater functional recovery than either of these interventions alone [28].

While Xenon's neuroprotective properties have been predominantly demonstrated in animal experiments, its effects on cardiac function have been extensively investigated in clinical trials, where Xenon proves to preserve arterial pressures and heart-rate variability in hemodynamically unstable patients [29, 30]. Xenon is known as a safe anesthetic with rapid recovery characteristics and only minor side-effects on hemodynamics [30, 31]. Although Xenon's minimal impact on myocardial function may also be particularly desirable for patients recovering from cardiac arrest, its high price, and the rarely available equipment needed for its application have precluded its widespread use in the field of post-arrest care.

17.4.2 Argon

In contrast to Xenon, the noble gas Argon is much more abundant in the atmosphere and available at a significantly lower price. Interestingly, accumulating data from preclinical studies provide evidence that Argon, albeit lacking of an anesthetic effect, has also organ-protective properties.

While several in vitro studies suggested Argon's potency to protect renal and nervous tissues against hypoxic-ischemic insults in the past several years [17, 18, 32, 33] there was only little evidence if these promising results are also present in vivo [33, 34].

However, our own group recently showed that Argon's neuroprotective properties are not limited to traumatic brain injury, transient middle cerebral artery occlusion, and neonatal asphyxia, but can also be observed after CA. Rats exposed to a single 1 h administration of 70 % Argon demonstrated significant and persistent reductions in cardiac arrest-induced neurological dysfunction which were accompanied by a concomitant decrease in the number of damaged neurons in hippocampal and cortical regions of the brain [35]. However, if these beneficial effects could be transferred into large animal models, and if they are dose- or time-dependent, they have to be proven in future studies. Further research is also necessary to elucidate whether Argon, like Xenon, would also enhance MTH-mediated neuroprotection. Furthermore, the mechanisms involved in Argon's neuroprotective properties are poorly understood [34, 36] and have to be investigated in future studies.

17.4.3 Hydrogen Sulfide

With a characteristic odor of rotten eggs and a significant toxicity, hydrogen sulfide (H_2S) and its donor compounds were for a long time not considered to play a significant role in physiology, only to be very recently discovered as the third endogenous gaseous transmitter. Besides its effects on vasotonus, H_2S surprisingly led to a hibernation-like state in rodents when inhaled in very low doses [37], protecting mice from otherwise lethal asphyxia [38]. This gave rise to the idea that this agent could be used as a neuroprotective drug in post-arrest care. Unfortunately, results from small animal models of hemorrhagic shock or CPR could not be easily transferred to large mammals [39]. Despite certain drawbacks in the recent history of research on this compound, more and more highly unanticipated roles in physiology are revealed for H_2S [39]. However, further research is necessary to elucidate the question whether H_2S may serve a significant role in organ-protection in the future.

17.4.4 Nitric Oxide

The most recent addition to the family of potential neuroprotective agents is nitric oxide (NO). NO is known to prevent lesions due to ischemia–reperfusion injury including models of myocardial infarction [40]. Due to its ability to induce systemic vasodilation, intravenous NO-donor compounds may exert undesired side-effects during or after CPR. Inhaled NO however circumvents these limitations, while still having beneficial effects on outcomes in a mouse model of cardiac arrest [41]. In addition to its myocardial and neuroprotective effects inhaled NO may also have desirable effects on transpulmonary blood flow and oxygenation when given during CPR. Whether this theoretical advantage translates into improved ROSC and long-term survival is yet to be proven in large animal experiments and clinical trials.

17.4.5 Erythropoietin

Besides its well-described role as erythropoietic mediator, erythropoietin (EPO) does appear to have certain cytoprotective effects, first described in myocardial ischemia–reperfusion injury [42]. Without significant data on EPO's neuroprotective properties from animal studies, some intriguing small-scale clinical trials have shed light on this novel drug in peri-arrest care [43]. These studies not only showed an increase in ROSC rates, but also increased survival to hospital discharge in EPO-treated patients. Further studies focusing on long-term survival, neurocognitive outcome, and setups within large clinical trials (NCT00999583) will have to prove whether this novel treatment may become a new standard in post-arrest care.

17.5   Cardiocirculatory Support

A novel approach to improve post-arrest care is optimizing intra- and post-arrest hemodynamics. It is well described that chest compressions can only account for 20–30 % of baseline cardiac output. In addition, myocardial lesions often result in insufficient circulation even after a spontaneous circulation has been achieved. Hence, improving the circulation during and after CPR may improve ROSC numbers as well as potentially long-term clinical outcomes.

An investigation looking at in-hospital cardiac arrest was able to demonstrate that circulatory support from an extracorporeal membrane oxygenator can help to improve the clinical outcome by optimizing peri-arrest hemodynamics [44]. However, due to the invasive nature of this procedure, this intervention will be only available for a limited population of patients in cardiac arrest. Other approaches to optimize peri-arrest hemodynamics with less-invasive procedures are needed to provide similar results in more settings of CA and CPR. One possible option might be the use of intravascular devices that are advanced percutaneously into the left ventricle.

The use of left ventricular assist devices is quite reasonable, as cardiac dysfunction following CA is frequently observed and often results in left ventricular pump-failure. It is obvious that optimizing the circulation during CPR by supporting or replacing cardiac function during and after CPR is the single most important action to improve brain resuscitation, and therefore the patient's prognosis. A goal that recent CPR guidelines try to achieve by emphasizing on the importance of chest compressions [45], in favor of nearly any other intervention performed during CPR.

A possible device for this purpose is the Impella 2.5 percutaneous left ventricular assist device (LVAD). This LVAD is capable to pump 2.5 L/min through a miniature turbine at the tip of a 12F catheter, therefore restoring up to 74 % of baseline cardiac output. To pump blood from the left ventricle into the ascending aorta, the LVAD is introduced via a 13F sheath introducer into the femoral artery, and advanced into the left ventricle, thereby releasing the ventricle from filling pressure, and improving coronary and cerebral perfusion. Its use in the setting of CA and CPR has been recently described in two case reports [46, 47], and tested in three animal studies [48–50]. These animal studies revealed that the LVAD is capable of restoring up to 74 % of baseline myocardial and up to 65 % of cerebral perfusion during VF [50]. The maintenance of cerebral blood flow by the LVAD during VF prevented serum markers of cerebral ischemia to rise during 20 min of VF. After 40 min of VF, lactate was the only marker to be significantly elevated in the same investigation [48].

Furthermore, the same group compared the efficacy of the LVAD versus cardiac massage in an open chest model of cardiac arrest [49]. In this study, the LVAD was equal or superior to manual compressions in terms of organ perfusion and rates of successful defibrillation after 20 min of VF.

Further animal studies will have to show if these promising results will translate into improved ROSC rates and clinical outcome in comparison to conventional chest compressions. It will furthermore be interesting to see whether the procedure of introducing this device under CPR-conditions will be feasible and effective in patients at all.

17.6 Conclusions

New strategies to improve the outcome after cardiac arrest aim at preserving cerebral and myocardial tissues from ischemia–reperfusion injury. Several medical gases may help to augment the efficacy of mild therapeutic hypothermia in the future. Until then, MTH remains the gold standard in post-arrest care, eventually augmented by targeted intra-arrest cooling in the near future. Improving and optimizing hemodynamics during and following cardiac arrest may yield a dramatic increase in ROSC rates and long-term outcomes. Yet, the technical devices at hand still have to prove whether their use in the field is feasible and associated with better clinical outcomes.

References

1. Olasveengen TM, Sunde K, Brunborg C et al (2009) Intravenous drug administration during out-of-hospital cardiac arrest: a randomized trial. JAMA 302(20):2222–2229

2. Neumar RW, Nolan JP, Adrie C et al (2008) Post-cardiac arrest syndrome: epidemiology, pathophysiology, treatment, and prognostication. A consensus statement from the International Liaison Committee on Resuscitation (American Heart Association, Australian and New Zealand Council on Resuscitation, European Resuscitation Council, Heart and Stroke Foundation of Canada, Inter American Heart Foundation, Resuscitation Council of Asia, and the Resuscitation Council of Southern Africa); the American Heart Association Emergency Cardiovascular Care Committee; the Council on Cardiovascular Surgery and Anesthesia; the Council on Cardiopulmonary, Perioperative, and Critical Care; the Council on Clinical Cardiology; and the Stroke Council. Circulation 118(23):2452–2483

3. Woodhall B, Sealy WC, Hall KD et al (1960) Craniotomy under conditions of quinidine-protected cardioplegia and profound hypothermia. Ann Surg 152:37–44

4. Mild therapeutic hypothermia to improve the neurologic outcome after cardiac arrest (2002). N Engl J Med 346(8):549–556

5. Bernard SA, Gray TW, Buist MD et al (2002) Treatment of comatose survivors of out-of-hospital cardiac arrest with induced hypothermia. N Engl J Med 346(8):557–563

6. Bernard SA, Gray TW, Buist MD et al (2005) International consensus on cardiopulmonary resuscitation and emergency cardiovascular care science with treatment recommendations. Part 4: Advanced life support. Resuscitation 67(2–3):213–247

7. Peberdy MA, Callaway CW, Neumar RW et al (2010) Part 9: post-cardiac arrest care: 2010 American heart association guidelines for cardiopulmonary resuscitation and emergency cardiovascular care. Circulation 122(18 Suppl 3):S768–786

8. Ji X, Luo Y, Ling F et al (2007) Mild hypothermia diminishes oxidative DNA damage and pro-death signaling events after cerebral ischemia: a mechanism for neuroprotection. Front Biosci 12:1737–1747

9. Ooboshi H, Ibayashi S, Takano K et al (2000) Hypothermia inhibits ischemia-induced efflux of amino acids and neuronal damage in the hippocampus of aged rats. Brain Res 884(1–2):23–30

10. Zhao H, Yenari MA, Sapolsky RM et al (2004) Mild postischemic hypothermia prolongs the time window for gene therapy by inhibiting cytochrome C release. Stroke 35(2):572–577

11. Finley Caulfield A, Rachabattula S, Eyngorn I et al (2011) A comparison of cooling techniques to treat cardiac arrest patients with hypothermia. Stroke Res Treat 2011:690506

12. Tsai MS, Barbut D, Tang W et al (2008) Rapid head cooling initiated coincident with cardiopulmonary resuscitation improves success of defibrillation and post-resuscitation myocardial function in a porcine model of prolonged cardiac arrest. J Am Coll Cardiol 51(20):1988–1990

13. Castren M, Nordberg P, Svensson L et al (2011) Intra-arrest transnasal evaporative cooling: a randomized, prehospital, multicenter study (PRINCE: Pre-ROSC IntraNasal Cooling Effectiveness). Circulation 122(7):729–736

14. Lipton P (1999) Ischemic cell death in brain neurons. Physiol Rev 79(4):1431–1568

15. Derwall M, Timper A, Kottmann K et al (2008) Neuroprotective effects of the inhalational anesthetics isoflurane and xenon after cardiac arrest in pigs. Crit Care Med 36(11 Suppl):S492–S495

16. Fries M, Nolte KW, Coburn M et al (2008) Xenon reduces neuro histopathological damage and improves the early neurological deficit after cardiac arrest in pigs. Crit Care Med 36(8):2420–2426

17. Jawad N, Rizvi M, Gu J et al (2009) Neuroprotection (and lack of neuroprotection) afforded by a series of noble gases in an in vitro model of neuronal injury. Neurosci Lett 460(3):232–236

18. Loetscher PD, Rossaint J, Rossaint R et al (2009) Argon: neuroprotection in invitro models of cerebral ischemia and traumatic brain injury. Crit Care 13(6):R206

19. Hobbs C, Thoresen M, Tucker A et al (2008) Xenon and hypothermia combine additively, offering long-term functional and histopathologic neuroprotection after neonatal hypoxia/ischemia. Stroke 39(4):1307–1313

20. Derwall M, Coburn M, Rex S et al (2009) Xenon: recent developments and future perspectives. Minerva Anestesiol 75(1–2):37–45
21. Franks NP, Dickinson R, de Sousa SL et al (1998) How does xenon produce anaesthesia? Nature 396(6709):324
22. Gruss M, Bushell TJ, Bright DP et al (2004) Two-pore-domain K + channels are a novel target for the anesthetic gases xenon, nitrous oxide, and cyclopropane. Mol Pharmacol 65(2):443–452
23. Coburn M, Maze M, Franks NP (2008) The neuroprotective effects of xenon and helium in an in vitro model of traumatic brain injury. Crit Care Med 36(2):588–595
24. David HN, Leveille F, Chazalviel L et al (2003) Reduction of ischemic brain damage by nitrous oxide and xenon. J Cereb Blood Flow Metab 23(10):1168–1173
25. Schmidt M, Marx T, Gloggl E et al (2005) Xenon attenuates cerebral damage after ischemia in pigs. Anesthesiology 102(5):929–936
26. Fries M, Coburn M, Nolte KW et al (2009) Early administration of xenon or isoflurane may not improve functional outcome and cerebral alterations in a porcine model of cardiac arrest. Resuscitation 80(5):584–590
27. Fries M, Brucken A, Cizen A et al (2012) Combining xenon and mild therapeutic hypothermia preserves neurological function after prolonged cardiac arrest in pigs. Crit Care Med 40(4):1297–1303
28. Chakkarapani E, Dingley J, Liu X et al (2010) Xenon enhances hypothermic neuroprotection in asphyxiated newborn pigs. Ann Neurol 68(3):330–341
29. Baumert JH, Hecker KE, Hein M et al (2005) Haemodynamic effects of haemorrhage during xenon anaesthesia in pigs. Br J Anaesth 94(6):727–732
30. Wappler F, Rossaint R, Baumert J et al (2007) Multicenter randomized comparison of xenon and isoflurane on left ventricular function in patients undergoing elective surgery. Anesthesiology 106(3):463–471
31. Rossaint R, Reyle-Hahn M, Schulte Am Esch J et al (2003) Multicenter randomized comparison of the efficacy and safety of xenon and isoflurane in patients undergoing elective surgery. Anesthesiology 98(1):6–13
32. David HN, Haelewyn B, Degoulet M et al (2012) Ex vivo and in vivo neuroprotection induced by argon when given after an excitotoxic or ischemic insult. PLoS One 7(2):e30934
33. Ryang YM, Fahlenkamp AV, Rossaint R et al (2012) Neuroprotective effects of argon in an in vivo model of transient middle cerebral artery occlusion in rats. Crit Care Med 39(6):1448–1453
34. Zhuang L YT, Zhao H, Fidalgo A, Vizcaychipi, Sanders R, Yu B, Takata M, Johnson M, Ma D (2012) The protective profile of argon, helium, and xenon in a model of neonatal asphyxia in rats. Crit Care Med 40(6):1724–1730
35. Brücken A, Cizen A, Fera C et al (2013) Argon reduces neurohistopathological damage and preserves functional recovery after cardiac arrest in rats. Br J Anaesth 110(Suppl 1):i106–i112
36. Abraini JH, Kriem B, Balon N et al (2003) Gamma-aminobutyric acid neuropharmacological investigations on narcosis produced by nitrogen, argon, or nitrous oxide. Anesth Analg 2003 96(3):746–749
37. Blackstone E, Morrison M, Roth MB (2005) H_2S induces a suspended animation-like state in mice. Science 308(5721):518
38. Blackstone E, Roth MB (2007) Suspended animation-like state protects mice from lethal hypoxia. Shock 27(4):370–372
39. Derwall M, Westerkamp M, Lower C et al (2010) Hydrogen sulfide does not increase resuscitability in a porcine model of prolonged cardiac arrest. Shock 34(2):190–195
40. Nagasaka Y, Fernandez BO, Garcia-Saura MF et al (2008) Brief periods of nitric oxide inhalation protect against myocardial ischemia-reperfusion injury. Anesthesiology 109(4):675–682

41. Minamishima S, Kida K, Tokuda K et al (2011) Inhaled nitric oxide improves outcomes after successful cardiopulmonary resuscitation in mice. Circulation 124(15):1645–1653
42. Fiordaliso F, Chimenti S, Staszewsky L et al (2005) A nonerythropoietic derivative of erythropoietin protects the myocardium from ischemia-reperfusion injury. Proc Natl Acad Sci USA 102(6):2046–2051
43. Grmec S, Strnad M, Kupnik D et al (2009) Erythropoietin facilitates the return of spontaneous circulation and survival in victims of out-of-hospital cardiac arrest. Resuscitation 80(6):631–637
44. Chen YS, Lin JW, Yu HY et al (2008) Cardiopulmonary resuscitation with assisted extracorporeal life-support versus conventional cardiopulmonary resuscitation in adults with in-hospital cardiac arrest: an observational study and propensity analysis. Lancet 372(9638):554–561
45. Nolan JP, Soar J, Zideman DA et al (2010) European Resuscitation Council Guidelines for Resuscitation 2010 Section 1 Executive summary. Resuscitation 81(10):1219–1276
46. Keilegavlen H, Nordrehaug JE, Faerestrand S et al (2010) Treatment of cardiogenic shock with left ventricular assist device combined with cardiac resynchronization therapy: a case report. J Cardiothorac Surg 5:54
47. Manzo-Silberman S, Fichet J, Leprince P et al (2010) Cardiac arrest caused by coronary vasospasm treated with isosorbide dinitrate and left ventricular assistance. Resuscitation 81(7):919–920
48. Tuseth V, Pettersen RJ, Epstein A et al (2009) Percutaneous left ventricular assist device can prevent acute cerebral ischaemia during ventricular fibrillation. Resuscitation 80(10):1197–1203
49. Tuseth V, Pettersen RJ, Grong K et al (2010) Randomised comparison of percutaneous left ventricular assist device with open-chest cardiac massage and with surgical assist device during ischaemic cardiac arrest. Resuscitation 81(11):1566–1570
50. Tuseth V, Salem M, Pettersen R et al (2009) Percutaneous left ventricular assist in ischemic cardiac arrest. Crit Care Med 37(4):1365–1372

New Methods to Induce Localized Brain and General Hypothermia

18

Guy H. Fontaine, Frédéric Lapostolle, Jean-Philippe Didon,
Johann-Jakob Schmid, Xavier Jouven
and Juan-Carlos Chachques

Sudden Cardiac Death is a major concern in industrialized countries [1]. In France, it is the cause of death of 40–60,000 cases per year. This figure may seem sketchy because a precise definition of sudden death has only recently been clarified and is not always properly reported by medical examiners.

Despite efforts made over decades to promote cardiac resuscitation science, education, and the arrival of automatic external defibrillators (AEDs), less than 50 % of cardiac arrest victims are likely to reach recovery of stable circulation (ROSC) and the percentage decreases even for patients who suffer a severe rhythm disorder that cannot be defibrillated (such as asystole or pulseless cardiac rhythm) [2–8]. This percentage is less than 20 % in rural areas. The vast majority of

G. H. Fontaine (✉)
Unité de rythmologie, Institut de Cardiologie, Hôpital de la Salpêtrière,
47 Boulevard de l'Hôpital, 75013, Paris, France
e-mail: guy.fontaine2@numericable.fr

F. Lapostolle
Emergency medical Service, Hopital Avicenne, 125, rue de Stalingrad,
93009, Bobigny, France

J.-P. Didon
Schiller Médical SAS, 4, Rue Louis Pasteur, ZAE Sud BP9005067162,
Wissembourg Cedex, France
e-mail: jean-philippe.didon@schiller.fr

J.-J. Schmid
Schiller AG, Altgasse 68, P.O. Box 1052, CH-6341, Baar, Switzerland
e-mail: JJ.Schmid@schiller.ch

X. Jouven · J.-C. Chachques
Hôpital Européen Georges Pompidou, 20 Rue Leblanc, 75015, Paris, France

A. Gullo and G. Ristagno (eds.), *Resuscitation*,
DOI: 10.1007/978-88-470-5507-0_18, © Springer-Verlag Italia 2014

patients leaving alive from the hospital after outdoor cardiac arrest bear irreversible brain damage.

However, the authors are convinced of the possibility of improving this situation through a better understanding of sudden death by screening high-risk individuals and a better organization of care through cooperation skills of the first responders, which has been called the "Chain of Survival." These are the main reasons for the creation of the first University Center of Expertise and Research on Sudden Cardiac Death (Research Center of European Georges Pompidou Hospital) in Paris.

Till date, all of the attempts to improve the situation by drug treatments such as vasopressin, epinephrine at high concentration, and thrombolysis have failed. Therefore, a more "physiological" approach needs to be investigated for brain and tissue protection and to increase blood flow.

One of the most promising methods involves therapeutic hypothermia. This chapter will review the main historical steps and will propose a new method of brain protection by localized hypothermia now under development.

18.1 Milestones

For many years, scientists and physicians have been working hard to explore the benefits of moderate hypothermia. Already in the 1950s, it was used to protect the brain against global ischemia occurring during open heart surgery. But, only recently and after positive experimental studies hypothermia has been used to protect the brain for out-of-hospital cardiac arrest (OHCA).

These investigations have suggested that induced hypothermia during cardiac arrest before ROSC improves neurological outcome compared to animals that were cooled after ROSC [9–13]. These studies also suggest that damage after resuscitation begins immediately after ROSC, and cooling during cardiac arrest may be a useful therapeutic approach to improve survival.

Two recent studies have demonstrated that use of therapeutic hypothermia improves neurological status after cooling to 33–34 °C within 8 h after ROSC in patients who had ventricular fibrillation (VF) [14, 15]. Based on these results, the International Liaison Committee has published guidelines recommending the use of moderate hypothermia on the routine treatment in patients after ROSC [16].

Specifically, these guidelines suggest that all patients who recover ROSC after VF must be cooled down as soon as possible and those recovering good circulation after nonshockable rhythm could also benefit from cooling down.

This is what led to the inclusion of this concept shortly later in the recommendations of the American Heart Association and the European Resuscitation Council [17, 18].

In one of these randomized trials, the cooling was started in the ambulance with ice plaques implemented by paramedical staff [15], whereas in another study the cooling began at arrival to the hospital [19]. The first trial was able to target low temperature quickly after arrival in the intensive care unit while the second one managed to do it 8 h later. The first study suggested a benefit due to rapid cooling and showed a higher percentage of those who had a favorable outcome compared with those who were not cooled with an odds ratio of 5.25.

Two additional studies have recently reassessed the relative efficiency of cooling by the administration of iced saline solution after returning to a stable situation obtained in the field. The first one was a "feasibility" study showing a trend toward improved survival to hospital discharge for patients cooled early after ventricular fibrillation [8]. This study shows that 85 % of subjects who received early cooling survived until arrival at the hospital and then 73 % survived. On the other hand, from the uncooled patients group, only 52 % survived (see Table 18.1).

However, the 21 % improvement was not enough to reach the level of statistical significance for improved survival. For those who had a nonshockable arrhythmia (but had reached a good spontaneous circulation) the trend was reversed. In fact, only 6 % instead of 20 % of uncooled patients survived until discharge. The two shockable rhythms are VF and pulseless ventricular tachycardia while the two nonshockable rhythms are asystole and pulseless electrical activity.

The second study was designed to detect an increase of 15 % favorable outcome up to discharge of those who were cooled out-of-hospital (in the field) after ROSC [14].

A recent French study performed on a large population showed, undoubtedly, the benefit of in-hospital hypothermia but only in patients with a shockable rhythm [20].

Focusing on methods of hypothermia for protection of the nervous system, in the light of previous studies, it appears that there are two methods to perform.

The first method consists in using externally cooled plates and chilling blankets or cool air. The second is by internal injection of cold fluids and more recently by intravascular cooling via a specific central venous balloon catheter, which is filled with saline solution and is continuously cooled via an external device.

External methods cool the body, starting by cooling the skin and peripheral components, while internal methods cool the blood and hence the entire body.

However, these methods are slow for brain cooling because they are focused on body's cooling rather than cooling the brain itself.

Table 18.1 Preliminary study suggesting efficacy of prehospital induction of mild hypothermia in out-of-hospital cardiac arrest patients with a rapid infusion of 4 °C normal saline

	Early cooling (%)	No cooling (%)	P
Hospital arrival	85	86	0.8
Survival	73	52	0.0007
Survival in ROSC	66	45	0.001

In addition, the cooling rate through the blood depends directly on patient cardiac output. This is why patients who are in hemodynamic failure with low cardiac output or in complete cardiac arrest are more difficult to cool.

For use in the field, chilling blankets are unsuitable because they require significant electrical energy. Ice packs have a limited cooling capacity.

Other methods have also been considered and tested on anesthetized healthy volunteers:

- Gastric washing produced abdominal cramps and diarrhea, for these reasons the first voluntary testing was interrupted [21].
- Washing the urinary bladder and filling the mattress with cold air were used both for freezing. These experiments demonstrated a slow cooling rate of 1.7 ± 0.5, and 1.6 ± 1.1 °C/h [21].
- Immersion of the whole body in ice water is the fastest method reducing the core temperature of 36.2 ± 0.3 to 34 °C in only 20 min [21, 22]. However, it is not possible to be performed outside the hospital and even within, it is not easy to implement. Patients who underwent neurosurgery were cooled through the skin and also by using a large diameter catheter administering a solution of 5 % albumin (1–6 °C) at a rate of 5 ml/kg for 5 or 30 min [23].
- The most powerful techniques for inducing hypothermia pass through the cooling of the blood itself. In extracorporeal circulation to which we have already alluded, cooling the blood has been studied and it is indeed possible when the cannulae are in place. It has been successfully used for the whole body cooling in dogs [10], pigs [24], and patients [25], but it needs to be performed in the hospital environment. It is necessary to make a significant and prolonged vascular access that requires a bulky equipment, which is a limiting factor on the ground.

New equipment for endovascular cooling has emerged using a cooled fluid through a balloon inserted into the vena cava, already in clinical use [26–28]. This method seems to be somewhat dangerous with the advantage of not overloading the circulation. Cooling of 1.1 °C/h was observed in resuscitated cardiac arrest. However, this method requires the introduction of catheters into the femoral vein; moreover, it requires an external pump, a heat exchanger, and a compressor generator cold, thus important source of electrical energy. These constraints make it impractical in an emergency situation on the ground.

To hasten brain cooling and prevent the complications inherent to whole body cooling (ventricular fibrillation, bleeding, pneumonia, infection), many researchers have attempted to refresh the brain while keeping the rest of the body at a temperature close to normal [29]. External methods to cool have shown their efficiency in cardio protection [30], cardiac and brain protections in experimental studies [31–34], but none has demonstrated its efficiency in patients [35–37].

18.2   Outlook

The need for effective and early hypothermia requires new approaches applicable in the field such as "intra-arrest cooling" inside the skull through the nose. In this case, the cold is produced by evaporation of a volatile fluid in the nasal cavity [38]. This initial work shows that this approach is feasible and safe, even in the sub-group of survivors of VF. However, we have seen that a profit of 15 % does not reach a significant level. This was considered as the consequence of lost time of 23 min on average between syncope and initiation of nasal cooling [38].

We think that this obstacle can be overcome by shortening the time of implementation of cooling and using a new approach based on the adiabatic expansion of gas pressure (patent pending). Experimental studies performed in our laboratory since October 2010 and then simulated on isolated pig head cooling through the nose, showed that it should be more powerful, simpler, and therefore faster to develop nasal cooling than previous investigated procedures.

In our approach, a compressed gas cylinder of one liter is connected to a flexible tube transmitting the pressurized gas to an introducer whose distal port is calculated to produce cold in greater quantity than that obtained with PFC. This method of PFC evaporation possesses several disadvantages, in particular complexity and cost.

Demonstration of the efficiency of our technique for humans requires a prospective, randomized, multicenter study that we are organizing. It will be started as soon as these promises have been strengthened by experimental data. Because of the novelty of this technique, basic aspects have been experimentally evaluated, in the following studies.

18.3   Study 1. Comparison of Oxygen, Air, and Carbon Dioxide for In Vitro Hypothermia

Several medical gases can be candidates for cold production. The purpose of this study was to compare cooling produced by expansion of oxygen (O_2), compressed air (CA), and carbon dioxide (CO_2) in vitro.

Method: Comparative experimental studies have been performed in which a given amount of 200 ml of water was cooled for 5 min by expansion of O_2, CA, and CO_2 at a pressure of 435 psi delivered at the exit of a semi-rigid polyamide injector. Temperatures in degree Celsius (precision 0.1 °C) were measured by a thermocouple probe type "K." Calories extraction was calculated from the drop in temperature. Data were processed by Statistica v6.0. A p value ≤ 0.05 was considered as significant 18.2.

Discussion: As suspected by physical principles, the stronger drop of temperature was observed with CO_2 when compared with O_2 and CA. The difference in calorie extraction with O_2 and CA is similar and therefore makes a specific study of N_2 alone unnecessary. This in vitro study demonstrates that carbon dioxide is

Table 18.2 Comparison of the cooling power of three compressed gases: Oxygen (O_2), compressed air (CA), and carbon dioxide (CO_2)

	O_2	CA	CO_2
N	10	25	11
Mean	140 ± 37.7 SD (100–220)	134 ± 49 (80–260	229 ± 89 (160–460)

Carbon dioxide is always the most effective gas. Compressed air and oxygen are equivalent
CA *versus* CO_2: $p = 0.00002$
O_2 *versus* CO_2: $p = 0.008$
O_2 *versus* CA: $p = 0.74$

the most effective gas for brain and body hypothermia. However, pure CO_2 cannot be used to ensure proper respiration. Therefore, it can be used for oral or nasal cooling while the patient is ventilated by an independent cuffed tracheal tube. In addition, an important property of CO_2 is to be stored in its liquid condition with a constant vapor pressure above the liquid of 830 psi under normal conditions of temperature and pressure, providing a reserve of high pressure gas larger than for O_2 or CA. However, CO_2 can be used in combination with O_2 as replacement for nitrogen.

Conclusion: CO_2 was the best gas for cooling by adiabatic expansion. Used alone it needs intubation for O_2 administration. It can replace nitrogen to keep proper O_2 concentration for respiration. Storage in its liquid phase is an important independent physical parameter.

18.4   Study 2. Comparison of O_2 and CO_2 for Brain and General Hypothermia in a Rabbit Model

Method: The study population consisted of 11 New Zealand rabbits (3.5 kg) studied under ketamine anesthesia without ventilation. Temperatures in degree Celsius were measured every minute by thermocouples; close to the injector exit inside a 12 mm Ø PVC 2 mm thick blind cannula inserted in the mouth up to the oropharynx, close to the cannula, in the nasopharynx and in the rectum. After stabilization of temperatures, gases were expanded in the cannula at the exit of the injector. Pressure was regulated at 507.5 psi (35 bar) and delivered during a period of mean 14 min $\pm$ 1.9 SD. Eight rabbits in Group 1 were submitted to CO_2 and three rabbits in Group 2 to O_2 expansion.

Results: No adverse side effect was observed during as well as after these experiments, especially no throat injury was observed by direct visual inspection. All rabbits recovered quickly (Table 18.3).

Discussion: The strongest drop in temperature (51.6) was observed close to the injector exit with CO_2 when compared to O_2 (27.3). This difference is strongly significant ($p = 0.0002$). Similarly, the strongest drop in temperature was observed in the oropharynx at 6.8 with CO_2 as compared to 4.9 with O_2. However, this difference did not reach significance ($p = 0.69$).

Table 18.3 Comparison of the cooling power of two compressed gases on a rabbit model with type "K" probes located near the injector, oral, nasal, and rectal using CO_2 in group 1 versus O_2 expansion in group 2

	G1	G2	p
Injector	51.6 ± 4.42	27.3 ± 12.2	$p = 0.0002$
Oral	6.8 ± 7.76	4.9 ± 1.82	$p = 0.69$
Nasal	1.12 ± 0.5	0.73 ± 0.15	$p = 0.23$
Rectal	0.21 ± 0.15	0.13 ± 0.15	$p = 0.36$

No significant difference is obtained except at the injector exit. However, as expected, a tendency of higher cooling is obtained in the nasal position

The same phenomenon was also observed in the nasopharynx as well as in the rectum, $p = 0.36$ and 0.23, respectively. Nevertheless, in all the cases the drop in temperature was always stronger with CO_2 when compared to O_2, 6.8 in the oropharynx, 1.12 in the nasopharynx, and 0.21 in the rectum. Core temperature drop was similar to that reported in pigs after fossa nasalis PFC evaporation (Yu et al. Crit. Care Medicine 2010). Therefore, CO_2 looks like the best gas to use for brain and general hypothermia. In addition, an important property of CO_2 is to be stored in its liquid phase with a constant vapor pressure above the liquid of 830 psi at 20 °C and "normal pressure" providing a reserve of high pressure gas larger than for O_2.

This study demonstrates that carbon dioxide is the most effective gas for brain and body hypothermia in a rabbit model. Its storage in its liquid phase is an important independent physical parameter [39].

18.5   Study 3. Physics of CO_2 Expansion with No Neurological Defect in the First OHCA Patient

A 74-year-old woman, Psychiatrist MD, experienced 6 min of cardiac arrest (CA) at home. She was treated by CPR: chest compression, insufflation, defibrillation, and the new technique of CO_2 adiabatic expansion. CO_2 was injected and expanded in the nasopharynx after ROSC. Four more episodes of documented VF were recorded in the intensive care unit at Salpêtrière hospital in Paris. At that time the troponin level was normal as well as in the "Institut de Cardiologie." FEVG was at 30 % a few days after the event. An ICD was implanted and a combination of amiodarone and bisoprolol was initiated. No further episode of arrhythmia was observed during a recovery period of 1 month and LVEF improved up to 43 % (Simpson) with NYHA Class I. The follow-up is now of 27 months (amiodarone has been interrupted after 2 years) and no arrhythmia has been recorded by the ICD teletransmission system. Absolutely no neurological defects were detected.

18.6   Study 4

The purpose of the following work was to reproduce on 10 subsequent in vitro experiments the physical parameters involved in this new form of localized therapeutic hypothermia in order to document its dynamics, safety, efficacy, and calories extraction.

Method: The same prototype high pressure bottle of 740 ml equipped with a 435 psi regulator was filled with CO_2 in 45 s at 841 psi (saturation vapor pressure). A semi-rigid flexible polyamide injector, connected to the bottle, was inserted in the pseudo (*ps*) nasal cavity of a mock-up of the fossa nasalis (23 ml) and adjacent tissues made with agar–agar (1400 g). Measures:

- Thermometry: Temperatures in degree Celsius (precision 0.1 °C) were measured automatically, recorded, and processed every minute by four "K" thermocouple probes located near the injector exit, at the site of expansion, in the adjacent 2 and 4 cm area and at the pseudo nostril exit.
- Dynamics: Speed of temperature decreases up to 90 % of maximal value and duration of drop of temperature up to 90 % of return to baseline were measured.
- Thermodynamics: The same protocol was repeated with expansion of CO_2 in 200 ml of H_2O.

Results: Thermometry minimal temperatures:

Injector; mean 4.4 ± 1.2 SD, 2 cm; 5.2 ± 1.8, 4 cm; 6 ± 1.8, *ps*n ostril exit; 18 ± 3 Speed; 2 ± 0.5 min Duration; 13 ± 3 Thermodynamics: A drop in temperature 6.25 ± 0.7 (5.2–7.6) after 7.7 ± 0.8 min and came back to 90 % lab temp in around 30 min. Calories extraction was 1240 ± 129 (1040–1400).

Discussion: These results demonstrate that CO_2 expansion produces fast, major, and localized hypothermia with a protocol mimicking the intra-arrest situation. Despite the short duration of this form of treatment a remarkable clinical result was obtained after ROSC.

Limitation: This work deals with a unique case; however, it can lay the foundation for further studies in- and out-of-hospital treatment of CA.

Conclusion: We have presented in this chapter an ideal clinical case of pure shockable rhythm, which can be the basis for further studies and opens new vistas for the development of a simple, easy to use apparatus for the emergency treatment of OHCA in the field which can be started intra-arrest before CPR. [1]

18.7   Future Directions

The results reported here are very preliminary. However, the outcome obtained on the first clinical case is encouraging. It is strongly suggested that adiabatic CO_2 expansion produces a significant cooling which can be beneficial for localized

---

[1] Addendum: Since the writing of this chapter further studies on a pig model have shown adverse side effects observed with large amount of CO_2 delivered to check the limit of this technique (extraction of more than 100 kcal in around 4 h).

brain hypothermia as well as general hypothermia produced by a relatively simple apparatus close to a fire extinguisher in terms of size, weight, easiness of use, and low cost.

Because of its simplicity it can be easily used in the field by the first responder. Intra-arrest cooling through the mouth is so easy that many people can use it with minimal or even no training at all. Drawings should be printed on the bottle to follow three steps: (1) Put the injector in the mouth; (2) Maintain it by the rubber band around the head; (3) Open the valve by counter clock rotation. In addition, start chest compression or depending on the delay from the fall, perform chest compression before cooling. Perform defibrillation if AED is available or call the emergency medical system.

The same method of hypothermia can be continued from a larger bottle in the ambulance until arrival to the hospital environment. Furthermore, the same technique can be also considered in the early treatment of stroke. Because of its simplicity and low price, the bottle can be the companion of any AED and even available at home.

References

1. Zheng ZJ, Croft JB, Giles WH (1999) State-specific mortality from sudden cardiac death-United States. Morb Mortal Wkly Rep 2002 5 l:123–126
2. Kass LE, Eitel DR, Sabulsky NK et al (1994) One-year survival after pre-hospital cardiac arrest: The Utstein style applied to a rural-sub-urban system. Am J Emerg Med 12:17–20
3. Kette F, Sbrojavacca R, Rellini G et al (1998) Epidemiology and survival rate of out-of-hospital cardiac arrest in North-east Italy: the F.A.C.S. study. friuli venezia giulia cardiac arrest cooperative study. Resuscitation 36:153–159
4. Skogvoll E, Sangolt GK, Isern E et al (1999) Out-of-hospital cardiopulmonary resuscitation: a population-based Norwegian study of incidence and survival. Eur J Emerg Med 6:323–330
5. Layon AJ, Gabrielli A, Goldfeder BW et al (2003) Utstein style analysis of rural out-of-hospital cardiac arrest [OOHCA]: total cardiopulmonary resuscitation (CPR) time inversely correlates with hospital discharge rate. Resuscitation 56:59–66
6. Ong Meh, Ornato JP, Edwards DP et al (2006) Use of an automated, load-distributing band chest compression device for out-of-hospital cardiac arrest resuscitation. JAMA 295:2629–2637
7. Fairbanks RJ, Shah MN, Lerner EB et al (2007) Epidemiology and outcomes of out-of-hospital cardiac arrest in Rochester. New York. Resuscitation 72:415–424
8. Kim F, Olsufka M, Longstreth WT Jr et al (2007) Pilot randomized clinical trial of prehospital induction of mild hypothermia in out-of-hospital cardiac arrest patients with a rapid infusion of 4 °C normal saline. Circulation 115:3064–3070
9. Sterz F, Safar P, Tisherman S et al (1991) Mild hypothermic cardiopulmonary resuscitation improves outcome after prolonged cardiac arrest in dogs. Crit Care Med 19:379–389
10. Kuboyama K, Safar P, Radovsky A et al (1993) Delay in cooling negates the beneficial effect of mild resuscitative cerebral hypothermia after cardiac arrest in dogs: a prospective, randomized study. Crit Care Med 21:1348–1358
11. Abella BS, Zhao D, Alvarado J et al (2004) Intra-arrest cooling improves outcomes in a murine cardiac arrest model. Circulation 109:2786–2791

12. Nozari A, Safar P, Stezoski SW et al (2006) Critical time window for intra-arrest cooling with cold saline flush in a dog model of cardiopulmonary resuscitation. Circulation 1:2690–2696

13. Zhao D, Abella BS, Beiser DG et al (2008) Intra-arrest cooling with delayed reperfusion yields higher survival than earlier normothermic resuscitation in a mouse model of cardiac arrest. Resuscitation 77(2):242–249

14. The HACA Study group (2002) Mild therapeutic hypothermia to improve the neurologic outcome after cardiac arrest. N Engl J Med 346:549–556

15. Bernard SA, Gray TW, Buist MD et al (2002) Treatment of comatose survivors of out-of-hospital cardiac arrest with induced hypothermia. N Engl J Med 346:557–563

16. Nolan JP, Morley PT, Hoek TL et al (2003) Therapeutic hypothermia after cardiac arrest: an advisory statement by the advancement life support task force of the international liaison committee on resuscitation. Resuscitation 57:231–235

17. American Heart Association (2005) American Heart Association guidelines for cardiopulmonary resuscitation and emergency cardiovascular care, part 7.5: postresuscitation support. Circulation 112(Suppl I):IV-84–IV-88

18. Nolan JP, Deakin CD, Soar J et al (2005) European Resuscitation Council guidelines for resuscitation section 4: Adult advanced life support. Resuscitation 67S1:S39-S86

19. Bernard SA, Smith K, Cameron P et al (2010) Rapid infusion of cold hartmanns (RICH) investigators: induction of therapeutic hypo-thermia by paramedics after resuscitation from out-of-hospital ventricular fibrillation cardiac arrest: a randomized controlled trial. Circulation 122:737–742

20. Dumas F, Grimaldi D, Zuber B et al (2011) Is hypothermia after cardiac arrest effective in both shockable and nonshockable patients? Circulation 123:877–886

21. Plattner O, Kurz A, Sessler DI et al (1997) Efficacy of intraoperative cooling methods. Anesthesiol 87:1089–1095

22. Lopez M, Sessler DI, Walter K et al (1994) Rate and gender dependence of the sweating, vasoconstriction, and shivering thresholds in humans. Anesthesiol 80:780–788

23. Baumgardner JE, Baranov D, Smith DS et al (1999) The effectiveness of rapidly infused intravenous fluids for inducing moderate hypothermia in neurosurgical patients. Anesth Analg 89:163–169

24. Janata A, Holzer M, Bayegan K et al (2006) Rapid induction of cerebral hypothermia by aortic flush during normovolemic cardiac arrest in pigs. Crit Care Med 34:1769–1774

25. Nagao K, Hayashi N, Kanmatsuse K et al (2000) Cardiopulmonary cerebral resuscitation using emergency cardiopulmonary bypass, coronary reperfusion therapy and mild hypothermia in patients with cardiac arrest outside the hospital. J Am Coll Cardiol 36:776–783

26. De Georgia MA, Krieger DW, Abou-Chebl A et al (2004) Cooling for Acute Ischemic Brain Damage (COOL AID): a feasibility trial of endovascular cooling. Neurology 63:312–317

27. Guluma KZ, Hemmen TM, Olsen SE et al (2006) A trial of therapeutic hypothermia via endovascular approach in awake patients with acute ischemic stroke: methodology. Acad Emerg Med 13:820–827

28. Arrich J (2007) European council HACA registry study group: clinical application of mild therapeutic hypothermia after cardiac arrest. Crit Care Med 35:1041–1047

29. Polderman KH (2004) Application of therapeutic hypothermia in the ICU: opportunities and pitfalls of a promising treatment modality part 2: practical aspects and side effects. Intensive Care Med 30:757–769

30. Shao ZH, Chang WT, Chan KC et al (2007) Hypothermia-induced cardioprotection using extended ischemia and early reperfusion cooling. Am J Physiol Heart Circ Physiol 292:H1995–H2003

31. Kuluz JW, Gregory GA, Yu AC et al (1992) Selective brain cooling during and after prolonged global ischemia reduces cortical damage in rats. Stroke 23:1792–1796

32. Kuluz JW, Prado R, Chang J et al (1993) Selective brain cooling increases cortical cerebral blood flow in rats. Am J Physiol 265(3):H824–H827
33. Tadler SC, Callaway CW, Menegazzi JJ (1998) Noninvasive cerebral cooling in a swine model of cardiac arrest. Acad Emerg Med 5:25–30
34. Yannopoulos D, Zviman M, Castro V et al (2009) Intra-cardiopulmonary resuscitation hypothermia with and without volume loading in an ischemic model of cardiac arrest. Circulation 120:1426–1435
35. Mellergard P (1992) Changes in human intracerebral temperature in response to different methods of brain cooling. NeurosurgERY 31:671–677
36. Callaway CW, Tadler SC, Katz LM et al (2002) Feasibility of external cranial cooling during out-of-hospital cardiac arrest. Resuscitation 52:159–165
37. Hachimi-Idrissi S, Come L, Ebinger G et al (2001) Mild hypothermia induced by a helmet device: a clinical feasibility study. Resuscitation 51:275–281
38. Castren M, Nordberg P, Svensson L et al (2010) Intra-arrest transnasal evaporative cooling: a randomized, prehospital, multicenter study (PRINCE: pre-ROSC intranasal cooling effectiveness). Circulation 122:729–736
39. Fontaine GH, Lapostolle F, Pages A, Piquet J, Lalot A, Didon JP, Schmid JJ, Jouven X, Chachques JC. New technique of gas adiabatic expansion for brain and general hypothermia in rabbit. In:American Heart Association Scientific Sessions 2012; Resuscitation science symposium. Los Angeles (USA); 3–7 November 2012

Predicting Outcome After Cardiac Arrest

19

Stefan Braunecker and Bernd W. Böttiger

19.1 Introduction

Patients with return of spontaneous circulation (ROSC) after cardiac arrest are a challenge for the modern intensive care. Approximately 350,000 EU citizens are resuscitated after cardiac arrest each year. At least every second patient has a ROSC during cardiopulmonary resuscitation (CPR). Of these patients, however, up to 70 % die in the post-resuscitation period. The major reason is the development of a neurological injury, which has been shown in both with [1] and without [2] therapeutic hypothermia.

Brain damage is one of the major causes of morbidity and mortality after cardiac arrest. Early assessment of brain damage and prediction of cerebral outcome after CPR, therefore, may influence post-arrest treatment strategies. In the past decade, several factors for poor outcome could be identified. Various attempts, including neurological evaluation, cranial CT, electroencephalogram, somatosensory evoked potentials, and measurement of cerebral oxygen consumption, have been made to assess brain damage in comatose patients soon after cardiac arrest. Already 10 years ago, it has been shown that 24 h of hypothermia (body temperature between 32 and 34 °C) might improve the prognosis in patients with ROSC. Since then, therapeutic hypothermia has been increasingly used in patients after CPR and is now an integral part of the resuscitation guidelines [3].

S. Braunecker (✉) · B. W. Böttiger
Department of Anaesthesiology and Intensive Care Medicine, University Hospital of Cologne,
Kerpener Straße 62, 50937, Cologne, Germany
e-mail: stefan.braunecker@uk-koeln.de

B. W. Böttiger
e-mail: bernd.boettiger@uk-koeln.de

A. Gullo and G. Ristagno (eds.), *Resuscitation*,
DOI: 10.1007/978-88-470-5507-0_19, © Springer-Verlag Italia 2014

The therapeutic hypothermia is used today not only when the initial cardiac arrest rhythm is ventricular fibrillation. Even patients with other rhythms or in-hospital cardiac arrest may benefit by such cooling. The question arises whether the previous indicators for assessing the prognosis of patients with ROSC are also reliable after therapeutic hypothermia. A large number of studies on this topic have been published after admitting therapeutic hypothermia to the guidelines. However, it remains unclear the extent to which hypothermia affects the validity of the discovered indicators of unfavorable prognosis.

19.2 Prognostication

Many studies have focused on prediction of poor long-term outcome to allow physicians to limit care or withdraw organ support. A major problem in comparing studies is the lack of a uniform definition of what constitutes a poor prognosis. In most cases death, persistent vegetative state, and severe disability with permanent dependence on care are viewed as unfavorable outcomes, corresponding to Cerebral Performance Category (CPC) 3–5 or Glasgow Outcome Scale (GOS) 1–3. A few publications define only death and persistent vegetative state as unfavorable (CPC 4–5, GOS 1–2). Another limitation for such tests is the required 100 % specificity and zero false positive rate (FPR). Achieving this goal is often very difficult, because many studies include only a small number of patients.

19.2.1 In Normothermic Patients

Several parameters are reliable for a poor prognosis in normothermic patients [4–7], provided that the influence of sedative substances such as midazolam, thiopental, or fentanyl is ruled out (Box 1). These parameters are based on different studies and include only one prospective class 1 study.

Box 1 Indicators of poor outcome in normothermic patients
Generalized seizures and early myoclonus within the first 24 h after ROSC.
Absence of pupillary reaction to light on the third day after ROSC.
Absence of corneal reflex on the third day after ROSC.
Absence of motor reaction to pain on the third day after ROSC.
Absence of somatosensory evoked potentials within the first 3 days after ROSC.
Burst-suppression EEG within the first 3 days after ROSC.
Isoelectric EEG within the first 3 days after ROSC.
Continuous generalized epileptiform discharges within the first 3 days after ROSC.

19.2.2 Impact of Therapeutic Hypothermia

To date, there are only limited data available on prognostication in therapeutic hypothermia. Most prognostication studies have been carried out before therapeutic hypothermia was implemented in the guidelines. There is evidence that the use of therapeutic hypothermia makes the well-established tests in normothermic patients less reliable. Since the 2010 guidelines, studies show no clear applicability of clinical neurological signs, electrophysiological examinations, biochemical markers, or imaging modalities to predict neurological outcome within the first 72 h after ROSC. A reliable prediction in therapeutic hypothermia is therefore quite difficult. Likewise, a residual effect of sedative and analgesic substances must be excluded. For this, it must be considered that metabolism during therapeutic hypothermia is reduced, so the half-life is longer than in normothermic patients. Nevertheless, there are a variety of factors that may indicate a poor neurological outcome. Preliminary findings indicate that hypothermia has no effect on how long it takes for patients with a good prognosis to become conscious. Normothermic and hypothermic patients with a favorable prognosis predominantly regain consciousness within 3 days [8]. A significantly delayed awaking in patients treated with therapeutic hypothermia, however, could be observed in some cases [9]. For this reason, the early termination of life support 72 h after rewarming needs to be reconsidered critically and is not indicated. Most likely, a prolonged support may lead to an increase in the number of survivors.

19.2.3 Clinical Examination

The clinical-neurological examination is an important component in predicting outcome. Advantage of the clinical examination is a simple and fast feasibility without great expense. It is independent of existing infrastructure, such as laboratory or EEG, and can be performed at any ICU. The examinated parameters include myoclonus, pupillary reaction to light, corneal reflex, and response to pain at 72 h after ROSC. While these parameters are well validated in normothermic patients, the question arises about the validity during therapeutic hypothermia. To date there is only limited information on this issue. Although some of these clinical indicators show a poor outcome, there are no reliable parameters to predict outcome less than 24 h after cardiac arrest.

19.2.3.1 Pupillary Light Reflex and Corneal Reflex

The pupillary reflex is used to adapt the diameter of the pupil in response to the intensity of the light that falls on the retina. The reflex consists of an interconnection of the optic nerve and the oculomotor nerve. The pupil reaction to light seems to be a valid parameter at least after excluding hypothermia, hypotension, sedatives, or relaxants. The absence of both pupillary light and corneal reflex 72 h after CPR indicates no good outcome with a zero FPR. Whether these tests are reliable during hypothermia is unknown. Other signs are far less reliable.

19.2.3.2 Myoclonus and Status Epilepticus

The significance of such events is controversial in patients with therapeutic hypothermia. In contrast to normothermia the appearance of myoclonus during hypothermia seems to be limited. Meanwhile, there are several case reports [10, 11] with a good neurological outcome of patients despite the occurrence of myoclonus status epilepticus. On the other hand, an absence of myoclonus cannot make a definitive statement about the outcome. Myoclonus could be suppressed by sedatives or muscle relaxants.

19.2.3.3 Reaction to Pain

The absence of pain response can be regarded as unsafe test. However, far more false-positive results are reported [8, 12] in hypothermic than in normothermic patients. This may be due to the use of analgesics and sedatives during the therapeutic hypothermia.

In addition, drugs are metabolized more slowly during the hypothermia state. As a result, sedatives and analgesics might show higher drug levels at the end of hypothermia and thus have a prolonged time of action. For this reason, clinical examination should not be evaluated as a prognostic factor until 72 h after resuscitation and at least 24 h after last drug administration [12].

19.2.4 Electrophysiological Indicators

Electrophysiological examinations are another cornerstone in prediction of outcome. Also, when these types of investigations are considered to be simple and noninvasive, they are not widely available and are difficult to interpret. Although there are studies that show a good validity in normothermic patients, the influence of hypothermia is yet not sufficiently tested.

19.2.4.1 Somatosensory Evoked Potentials

Somatosensory evoked potentials (SEPs) are a record of the electrical response of fast conducting sensitive nerve fibers. They are derived by repeated electrical stimulation of peripheral nerves at various points. SEP in patients not treated with hypothermia are well validated with an FPR of 0.7 % [5]. Initial investigations suggest that the FPR is increased by multiples during and after hypothermia [13]. The use of sedatives and analgesics during hypothermia complicates the use of SEP. The use of SEP is therefore suitable only in rewarmed patients more than 72 h after termination sedation.

19.2.4.2 Electroencephalography

Electroencephalography (EEG) is a method of medical diagnostics to measure the summed electrical activity of the brain. As the SEP, the EEG is highly influenced by the administration of sedatives and analgetics. Moreover, all EEG studies were made while the patients were taking midazolam and fentanyl, so these drugs may have affected the results [14]. Recent studies indicate that the special EEGs (generalized suppression less than 20 µV or burst suppression pattern) observed between 24 and 72 h after ROSC predict a poor outcome with an FPR of 3 % [5].

To this day, there is insufficient evidence to support the routine use of EEG or SEP for prognostication of poor outcome in comatose cardiac arrest survivors.

19.2.5 Biochemical Markers

Meanwhile, several biomarkers for assessing neuronal damage are known. Biochemical markers of brain injury are logical choices as prognostic markers of neurological outcome. Of these biomarkers neuron-specific enolase (NSE) and Protein S-100 (S100) are among the most widely studied and used.

19.2.5.1 Neuron-Specific Enolase

NSE is a neuron-derived enzyme, which is released after stroke and cardiac arrest and can be detected in the blood. Its level in serum correlates with the extent of the neurological damage. The predictive value of NSE in patients with ROSC has been shown in several trials prior to the use of hypothermia [15, 16]. An elevation of NSE is associated with poor outcome for comatose patients after cardiac arrest [17]. However, a subgroup analysis of the Hypothermia after Cardiac Arrest (HACA) trial [18] showed a decreased prognostic value of NSE in patients treated with hypothermia. Since the introduction of the 2010 guidelines, various studies have dealt with NSE during hypothermia. Although an elevated NSE predicts a poor outcome, there are case reports of good neurological survival despite extremely high NSE levels in serum (<116 ng/ml) [17, 19]. It is therefore impossible to specify a cutoff.

19.2.5.2 Protein S-100

S100 is an astroglial protein, which is also released after stroke and cardiac arrest. As NSE, S100 is one of the best characterized biochemical markers for brain injury after ROSC. Studies have shown that S100 can be used to identify patients at risk of significant cognitive impairment [20]. However, the use of S100 for treatment limitation is controversial. Similar to the NSE, the definition of a cutoff is impossible.

Both NSE and S100 concentrations measured 24–48 h after cardiac arrest provide useful additional information. Although high serum levels argue against a good outcome, there are some case reports with good survival after extreme high serum level. A final decision can therefore never be made on the basis of NSE or S100.

19.3   Conclusions

Prognostic assessment of patients after cardiac arrest is and remains challenging. Meanwhile, there are various useful tests that help to identify patients after cardiac arrest with poor neurological outcome. However, none of these tests alone could make a reliable prediction. In particular, the use of sedatives and analgesics, and also the application of hypothermia with their influence on the metabolism, reduces the significance of the various tests and, therefore, must be ruled out. In order to avoid unnecessary prolongation of intensive care when good functional recovery is unlikely and, on the other hand, to avoid falsely pessimistic prognosis, which could lead to unjustified withdrawal of care, the prediction of unfavorable outcome must have a higher specificity. Such wide-reaching decisions should not be made based on the result of a single prognostication tool.

The time clinicians should wait before withdrawing supportive care for comatose patients after therapeutic hypothermia, may need to be extended beyond 72 h. Withdrawal of life support 72 h after rewarming may prematurely terminate life in at least 10 % of all potentially neurologically intact survivors [9].

References

1. Olasveengen TM, Sunde K, Brunborg C, Thowsen J, Steen PA, Wik L (2009) Intravenous drug administration during out-of-hospital cardiac arrest: a randomized trial. JAMA: J Am Med Assoc 302:2222–2229
2. Laver S, Farrow C, Turner D, Nolan J (2004) Mode of death after admission to an intensive care unit following cardiac arrest. Intensive Care Med 30:2126–2128
3. Deakin CD, Nolan JP, Soar J et al (2010) European resuscitation council guidelines for resuscitation 2010 section 4. Adult advanced life support. Resuscitation 81:1305–1352
4. Booth CM, Boone RH, Tomlinson G, Detsky AS (2004) Is this patient dead, vegetative, or severely neurologically impaired? Assessing outcome for comatose survivors of cardiac arrest. JAMA: J Am Med Assoc 291:870–879
5. Wiese CH, Bahr J, Popov AF, Hinz JM, Graf BM (2009) Influence of airway management strategy on "no-flow-time" in a standardized single rescuer manikin scenario (a comparison between LTS-D and I-gel). Resuscitation 80:100–103
6. Zandbergen EG, de Haan RJ, Hijdra A (2001) Systematic review of prediction of poor outcome in anoxic-ischaemic coma with biochemical markers of brain damage. Intensive Care Med 27:1661–1667
7. Zandbergen EG, de Haan RJ, Stoutenbeek CP, Koelman JH, Hijdra A (1998) Systematic review of early prediction of poor outcome in anoxic-ischaemic coma. Lancet 352:1808–1812
8. Fugate JE, Wijdicks EF, White RD, Rabinstein AA (2011) Does therapeutic hypothermia affect time to awakening in cardiac arrest survivors? Neurology 77:1346–1350
9. Lurie K, Davis S, Olsen J et al (2011) Awakening after cardiac arrest and post-resuscitation hypothermia: Are we pulling the plug too early? Circulation 122
10. Rossetti AO, Oddo M, Liaudet L, Kaplan PW (2009) Predictors of awakening from postanoxic status epilepticus after therapeutic hypothermia. Neurology 72:744–749
11. Thomke F, Marx JJ, Sauer O et al (2005) Observations on comatose survivors of cardiopulmonary resuscitation with generalized myoclonus. BMC Neurology 5:14

12. Samaniego EA, Mlynash M, Caulfield AF, Eyngorn I, Wijman CA (2011) Sedation confounds outcome prediction in cardiac arrest survivors treated with hypothermia. Neurocrit Care 15:113–119
13. Leithner C, Ploner CJ, Hasper D, Storm C (2010) Does hypothermia influence the predictive value of bilateral absent N20 after cardiac arrest? Neurology 74:965–969
14. Rossetti AO, Carrera E, Oddo M (2012) Early EEG correlates of neuronal injury after brain anoxia. Neurology 78:796–802
15. Reisinger J, Hollinger K, Lang W et al (2007) Prediction of neurological outcome after cardiopulmonary resuscitation by serial determination of serum neuron-specific enolase. Eur Heart J 28:52–58
16. Zandbergen EG, Hijdra A, Koelman JH et al (2006) Prediction of poor outcome within the first 3 days of postanoxic coma. Neurol 66:62–68
17. Grubb NR, Simpson C, Sherwood RA et al (2007) Prediction of cognitive dysfunction after resuscitation from out-of-hospital cardiac arrest using serum neuron-specific enolase and protein S-100. Heart 93:1268–1273
18. Tiainen M, Roine RO, Pettila V, Takkunen O (2003) Serum neuron-specific enolase and S-100B protein in cardiac arrest patients treated with hypothermia. Stroke: A J Cereb Circ 34:2881–2886
19. Krumnikl JJ, Böttiger BW, Strittmatter HJ, Motsch J (2002) Complete recovery after 2 h of cardiopulmonary resuscitation following high-dose prostaglandin treatment for atonic uterine haemorrhage. Acta Anaesthesiol Scand 46:1168–1170
20. Rundgren M, Karlsson T, Nielsen N, Cronberg T, Johnsson P, Friberg H (2009) Neuron specific enolase and S-100B as predictors of outcome after cardiac arrest and induced hypothermia. Resuscitation 80:784–789

Circulating Cardiac Biomarkers and Outcome

20

Roberto Latini and Serge Masson

20.1 Background

Cardiac arrest is the final, catastrophic event of heart disease in most cases [1]. The arrest is abrupt and unexpected and cardiopulmonary resuscitation (CPR) maneuvres must be applied as early as possible according to the existing guidelines [1]. The sooner CPR is started the higher are the chances of restoring pulse and respiration. Resuscitation is achieved in approximately 2–39 % of the cases depending on the setting and underlying patient conditions [2]. However, brain injury often ensues leading to permanent deficits [3].

The question is why and when to use a biomarker in this extreme and rapidly evolving clinical condition?

Let us first define a biomarker; a biomarker is a characteristic that is objectively measured and provides information about normal biologic and pathologic processes, and about responses to interventions. According to this widely accepted definition, ECG and blood pressure are the two biomarkers generally used as a guide for CPR. In most disease states, circulating biomarkers are being routinely used to help the clinician in diagnosis, risk assessment, and to monitor disease progression and its response to treatments. Then the second question is: Does a circulating biomarker have a place in the context of cardiac arrest? The answer is not intuitively available, and that is why to date there are no validated circulating biomarkers in cardiac arrest.

R. Latini (✉) · S. Masson
Department of Cardiovascular Research, IRCCS—Istituto di Ricerche Farmacologiche Mario Negri, via Privata Giuseppe La Masa 19, 20156, Milan, Italy
e-mail: roberto.latini@marionegri.it

A. Gullo and G. Ristagno (eds.), *Resuscitation*,
DOI: 10.1007/978-88-470-5507-0_20, © Springer-Verlag Italia 2014

Few biomarkers have been assayed in resuscitated patients and only for research purposes. Potential use of circulating biomarkers could be (a) to predict outcomes, first neurological then cardiac, and (b) to individualize treatments, which to now is a wishful thought.

Regardless of the purpose of its use, a biomarker will be of clinical value if it can be measured accurately, reproducible by a cheap assay, acceptable to the patient, easy to interpret by the clinician, sensitive and specific for the disease process, explains a reasonable proportion of patient disease status and outcomes, on top of established clinical and instrumental variables, and at the end substantially contributes to patient management.

When interpreting the findings of the limited number of studies on circulating biomarkers in cardiac arrest, all the above conditions must be kept in mind. Two major methodological issues should also be adequately addressed to:

1. Representativeness of the population studied: Given the advancement in CPR leading to the use of therapeutic hypothermia (TH) as an effective intervention [4], contemporary studies on biomarkers should be conducted in patients undergoing TH, since this intervention may alter both outcomes and circulating levels of the biomarker.

2. Sample size: The correct assessment of the clinical value of a biomarker requires an adequate number of patients to be studied, in order to minimize the probability of a type-II error. In other words, it can be concluded that the biomarker is unrelated to disease or to its outcomes just because the sample was too small. Statistics offer methods to calculate the power of the study on predictive biomarker as it is commonly done when designing a clinical trial.

A survey of studies on biomarkers in resuscitated cardiac arrest reveals that often the patient did not undergo contemporary resuscitation maneuvres including TH, and that most studies are underpowered.

Given the objective difficulty in applying rigid blood sampling schedules in a quickly changing condition, blood samples should be collected as part of clinical trials or of large cohort studies in cardiac arrest.

In this way, as recently shown by the FINNRESUSCI Collaboration [5], biobanks from well-studied patients should be instituted. This would allow, as is commonly experienced in other fields, the systematic study of known molecules and the discovery of new biomarkers.

Since a new biomarker (or an old biomarker for a new application) that does not change patient management and consequently outcomes is not cost-effective, prospective studies will have to be conducted with the aim of assessing whether a biomarker-guided approach will improve patients' outcomes compared to an approach without biomarker.

20.2   Cardiac Biomarkers and Outcome

Troponins and natriuretic peptides are the two most widely used circulating markers in clinical cardiology, the first for the diagnosis of acute myocardial infarction, the second for the differential diagnosis of dyspnea of cardiac origin at the emergency department. Both are also excellent prognosticators of mortality in chronic cardiac conditions. Not surprisingly, the same two markers are those best studied in the context of cardiac arrest. Cardiac troponins are integral parts of the cardiac muscle infrastructure and play a critical role in the excitation–contraction coupling. Their release from the damaged cardiomyocytes into the bloodstream is the basis for estimating extent of cardiac damage [6]. Natriuretic peptides are secreted by ventricular and atrial myocytes under conditions of cell stretching and exert mainly diuretic and natriuretic actions, but they also have a role in opposing some neurohormonal systems and in lipolysis [7, 8].

There are few investigations on the role of cardiac troponins for the differential diagnosis of acute myocardial infarction (AMI) in patients successfully resuscitated after out-of-hospital cardiac arrest (OHCA). Early studies reported a substantial lack of sensitivity and specificity [9]. This may be due to the fact that procedures used for CPR (chest compression or defibrillation) or persistent circulatory shock may directly provoke myocardial damage and the release of cardiac markers, in absence of coronary artery occlusion [10]. Troponin elevation in patients resuscitated from OHCA but who do not have AMI is, however, lower and normalizes faster compared in those with AMI [11]. In a recent, single-center study, 163 patients resuscitated from OHCA were assessed with coronary angiography on admission for AMI, that was diagnosed in 37 % of the cases [12]. High circulating troponin concentrations were measured very early after cardiac arrest, even in patients with normal angiograms (median cTnI was 0.6 ng/mL in the latter group), indicative of nonischemic myocardial injury during chest compression. However, combined with ST-elevation on ECG, elevated troponin concentration on admission (cTnI > 2.5 ng/mL) showed a good performance to exclude the diagnosis of AMI (sensitivity 93 %, negative predictive value 94 %). The specificity remained low even in combination with ST-elevation on ECG (64 %).

International guidelines recommend considering emergent coronary angiography and percutaneous coronary intervention in patients with OHCA and return of spontaneous circulation (ROSC), even in the absence of STEMI [4]. Since clinical findings such as chest pain are often lacking and the predictive value of ECG for AMI is poor, troponin testing may provide a simple and objective selection of post-resuscitation patient candidate for immediate coronary angiography. This triage strategy has recently been tested in 422 cardiac arrest survivors without obvious extra-cardiac causes [13]. In this large study, a coronary angiography was systematically performed and cardiac troponin measured on admission. However, even if independently associated with coronary occlusion, elevation of cardiac troponin levels has a poor accuracy to identify a recent coronary lesion, precluding its use as the sole criteria for the decision to perform or not early coronary angiography in these patients.

Acute coronary artery occlusion is therefore difficult to diagnose in survivors of cardiac arrest using circulating markers alone, especially in case of ambiguous ECG. There are no data available to date on the diagnostic performance of cardiac troponins after cardiac arrest, when using high sensitivity assays that may readily detect concentrations in the order of few nanograms per liter, ten to hundred times lower than the conventional assays. However, one may speculate that specificity will become an even more critical issue since the recent introduction of this new generation of high sensitivity reagents has led to a substantial increase in the proportion of detectable troponin levels attributable to conditions distinct from acute coronary syndromes [14].

Natriuretic peptides have been tested for their relation to survival or neurological outcome after OHCA. Nagao et al. measured brain natriuretic peptide on arrival at emergency room in 401 patients with presumed cardiac origin of OHCA, according to the Utstein Style [15]. Primary outcome was survival to hospital discharge, and among the secondary outcomes was neurological evaluation according to the Pittsburgh Cerebral Performance Categories (CPC) scale. Mean brain natriuretic peptide (BNP) was significantly higher in the decedents (260 pg/mL) than in the 52 survivors (74 pg/mL). Survival decreased steeply across the quartiles of BNP concentration, being 34, 10, 7, and 1 %, respectively, from bottom to top. The same trends were observed in patients with witnessed arrest, CPR by bystander, with shockable rhythm, or with ROSC after arrival at emergency room. Higher BNP levels were significantly associated to death, even after adjustment for variables associated with survival (witnessed arrest and ROSC before hospital), suggesting a role of BNP for risk stratification of survival of patients with OHCA. The highest prognostic accuracy was observed at a BNP concentration of 100 pg/mL that corresponded to a negative predictive value of 96 % and a specificity of 66 %. Finally, the proportion of patients with favorable neurological outcome (good recovery or moderate disability) decreased from 33 % in the bottom quartile of BNP concentration to 0 % in the top one [15]. The same group evaluated more recently BNP to predict neurological outcome in comatose survivors of OHCA due to cardiac causes and treated with mild hypothermia by extracorporeal cooling [16]. The primary endpoint was a favorable neurological outcome at the time of hospital discharge. There was a rapid fall in the proportion of patients with favorable neurological outcome across the quartiles of BNP concentration, in all patients, and in those with witnessed arrest, bystander CPR, shockable rhythm, ROSC after arrival at emergency room or cardiac arrest due to acute coronary syndrome [16]. The fact that BNP levels measured on admission in comatose cardiac arrest survivors may predict neurological outcome has been confirmed in an independent study that enrolled 115 patients followed for 6 months [17]. In this setting, BNP was significantly associated with an adverse neurological outcome and mortality, independent of the pre-arrest health and cardiac conditions. Although natriuretic peptides provide invaluable information about the post-resuscitation cardiovascular function, and therefore indirectly on cerebral perfusion, it is clear that brain-specific markers, such as neuron-specific enolase (NSE) or S100B, are more promising candidates for the prediction of neurological outcome after OHCA and cardiopulmonary resuscitation [18].

20.3 Matrix Metalloproteinases

Other circulating biomarkers, not strictly of cardiac origin, have been evaluated for risk stratification after OHCA. Among them, matrix metalloproteinases (MMP) that play a major role in the turnover extracellular matrix components and cardiac remodeling after ischemia–reperfusion injury. They have been proposed as therapeutic targets in different organs, including the heart [19]. The clinical usefulness for risk stratification of MMP-9 has been assessed in 96 OHCA patients [20]. Circulating levels on admission were significantly higher in patients with failed (93 ng/mL) than with successful CPR (70 ng/mL). In addition, MMP-9 concentration on admission was the sole predictor of early mortality (odds ratio 1.50, $p < 0.001$), in multivariable models that included presence of asystole, mean duration of cardiac arrest, out-of-hospital CPR, electrolytes, and arterial pH. At optimal cutoff value, MMP-9 predicted failed CPR with a sensitivity of 88 % and a specificity of 98 %, suggesting that it might help in risk stratification of patients with cardiac arrest [20]. Elevation of different matrix metalloproteinases (MMP-7 and MMP-9) has been confirmed in 51 patients resuscitated form cardiac arrest at 24 h from ROSC [21]. In this study, therapeutic hypothermia was associated with reduced MMP-9 levels, suggesting an attenuation of inflammatory response by this treatment. The influence of hypothermia after cardiac arrest on the activation of circulating inflammatory markers and their role in tissue injury remains, however, controversial with conflicting data between human and animal studies [22–25].

20.4 The Kynurenine Pathway

More consistent data have been obtained very recently in a fully translational approach following cardiopulmonary resuscitation in rats, pigs, and humans [26]. Using untargeted metabolomics, the authors identified alterations in a major route of the tryptophan catabolism, namely the kynurenine pathway, in post-resuscitation circulating metabolites. The kynurenine pathway is mainly activated upon inflammatory stimulation and is implicated in the pathogenesis of numerous central nervous system disorders, as well as in sepsis development and profound hypotension during septic shock [27]. A significant increase in the plasma levels of 3-hydroxyanthranilic acid (3-HAA) and kynurenic acid in each species (rats, pigs, and humans) persisted up to 3–5 days post-cardiac arrest [26]. In addition, kynurenine pathway activation was significantly related to the severity of post-resuscitation myocardial dysfunction, cerebral injury, functional outcome, and survival. More efforts are currently under way to evaluate the clinical utility of the metabolites of the kynurenine pathway in larger cohorts of patients with OHCA.

References

1. Berg RA, Hemphill R, Abella BS, Aufderheide TP, Cave DM, Hazinski MF, Lerner EB, Rea TD, Sayre MR, Swor RA (2010) Part 5: adult basic life support: 2010 American heart association guidelines for cardiopulmonary resuscitation and emergency cardiovascular care. Circulation 122:S685–S705
2. Eisenberg M, White RD (2009) The unacceptable disparity in cardiac arrest survival among American communities. Ann Emerg Med 54:258–260
3. Nolan JP, Neumar RW, Adrie C, Aibiki M, Berg RA, Böttiger BW, Callaway C, Clark RS, Geocadin RG, Jauch EC, Kern KB, Laurent I, Longstreth WT, Merchant RM, Morley P, Morrison LJ, Nadkarni V, Peberdy MA, Rivers EP, Rodriguez-Nunez A, Sellke FW, Spaulding C, Sunde K, Hoek TV (2008) Post-cardiac arrest syndrome: epidemiology, pathophysiology, treatment, and prognostication a scientific statement from the international liaison committee on resuscitation; the American heart association emergency cardiovascular care committee; the council on cardiovascular surgery and anesthesia; the council on cardiopulmonary, perioperative, and critical care; the council on clinical cardiology; the council on stroke. Resuscitation 79:350–379
4. Peberdy MA, Callaway CW, Neumar RW, Geocadin RG, Zimmerman JL, Donnino M, Gabrielli A, Silvers SM, Zaritsky AL, Merchant R, Vanden Hoek TL, Kronick SL (2010) American heart association, part 9: post-cardiac arrest care: 2010 American heart association guidelines for cardiopulmonary resuscitation and emergency cardiovascular care. Circulation 122:S768–S786
5. Vaahersalo J, Hiltunen P, Tiainen M, Oksanen T, Kaukonen KM, Kurola J, Ruokonen E, Tenhunen J, Ala-Kokko T, Lund V, Reinikainen M, Kiviniemi O, Silfvast T, Kuisma M, Varpula T, Pettilä V; FINNRESUSCI Study Group (2013) Therapeutic hypothermia after out-of-hospital cardiac arrest in Finnish intensive care units: the FINNRESUSCI study. Intensive Care Med 39:826–837
6. Agewall S, Giannitsis E, Jernberg T, Katus H (2011) Troponin elevation in coronary vs non-coronary disease. Eur Heart J 32:404–411
7. Daniels LB, Maisel AS (2007) Natriuretic peptides. J Am Coll Cardiol 50:2357–2368
8. Moro C, Lafontan M (2013) Natriuretic peptides and cGMP signaling control of energy homeostasis. Am J Physiol Heart Circ Physiol 304:H358–H368
9. Müllner M, Hirschl MM, Herkner H, Sterz F, Leitha T, Exner M, Binder M, Laggner AN (1996) Creatine kinase-mb fraction and cardiac troponin T to diagnose acute myocardial infarction after cardiopulmonary resuscitation. J Am Coll Cardiol 28:1220–1225
10. Müllner M, Oschatz E, Sterz F, Pirich C, Exner M, Schörkhuber W, Laggner AN, Hirschl MM (1998) The influence of chest compressions and external defibrillation on the release of creatine kinase-MB and cardiac troponin T in patients resuscitated from out-of-hospital cardiac arrest. Resuscitation 38:99–105
11. Oh SH, Kim YM, Kim HJ, Youn CS, Choi SP, Wee JH, Kim SH, Jeong WJ, Park KN (2012) Implication of cardiac marker elevation in patients who resuscitated from out-of-hospital cardiac arrest. Am J Emerg Med 30:464–471
12. Voicu S, Sideris G, Deye N, Dillinger JG, Logeart D, Broche C, Vivien B, Brun PY, Capan DD, Manzo-Silberman S, Megarbane B, Baud FJ, Henry P (2012) Role of cardiac troponin in the diagnosis of acute myocardial infarction in comatose patients resuscitated from out-of-hospital cardiac arrest. Resuscitation 83:452–458
13. Dumas F, Manzo-Silberman S, Fichet J, Mami Z, Zuber B, Vivien B, Chenevier-Gobeaux C, Varenne O, Empana JP, Pène F, Spaulding C, Cariou A (2012) Can early cardiac troponin I measurement help to predict recent coronary occlusion in out-of-hospital cardiac arrest survivors? Crit Care Med 40:1777–1784
14. de Lemos JA (2013) Increasingly sensitive assays for cardiac troponins: a review. JAMA 309:2262–2269

15. Nagao K, Hayashi N, Kanmatsuse K, Kikuchi S, Kikushima K, Watanabe K, Mukouyama T (2004) B-type natriuretic peptide as a marker of resuscitation in patients with cardiac arrest outside the hospital. Circ J 68:477–482

16. Nagao K, Mukoyama T, Kikushima K, Watanabe K, Tachibana E, Iida K, Tani S, Watanabe I, Hayashi N, Kanmatsuse K (2007) Resuscitative value of B-type natriuretic peptide in comatose survivors treated with hypothermia after out-of-hospital cardiac arrest due to cardiac causes. Circ J 71:370–376

17. Sodeck GH, Domanovits H, Sterz F, Schillinger M, Losert H, Havel C, Kliegel A, Vlcek M, Frossard M, Laggner AN (2007) Can brain natriuretic peptide predict outcome after cardiac arrest? An observational study. Resuscitation 74:439–445

18. Shinozaki K, Oda S, Sadahiro T, Nakamura M, Hirayama Y, Abe R, Tateishi Y, Hattori N, Shimada T, Hirasawa H (2009) S-100B and neuron-specific enolase as predictors of neurological outcome in patients after cardiac arrest and return of spontaneous circulation: a systematic review. Crit Care 13:R121

19. Dejonckheere E, Vandenbroucke RE, Libert C (2011) Matrix metalloproteinases as drug targets in ischemia/reperfusion injury. Drug Discov Today 16:762–778

20. Turkdogan KA, Zorlu A, Guven FM, Ekinozu I, Eryigit U, Yilmaz MB (2012) Usefulness of admission matrix metalloproteinase 9 as a predictor of early mortality after cardiopulmonary resuscitation in cardiac arrest patients. Am J Emerg Med 30:1804–1809

21. Hästbacka J, Tiainen M, Hynninen M, Kolho E, Tervahartiala T, Sorsa T, Lauhio A, Pettilä V (2012) Serum matrix metalloproteinases in patients resuscitated from cardiac arrest. The association with therapeutic hypothermia. Resuscitation 83:197–201

22. Fairchild KD, Singh IS, Patel S, Drysdale BE, Viscardi RM, Hester L, Lazusky HM, Hasday JD (2004) Hypothermia prolongs activation of NF-kappaB and augments generation of inflammatory cytokines. Am J Physiol Cell Physiol 287:C422–C431

23. Callaway CW, Rittenberger JC, Logue ES, McMichael MJ (2008) Hypothermia after cardiac arrest does not alter serum inflammatory markers. Crit Care Med 36:2607–2612

24. Meybohm P, Gruenewald M, Albrecht M, Zacharowski KD, Lucius R, Zitta K, Koch A, Tran N, Scholz J, Bein B (2009) Hypothermia and postconditioning after cardiopulmonary resuscitation reduce cardiac dysfunction by modulating inflammation, apoptosis and remodeling. PLoS ONE 4:e7588

25. Fries M, Stoppe C, Brücken D, Rossaint R, Kuhlen R (2009) Influence of mild therapeutic hypothermia on the inflammatory response after successful resuscitation from cardiac arrest. J Crit Care 24:453–457

26. Ristagno G, Fries M, Brunelli L, Fumagalli F, Bagnati R, Russo I, Staszewsky L, Masson S, Volti GL, Zappalà A, Derwall M, Brücken A, Pastorelli R, Latini R (2013) Early kynurenine pathway activation following cardiac arrest in rats, pigs, and humans. Resuscitation. doi: 10.1016/j.resuscitation.2013.06.002 pii: S0300-9572(13)00309-2

27. Wang Y, Liu H, McKenzie G, Witting PK, Stasch JP, Hahn M, Changsirivathanathamrong D, Wu BJ, Ball HJ, Thomas SR, Kapoor V, Celermajer DS, Mellor AL, Keaney JF Jr, Hunt NH, Stocker R (2010) Kynurenine is an endothelium-derived relaxing factor produced during inflammation. Nat Med 16:279–285

Circulatory Shock: Definition, Assessment, and Management

21

Jean-Louis Vincent

21.1 Introduction

The key function of the cardiovascular system is to provide adequate perfusion of all organs and tissues to ensure transport of oxygen, carbon dioxide, nutrients, hormones, etc., in order to maintain local and global homeostasis. In conditions of circulatory shock, cardiovascular function is impaired resulting in inadequate perfusion with associated tissue hypoxia and buildup of metabolic waste, leading ultimately to cellular death and organ failure. The circulatory system is essentially composed of a pump (the heart) and a series of transport pipes (arteries, veins, capillaries). Circulatory shock can arise as a result of altered function of any or several parts of this circuit but the hallmark of all forms of circulatory shock is an imbalance in tissue oxygen demand and oxygen delivery, resulting in aerobic metabolism and increasing blood lactate levels. In this chapter, we will briefly describe the characteristics of the different types of shock, and approaches to the clinical assessment and management of the patient with circulatory shock.

21.2 Definition

Shock has been defined as a clinical syndrome characterized by signs of altered tissue perfusion, including pallor, a cold moist skin, altered mental status, oliguria, and arterial hypotension (systolic arterial pressure <90 mmHg or a decrease in arterial pressure by more than 50 mmHg from basal levels) [1]. Importantly,

J.-L. Vincent (✉)
Department of Intensive Care, Erasme Hospital, Université libre de Bruxelles,
Route de Lennik 808, 1070, Brussels, Belgium
e-mail: jlvincent@ulb.ac.be

A. Gullo and G. Ristagno (eds.), *Resuscitation*,
DOI: 10.1007/978-88-470-5507-0_21, © Springer-Verlag Italia 2014

although arterial hypotension is generally considered as one of the main signs of circulatory shock, it may not always be present because of the general vasoconstriction caused by the activated sympathetic nervous system, which can mask the fall in blood pressure [2]. Moreover, although the usual lower limit for systolic arterial pressure is considered as 90 mmHg, this may vary from one patient to another, e.g., the pressure threshold may be different in older compared to younger patients or in patients with chronic hypertension or on antihypertensive medication.

The classification of circulatory shock that is still widely used today was first introduced by Weil and Shubin more than 40 years ago [3]! In this system, the principal underlying mechanism is used to define four types of circulatory shock:

- Cardiogenic: resulting from primary failure of the cardiac pump because of physical or functional loss of myocardium. Cardiogenic shock is most often associated with acute myocardial infarction, end-stage cardiomyopathy, advanced valvular disease, severe myocarditis, or severe cardiac arrhythmias.
- Hypovolemic: resulting from external (exogenous) or internal (endogenous) fluid loss causing a decreased circulating blood volume. The most obvious cause of external hypovolemic shock is acute hemorrhage, but severe vomiting or diarrhea can also be implicated, particularly in children and the elderly. Internal fluid loss can occur as a result of tissue extravasation, for example in inflammation or anaphylaxis.
- Obstructive: resulting from an impediment to blood flow in the cardiovascular system outside of the heart itself. The main causes of obstructive shock are massive pulmonary embolism, cardiac tamponade, or tension pneumothorax.
- Distributive: resulting from widespread vascular dilatation associated with the release of inflammatory mediators, as typically observed in sepsis, but also occurring in anaphylaxis, spinal shock, and some endocrinological disorders, such as thyroid or adrenal crises.

Septic shock is the most common form of shock in the intensive care unit (ICU) patient, followed by cardiogenic and hypovolemic shock; obstructive shock is relatively rare. In a trial comparing dopamine to norepinephrine for the treatment of shock in 1,600 patients, 62 % had septic (distributive) shock, 17 % cardiogenic shock, and 16 % hypovolemic shock [4].

In all types of circulatory shock, the end-result is inadequate tissue oxygenation. In the first three mechanisms, the cause is inadequate oxygen transport as a result of a low cardiac output. In contrast, in distributive forms of shock, the main cause is altered tissue oxygen extraction; indeed, in these patients, cardiac output is typically high, even if there is associated myocardial depression.

Importantly, a patient may have several types of shock present simultaneously: for example, a patient with septic shock will initially have distributive shock but may also then develop hypovolemic (sweating, diarrhea, extravasation…) and cardiogenic (sepsis-induced myocardial depression) forms; a patient with anaphylactic shock may have a similar pattern with distributive, hypovolemic (extravasation), and cardiogenic forms all present.

21.3   Assessment

Assessment of the patient with presumed circulatory shock involves a combination of clinical, hemodynamic, and biochemical signs:

- Clinical signs of shock: these are largely related to poor perfusion, and include cold, clammy skin as a result of vasoconstriction with cyanosis also generally present in low flow states; decreased urine output to less than 0.5 mL/kg/h; and obtundation, disorientation, and confusion as a result of decreased cerebral perfusion. These areas have been called the three "windows" of the body [2] (Fig. 21.1). A possible fourth window is the sublingual microcirculation. Although still experimental, observation of the sublingual microcirculation using orthogonal polarization spectral (OPS) or, more recently, sidestream darkfield (SDF) imaging is providing interesting insight into the effects of shock on microcirculatory perfusion. Shock is associated with characteristic and semi-quantifiable [5] changes in the microcirculation, including increased hetero-geneity of flow, which are related to severity and outcome and can be influenced by therapy [6–10]. Repeated observation of the sublingual microcirculation could, therefore, be a useful additional point of assessment for diagnosis and follow-up of patients with shock although further clinical studies are needed to confirm that microcirculatory-guided therapies do indeed improve outcomes.

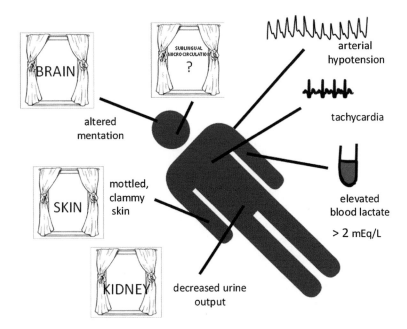

Fig. 21.1 The assessment of the patient with shock, showing the three "windows" of the body

- Hemodynamic signs of shock: as mentioned earlier, although hypotension is perhaps considered the hallmark of acute circulatory shock, it may in fact only be moderate, especially in patients with chronic hypertension. Tachycardia is usually present. Other hemodynamic variables differ according to the type of shock: for example, cardiac output will be reduced in cardiogenic, hypovolemic, and obstructive shock but normal or high in distributive shock; similarly systemic vascular resistance is typically increased in distributive shock but reduced in all other forms; pulmonary artery occlusion pressure will be reduced in hypovolemic shock, but increased in other forms of shock.
- Biochemical signs of shock: The biochemical changes associated with circulatory shock will again vary according to the type of shock, but one biochemical sign that is present in all forms of shock is hyperlactatemia. The importance of blood lactate concentrations in patients with shock was highlighted by Dr Weil and colleagues almost 50 years ago and blood lactate concentrations remain very relevant today [11, 12]. The reduced tissue oxygenation results in anaerobic metabolism and hence in raised blood lactate concentrations. Normal lactate concentrations are around 1 mEq/L and a value greater than 2 mEq/L is generally considered to reflect the presence of shock in the absence of other potentially causative factors, such as excessive aerobic glycolysis (e.g., during shivering, seizures, hyperventilation) and/or decreased utilization (e.g., liver failure, mitochondrial inhibition). In patients with shock, the severity of hyperlactatemia is directly related to outcome [13, 14]. Changes in lactate concentrations over time are particularly useful in predicting prognosis [15, 16].

21.4 Management

Circulatory shock is a medical emergency and early and adequate hemodynamic support is crucial to avoid worsening organ dysfunction. It is important to determine the underlying cause of the shock so that it can be managed accordingly, but this should not delay appropriate resuscitation, which must be started immediately. Once a cause is identified, specific management can be added, for example, control of bleeding, percutaneous coronary intervention, thrombolytic agent, administration of antibiotics, etc.

The goals of resuscitation are essentially to restore adequate tissue perfusion and oxygenation but these targets are currently difficult to define and monitor. An appropriate initial mean systemic arterial pressure target of 65–70 mmHg is often quoted [17], but this level should be adjusted according to signs of tissue perfusion, such as the mental status, cutaneous signs, and urine output described earlier. Moreover, a lower blood pressure may initially be acceptable in an acutely bleeding patient who has no major neurological problems, because this may help limit blood losses. Similarly, optimal cardiac output is difficult to define and will vary in different patients and in the same patient over time. Mixed venous oxygen saturation (SvO_2) can help to indicate whether the balance between oxygen demand and supply is adequate, but requires invasive monitoring. Central venous oxygen saturation ($ScvO_2$), measured in the superior vena cava using a central venous catheter, can be used as a surrogate but reflects the oxygen saturation of the venous blood from the upper half of the body only. Nevertheless, in patients presenting to an emergency department with septic shock, a treatment algorithm targeting an $ScvO_2$ of at least 70 % during the first 6 h was associated with decreased mortality rates [18]. This approach is currently being evaluated in multicenter trials. Changes in blood lactate concentrations can also be used to indicate response to therapy although they take place more slowly than changes in systemic arterial pressure or cardiac output. In ICU patients with shock and a blood lactate concentration >3 mEq/L, targeting a decrease in blood lactate level of at least 20 % over 2 h was associated with reduced hospital mortality [19]. The latest guidelines for management of patients with severe sepsis and septic shock suggest (grade 2C) that therapy should be targeted to normalize blood lactate levels [17].

The initial management of the patient with shock can be conducted according to the VIP (Ventilate, Infuse, Pump) mnemonic [20]:

- **Ventilate:** Oxygen should be administered immediately to correct hypoxemia and increase oxygen delivery. Noninvasive mechanical ventilation has a limited place in these patients as failure can rapidly result in respiratory arrest. Hence, there should be a low threshold for performing endotracheal intubation and starting mechanical ventilation. Moreover, in addition to optimizing oxygen delivery, invasive mechanical ventilation can reduce respiratory muscle oxygen demand and, by increasing intrathoracic pressures, can decrease left ventricular afterload.

  In the acute resuscitation period, adequate oxygenation is essential and oxygen can generally be given fairly liberally; nevertheless, there are some concerns about the microvascular risks associated with high PaO_2 over longer periods, particularly after cardiac arrest [21]. In patients with shock, pulse oximetry can be unreliable because of decreased cutaneous perfusion, and insertion of an arterial catheter is often required to facilitate arterial blood sampling and titration of oxygen.

- **Infuse:** Fluid administration is another cornerstone in the management of patients with shock aimed at increasing cardiac output and improving tissue perfusion. Importantly, fluids should not be restricted in patients with shock who have edema as this may be the result of extravasation, which can decrease intravascular blood volume [22].

  The choice of fluid remains controversial. Essentially, there are two main groups of fluid—the crystalloids and the colloids. The perceived benefit of colloid solutions over crystalloids lies in the fact that colloids remain more and longer in the intravascular space than crystalloids and thus maintain plasma oncotic pressure better, although this difference may be less marked in patients with altered membrane permeability, such as those with sepsis. Nevertheless, in general, less colloid is needed to achieve the same resuscitation endpoints as crystalloid, thus potentially reducing the risks of fluid overload. No study in heterogeneous groups of critically ill patients has demonstrated a beneficial effect on survival of resuscitation with colloid over crystalloid solutions.

The latest Surviving Sepsis Campaign (SSC) guidelines [17] recommend (grade 1B) use of crystalloids as the initial fluid of choice in the resuscitation of patients with sepsis. Although there is some debate about the use of saline solutions in the presence of severe metabolic acidosis because of the chloride load, the clinical impact of this effect is unclear. Recent evidence has suggested that hydroxyethyl starch solutions have no benefit over other crystalloid solutions and may have negative effects on risks of renal failure [23–26], such that these solutions are no longer recommended as first-line fluids [17]. Some studies have suggested that 4 % albumin solutions may be of benefit compared to normal saline in patients with sepsis [27]. Currently, the optimal approach would seem to be to start with balanced crystalloid solutions and then to prescribe further fluids much as one prescribes other drugs, taking into account individual patient characteristics and the beneficial and adverse effects of each fluid type. Although blood transfusions may be required in certain patients, detailed consideration of the indications, benefits, and risks associated with transfusion is beyond the scope of this chapter.

Whichever fluid type is selected, fluid administration needs to be closely monitored to avoid fluid overload. However, assessing fluid requirements can be difficult. The ultimate objective of fluid administration is for cardiac output to become preload independent (i.e., on the plateau portion of the Frank-Starling curve), but static values of effective filling (pressures or volumes) are poor predictors of the response to fluids [28, 29] and should not be used to guide fluid administration. Dynamic measures of fluid responsiveness are increasingly used, including pulse pressure variation and stroke volume variation during mechanical ventilation or after passive leg-raising [29, 30], but each has its limitations.

Fluid challenges should therefore be used to determine the need for ongoing fluid infusion [31]. A fluid challenge incorporates four elements that must be defined in advance:

1. The type of fluid (see earlier).
2. The rate of fluid administration: Typically 300–500 mL are given over 20–30 min [17].
3. The objective: This is generally an increase in arterial pressure in patients in shock, but a decrease in heart rate or an increase in urine output may be alternatives in certain patients.
4. The safety limits: A central venous pressure (CVP) limit slightly above the baseline value is usually set to avoid risks of fluid overload [17].
   Fluid challenges can be repeated as necessary to ensure patients receive adequate fluid administration, but must be stopped if the safety limits are breached or there is no response.

- **Pump:** In the vast majority of patients with circulatory shock, vasoactive agents will be required to help restore adequate perfusion pressure. Vasopressors should be given first and can be started while fluid resuscitation is ongoing, with the aim of reducing doses if possible once normovolemia is established.

Norepinephrine is the preferred vasopressor agent, being associated with lower mortality rates than dopamine in cardiogenic [4] and in septic [32] shock. The usual dose ranges between 0.1 and 2 µg/kg/min. If inotropic agents are needed to increase cardiac output, dobutamine is preferred and should be titrated according to individual patient response.

21.5 Conclusion

Circulatory shock of whatever cause is a life-threatening condition that requires immediate and intensive treatment. Invasive monitoring will likely be necessary to guide resuscitation. The initial management of shock has the same aim regardless of the underlying etiology, i.e., to restore tissue oxygenation. Monitoring of shock relies on assessment of arterial pressure, cardiac output, tissue perfusion abnormalities, and blood lactate concentrations. Monitoring of the microcirculation may help, but further study is needed to confirm this.

References

1. Weil MH, Henning RJ (1979) New concepts in the diagnosis and fluid treatment of circulatory shock. Thirteenth Annual Becton, Dickinson and Company Oscar Schwidetsky Memorial Lecture. Anesth Analg 58:124–132
2. Vincent JL, Ince C, Bakker J (2012) Circulatory shock: an update—a tribute to Professor Max Harry Weil. Crit Care 16:239
3. Weil MH, Shubin H (1971) Proposed reclassification of shock states with special reference to distributive defects. Adv Exp Med Biol 23:13–23
4. De Backer D, Biston P, Devriendt J, Madl C, Chochrad D, Aldecoa C, Brasseur A, Defrance P, Gottignies P, Vincent JL (2010) Comparison of dopamine and norepinephrine in the treatment of shock. N Engl J Med 362:779–789
5. De Backer D, Hollenberg S, Boerma C, Goedhart P, Buchele G, Ospina-Tascon G, Dobbe I, Ince C (2007) How to evaluate the microcirculation: report of a round table conference. Crit Care 11:R101
6. De Backer D, Creteur J, Dubois MJ, Sakr Y, Vincent JL (2004) Microvascular alterations in patients with acute severe heart failure and cardiogenic shock. Am Heart J 147:91–99
7. Sakr Y, Dubois MJ, De Backer D, Creteur J, Vincent JL (2004) Persistent microcirculatory alterations are associated with organ failure and death in patients with septic shock. Crit Care Med 32:1825–1831
8. Trzeciak S, McCoy JV, Phillip DR, Arnold RC, Rizzuto M, Abate NL, Shapiro NI, Parrillo JE, Hollenberg SM (2008) Early increases in microcirculatory perfusion during protocol-directed resuscitation are associated with reduced multi-organ failure at 24 h in patients with sepsis. Intensive Care Med 34:2210–2217
9. Trzeciak S, Dellinger RP, Parrillo JE, Guglielmi M, Bajaj J, Abate NL, Arnold RC, Colilla S, Zanotti S, Hollenberg SM (2007) Early microcirculatory perfusion derangements in patients with severe sepsis and septic shock: relationship to hemodynamics, oxygen transport, and survival. Ann Emerg Med 49(88–98):98
10. den Uil CA, Lagrand WK, van der EM, Jewbali LS, Cheng JM, Spronk PE, Simoons ML (2010) Impaired microcirculation predicts poor outcome of patients with acute myocardial infarction complicated by cardiogenic shock. Eur Heart J 31:3032–3039

11. Broder G, Weil MH (1964) Excess lactate: an index of reversibility of shock in human patients. Science 143:1457–1459
12. Weil MH, Afifi AA (1970) Experimental and clinical studies on lactate and pyruvate as indicators of the severity of acute circulatory failure (shock). Circulation 41:989–1001
13. Vincent JL, Dufaye P, Berre J, Leeman M, Degaute JP, Kahn RJ (1983) Serial lactate determinations during circulatory shock. Crit Care Med 11:449–451
14. Bakker J, Coffernils M, Leon M, Gris P, Vincent JL (1991) Blood lactate levels are superior to oxygen-derived variables in predicting outcome in human septic shock. Chest 99:956–962
15. Nichol AD, Egi M, Pettila V, Bellomo R, French C, Hart G, Davies A, Stachowski E, Reade MC, Bailey M, Cooper DJ (2010) Relative hyperlactatemia and hospital mortality in critically ill patients: a retrospective multi-centre study. Crit Care 14:R25
16. Nichol A, Bailey M, Egi M, Pettila V, French C, Stachowski E, Reade MC, Cooper DJ, Bellomo R (2011) Dynamic lactate indices as predictors of outcome in critically ill patients. Crit Care 15:R242
17. Dellinger RP, Levy MM, Rhodes A, Annane D, Gerlach H, Opal SM, Sevransky JE, Sprung CL, Douglas IS, Jaeschke R, Osborn TM, Nunnally ME, Townsend SR, Reinhart K, Kleinpell RM, Angus DC, Deutschman CS, Machado FR, Rubenfeld GD, Webb SA, Beale RJ, Vincent JL, Moreno R (2013) Surviving sepsis campaign: international guidelines for management of severe sepsis and septic shock: 2012. Crit Care Med 41:580–637
18. Rivers E, Nguyen B, Havstad S, Ressler J, Muzzin A, Knoblich B, Peterson E, Tomlanovich M (2001) Early goal-directed therapy in the treatment of severe sepsis and septic shock. N Engl J Med 345:1368–1377
19. Jansen TC, van Bommel J, Schoonderbeek FJ, Sleeswijk Visser SJ, van der Klooster JM, Lima AP, Willemsen SP, Bakker J (2010) Early lactate-guided therapy in intensive care unit patients: a multicenter, open-label, randomized controlled trial. Am J Respir Crit Care Med 182:752–761
20. Weil MH, Shubin H (1969) The "VIP" approach to the bedside management of shock. JAMA 207:337–340
21. Kilgannon JH, Jones AE, Shapiro NI, Angelos MG, Milcarek B, Hunter K, Parrillo JE, Trzeciak S (2010) Association between arterial hyperoxia following resuscitation from cardiac arrest and in-hospital mortality. JAMA 303:2165–2171
22. da Luz PL, Weil MH, Liu VY, Shubin H (1974) Plasma volume prior to and following volume loading during shock complicating acute myocardial infarction. Circulation 49:98–105
23. Brunkhorst FM, Engel C, Bloos F, Meier-Hellmann A, Ragaller M, Weiler N, Moerer O, Gruendling M, Oppert M, Grond S, Olthoff D, Jaschinski U, John S, Rossaint R, Welte T, Schaefer M, Kern P, Kuhnt E, Kiehntopf M, Hartog C, Natanson C, Loeffler M, Reinhart K (2008) Intensive insulin therapy and pentastarch resuscitation in severe sepsis. N Engl J Med 358:125–139
24. Perner A, Haase N, Guttormsen AB, Tenhunen J, Klemenzson G, Aneman A, Madsen KR, Moller MH, Elkjaer JM, Poulsen LM, Bendtsen A, Winding R, Steensen M, Berezowicz P, Soe-Jensen P, Bestle M, Strand K, Wiis J, White JO, Thornberg KJ, Quist L, Nielsen J, Andersen LH, Holst LB, Thormar K, Kjaeldgaard AL, Fabritius ML, Mondrup F, Pott FC, Moller TP, Winkel P, Wetterslev J (2012) Hydroxyethyl starch 130/0.42 versus Ringer's acetate in severe sepsis. N Engl J Med 367:124–134
25. Guidet B, Martinet O, Boulain T, Philippart F, Poussel JF, Maizel J, Forceville X, Feissel M, Hasselmann M, Heininger A, Van Aken H (2012) Assessment of hemodynamic efficacy and safety of 6% hydroxyethylstarch 130/0.4 vs. 0.9% NaCl fluid replacement in patients with severe sepsis: The CRYSTMAS study. Crit Care 16:R94
26. Myburgh JA, Finfer S, Bellomo R, Billot L, Cass A, Gattas D, Glass P, Lipman J, Liu B, McArthur C, McGuinness S, Rajbhandari D, Taylor CB, Webb SA (2012) Hydroxyethyl starch or saline for fluid resuscitation in intensive care. N Engl J Med 367:1901–1911

27. Finfer S, McEvoy S, Bellomo R, McArthur C, Myburgh J, Norton R (2011) Impact of albumin compared to saline on organ function and mortality of patients with severe sepsis. Intensive Care Med 37:86–96
28. Osman D, Ridel C, Ray P, Monnet X, Anguel N, Richard C, Teboul JL (2007) Cardiac filling pressures are not appropriate to predict hemodynamic response to volume challenge. Crit Care Med 35:64–68
29. Marik PE, Cavallazzi R, Vasu T, Hirani A (2009) Dynamic changes in arterial waveform derived variables and fluid responsiveness in mechanically ventilated patients: a systematic review of the literature. Crit Care Med 37:2642–2647
30. Cavallaro F, Sandroni C, Marano C, La Torre G, Mannocci A, de Waure C, Bello G, Maviglia R, Antonelli M (2010) Diagnostic accuracy of passive leg raising for prediction of fluid responsiveness in adults: systematic review and meta-analysis of clinical studies. Intensive Care Med 36:1475–1483
31. Vincent JL, Weil MH (2006) Fluid challenge revisited. Crit Care Med 34:1333–1337
32. De Backer D, Aldecoa C, Njimi H, Vincent JL (2012) Dopamine versus norepinephrine in the treatment of septic shock: a meta-analysis. Crit Care Med 40:725–730

Resuscitation and Ethics: How to Deal with the "Do not Resuscitate Order"?

22

Cristina Santonocito, Filippo Sanfilippo, Giuseppe Ristagno and Antonino Gullo

22.1 Introduction

Resuscitation has the ability to reverse death, but it can also prolong terminal illness, and cause patient's discomfort [1]. A "do not resuscitate" (DNR) order is one of the most important patient care directives. It is a written medical option that documents patient's wishes regarding resuscitation and patient's desire to avoid overtreatment [2]. Indeed, DNR has irreversible consequences.

There are a few important concepts for a better DNR understanding: "medical futility," "informed consent," and "informed assent."

The definition and value of the "futility" principle in medical decision refers to treatments recognized as nonbeneficial or ineffective [3]. The principle of futility is currently being used in clinical practice. The informed consent should be obtained and signed directly by the person performing the procedure. Because the process

C. Santonocito (✉) · F. Sanfilippo
Cardiothoracic Critical Care, Oxford Heart Centre, John Radcliffe Hospital, Oxford University Hospitals, Oxford, Oxfordshire OX3 9DU, UK
e-mail: cristina.santonocito@gmail.com

F. Sanfilippo
e-mail: filipposanfi@yahoo.it

G. Ristagno
IRCCS, Istituto di Ricerche Farmacologiche "Mario Negri", Via La Masa 19, 20156, Milan, Italy
e-mail: gristag@gmail.com

A. Gullo
Department of Anaesthesia and Intensive Care, Medical School of Catania "Policlinico-Vittorio Emanuele", Via S.Sofia, 78, 95123, Catania, Italy
e-mail: a.gullo@policlinico.unict.it

A. Gullo and G. Ristagno (eds.), *Resuscitation*,
DOI: 10.1007/978-88-470-5507-0_22, © Springer-Verlag Italia 2014

of obtaining "informed consent" may be stressful for the patient and his family, it has been agreed that obtaining "informed assent," by which the patient or family is explicitly invited to defer to clinician's judgment for treatment decision is an appropriate, ethical alternative [4]. Nevertheless, this alternative should not be offered when clinicians are uncertain about the patient's prognosis. It is recommended that clinicians should address careful attention to the particular wishes and needs of specific patients and families and should spend enough time with them during the consent obtaining process.

22.2 Ethics and Communication

Looking at the international policies, different attitudes are shown toward the so-called advanced directives (ADs) and often confusion remains on how they have to be followed. Indeed, European, Australian, and American healthcare systems are working on their implementation [5]. Regarding ADs, and especially the DNR order, it is important to consider that the motivating moral idea behind them is the same as the informed consent. DNR, in fact, in essence, represents a proactive informed refusal of therapies, and more specifically of resuscitation maneuvers, in a future state. It is well recognized that one of the moral bases for informed consent is respect for patient's autonomous wishes, according to the four cardinal ethical points reported in Table 22.1.

Although unlikely, ADs are frequently discussed and considered during stressful and urgent circumstances, in the Emergency Room and in the Intensive Care Unit. For this reason, discussions about DNR order should be considered and implemented as an essential part of the standard of care. The conversation ought also to continue after patients have filled out any forms, as the goal of the discussion is the development of a worldview regarding future medical care by the patient. People will be able to change their ADs over time, and this point should be clearly thought linked with good communication skills by the healthcare professionals dealing with patients potentially involved in DNR order. In the USA, the physician's attitude to discuss about this issue with patient is raising over time. It should be desirable that this discussion should take place not only when the patient is near to the end of his life, but in earlier times. The discussion is aimed at expressing the values that could help in guiding a decision-making process when

Table 22.1 The four cardinal ethical points

Autonomy	The right of the patient to accept or refuse any treatment
Not malefiency	Doing no harm or, even more appropriate, no further harm
Beneficial	Implies that healthcare providers must provide benefits in the best interest of the individual patient while balancing benefits and risks
Justice	Implies the concern and duty to distribute limited health resources equally within a society, and the decision of who gets what treatment (fairness and equality).

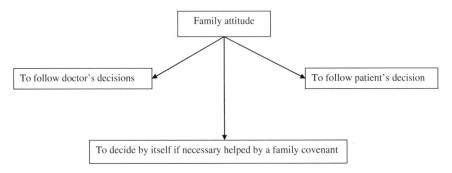

Fig. 22.1 Family attitude in case of end-of-life care

the patient is unable to make his own decisions. In the USA, it is, otherwise, possible to have a family covenant, an open healthcare agreement that can facilitate advance care planning. Since the individual values are the relevant features of ADs, making those values clear and explicit can greatly assist the family and physicians to achieve patient's benefit, as detailed in Fig. 22.1. It is also necessary to identify how nurses and physicians perceive end-of-life care so that their communication can be improved [6]. The most common attitude is that physicians are more likely to discuss DNR orders only when the patient's prognosis is poor. However, often, despite the short surviving time, cancer patients have no ADs and this may be an indicator of suboptimal doctor–patient communication [7]. Moreover, terminology often lacks full consensus, i.e., it has been proposed that "DNR" represents a problematic, especially from a legal point of view, sentence and should be replaced with "allow natural death" (AND) [8].

22.3   Legal Aspects

After the mid-1970s, the decision "not to resuscitate" was first legalized and in the USA the American Medical Association first recommended that decisions to forego resuscitation be formally documented. Importantly, it was emphasized that CPR was intended for the prevention of a sudden, unexpected death—not the treatment of a terminal, irreversible illness [9]. Explicit DNR policies soon followed. However, there was no clarity about the DNR order until the Cruzan case in USA, 1990. On that occasion, the Justice emphasized the importance of clear oral and written instructions prior to incapacity, as well as clear appointment of durable powers of attorney as means for the incompetent individual to exercise choices. After that case, the Patient Self-Determination Act (PSDA), with the intent to reduce the number of situations in which patients did not have written ADs went into effect, making ADs legally acceptable by statute in all 50 US states [10]. The DNR issue was considered not only in the out-of-hospital scene but also in perioperative time. However, after the 1990s, DNR orders were routinely suspended during the intraoperative and immediate postoperative periods. Finally, the American Society of Anesthesiologists formalized this policy in a set of guidelines approved in 1993 and updated in 1998 [11, 12].

At present, there is no standardized DNR policy for the whole healthcare system in USA. In several countries, this issue is faced in different ways depending on religious, cultural, historical, and ethical differences existing between people. There is evidence of a lack about a universal DNR order policy around the world as shown in Table 22.2 [13–18].

Table 22.2 DNR order around the world

Country	Policy
USA	signed consent policy witnessed verbal consent policy
South America	oral orders take preference ADs: physician thinks to share with the patient in decision making
UK	an advance refusal has legal force
Spain	DNR decisions are clearly indicated to limit the therapeutic effort
France	directives by the patient's family or a surrogate decision maker have only a consultative role care decisions are made after a collegial procedure
Belgium	law regulating euthanasia End-of-life decisions often occur within the context of multidisciplinary care
Norway	withholding and/or withdrawing life-sustaining treatment were taken in the aftermath of a DNR order
Netherlands	euthanasia and self-written ADs are legally binding
Italy	Guidelines (SIAARTI) but there is no law The doctors decide what to do trying to respect and giving a right interpretation of patient's will
Israel	No consensual practice strong ethnic and religious beliefs (e.g., Jewish religion considers the dying event as an uninterrupted, peaceful transition from life to death)
China	it is preferable that dying people exhale their last breath at home more DNR orders being written
Japan	The physicians could institute DNR order without consulting the family when the physician feels that a CPR is unjustified and futile (The Japan Society for Dying with Dignity)
Australia and New Zealand	most of the patients prefer DNR orders to 'good palliative care' orders and prefer written orders

22.4 Future Goals

The need for standardization appears clear in all countries and several contributions support the target for achieving a consensus in this critical issue [19, 20]:

1. *Good communication and discussion are essential* between patient, family, religious representative, and hospital staff to clarify the patient's preferences if him/her is still mentally competent. Formal physician education on this issue is urgently needed and should be considered as a part of the formative curriculum for undergraduate and postgraduate doctors and nurses.
2. *Provide psychosocial support so the patients feel comfortable in expressing their preferences.* Avoiding futile interventions would be an important step to increase trust between patient and healthcare system. If an intervention is determined to be ineffective, the physician is under no ethical obligation to offer, provide, or continue it, because it is important to respect patient's autonomy.
3. *Improving standards and quality of care in authorizing a DNR order.*
4. *Recognize that ADs (living wills) are associated with end-of-life expenditures and treatments*, particularly, with a significantly lower level of Medicare spending.
5. *Continuing education on professionalism.* Ethical values in clinical practice, especially patient autonomy, should be addressed during early stage of the medical curriculum. Education, scholarship, and ethical values are proclaimed by the Medical Professional in which among several concepts, also *respect for others and self-regulation*, are included.

22.5 Conclusions

Professional reflection is required on end-of-life care and the "DNR" order. Despite the ardent desire to sustain life, medical professionals should withstand the temptation to act when the patient's wish is to not be resuscitated. Rather than perceiving that they are doing nothing, something has indeed been done; the patient's wishes have been respected, their autonomy has been preserved, and they have been allowed to die with dignity. Complying with these wishes represents a real challenge for patients and their families, physicians, nurses, and also the community.

References

1. Vincent JL (2005) Outcome and ethics in severe brain damage. Prog Brain Res 150:555–563
2. Payne JK, Thornlow DK (2008) Clinical perspectives on portable do-not-resuscitate orders. J Gerontol Nurs 34(10):11–16
3. The Ethics Committee of the Society of Critical Care Medicine (1997) Consensus statement of the society of critical care medicine's ethics committee regarding futile and other possibly inadvisable treatments. Crit Care Med 25:887–891

4. Curtis JR, Burt RA (2007) Point: the ethics of unilateral "do not resuscitate" orders: the role of "informed assent". Chest 132(3):748–751
5. Kierzek G, Rac V, Pourriat JL (2010) Advance directives and surrogate decision making before death. N Engl J Med 363(3):295
6. Curtis JR, Vincent JL (2010) Ethics and end-of-life care for adults in the intensive care unit. Lancet 376(9749):1347–1353
7. Guo Y, Palmer JL, Bianty J et al (2010) Advance directives and do-not-resuscitate orders in patients with cancer with metastatic spinal cord compression: advanced care planning implications. J Palliat Med 13(5):513–517
8. Venneman SS, Narnor-Harris P, Perish M et al (2008) "Allow natural death" versus "do not resuscitate": three words that can change a life. J Med Ethics 34(1):2–6
9. National Conference on Cardiopulmonary Resuscitation (CPR) and Emergency Cardiac Care (ECC) (1986) Standards and guidelines for cardiopulmonary resuscitation (CPR) and emergency cardiac care (ECC). Part VIII: medicolegal considerations and recommendations. JAMA 255(21):2979–2984
10. Stephen SS, Doukas DJ (2009) Advance directives. The penn center guide to bioethics. Springer, pp 749–754
11. Truog RD (1991) Do-not-resuscitate orders during anesthesia and surgery. Anesthesiology 74:606–608
12. American society of anesthesiologists ethical guidelines for the anesthesia care of patients with do-not-resuscitate orders or other directives that limit care (1998) American Society of Anesthesiologists 1999 Directory of Members. American Society of Anesthesiologists, Park Ridge, pp 470–471
13. Holley A, Kravet SJ, Cordts G (2009) Documentation of code status and discussion of goals of care in gravely ill hospitalized patients. J Crit Care 24(2):288–292
14. Cohen RI, Lisker GN, Eichhorn A et al (2009) The impact of do-not-resuscitate order on triage decisions to a medical intensive care unit. J Crit Care 24(2):311–315
15. Vincent JL, Berré J, Creteur J (2004) Withholding and withdrawing life prolonging treatment in the intensive care unit: a current European perspective. Chron Respir Dis 1(2):115–120
16. Van den Block L, Deschepper R, Bilsen J et al (2009) Euthanasia and other end of life decisions and care provided in final three months of life: nationwide retrospective study in Belgium. BMJ 339:b2772
17. SIAARTI—Italian Society of Anaesthesia Analgesia Resuscitation and Intensive Care Bioethical Board (2006) End-of-life care and the intensivist: SIAARTI recommendations on the management of the dying patient. Minerva Anestesiol 72:927–963
18. Jaing TH, Tsay PK, Fang EC et al (2007) "Do-not-resuscitate" orders in patients with cancer at a children's hospital in Taiwan. J Med Ethics 33(4):194–196
19. Shetty P (2010) The parlous state of palliative care in the developing world. Lancet 376(9751):1453–1454
20. Nicholas LH, Langa KM, Iwashyna TJ et al (2011) Regional variation in the association between advance directives and end-of-life Medicare expenditures. JAMA 306(13):1447–1453

Translational Research: An Ongoing Challenge in Cardiac Arrest

23

Antonino Gullo

...time is necessary for teachers to teach, for learners to learn, and...for the education process to be long enough for major educational objectives to be met.

M. H. Weil (1927–2011).

23.1 Background

Cardiovascular disease is the first cause of mortality in developed countries. The heart responds to many pathological conditions with hypertrophic growth by enlarging individual myocytes to augment the cardiac pump function and to decrease ventricular wall tension. Initially, such cardiac elements are often compensatory, but as time progresses these changes evidence subclinical and/or symptomatic grading of dysfunction. Cardiac remodeling and hypertrophy are the major predictors leading to heart failure and dangerous arrhythmias, ultimately determining a condition of sudden cardiac death (SCA) [1].

Advances in medicine emerge from molecular and genetic studies of cardiovascular disease in experimental models and in patients at risk. In the last 20 years selected therapeutic targets have emerged and have a tangible translational potential given the available pharmacologic agents that could be readily evaluated in human observations and in clinical trials [2]. Indeed, there is growing evidence of the importance of translational science and medicine, according to the bench-bedside concept, in the improvement of patient outcome, even though the definitions of translational science, translational medicine, and clinical medicine need to be further clarified. In other words, clinical and translational medicine are expected to include scientific and regulatory investigations to translate preclinical research to clinical application with a specific emphasis on new biotechnologies, biomaterials, bioengineering, disease-specific biomarkers, cellular and molecular

A. Gullo (✉)

Dipartimento di Anestesia e Terapia Intensiva Catania, Scuola di Medicina, Università di Catania, Via Santa Sofia 78 (Padiglione 1), 95123, Catania, Italy
e-mail: gullounict@libero.it

A. Gullo and G. Ristagno (eds.), *Resuscitation*,
DOI: 10.1007/978-88-470-5507-0_23, © Springer-Verlag Italia 2014

medicine, 'omics science, bioinformatics, applied immunology, molecular imaging, drug discovery and development, and health policy regulation.

Translational medicine should meet the increasing demand for expanding the biomedical workforce and education programs that attract and retain young people to the translational biomedical science. In the present perspective we selected a series of contributions, a sort of decalogue about clinical and translational medicine, to support the efforts of scientists and clinicians to understand better the mechanisms of biological and cellular disorders in animal models, in human being studies, and in the clinical randomized controlled trials. This dynamic concept is maintained and supported by continuing education and training programs to save lives. The central pillar to implement guidelines and ultimately the clinical outcome is based on the importance of translation research to guide future directions and perspectives in the field of resuscitation science.

23.2 Sudden Cardiac Arrest

Cardiac arrest is a dramatic condition leading to sudden death if two determinant interventions, basic life support, and early defibrillation, cannot be performed on time. In coincidence with the decreased mortality from coronary artery disease, there is evidence pointing toward a decrease in rates of SCA in the United States during the second half of the twentieth century. However, the alarming rise in prevalence of obesity and diabetes in the first decade of the new millennium both in the United States and worldwide, would indicate that this favorable trend is unlikely to persist [3]. SCA is a complex phenotype, and determinants are likely to be multifactorial. More recently, an additional significant genetic component has been considered in the context of multiple cardiac conditions, comorbidities, as well as epidemiologic and environmental factors [4].

In real life, the critical time intervals, in part based on the Utstein templates for documenting the sequence of interventions [5], begins with the call for emergency assistance, documents arrival time of rescuers including bystander, the interventions performed by the emergency medical responders at the site of the victim, and the sequences of interventions that follow. In the instance of ventricular fibrillation (VF), automated external defibrillation (AED) has enfranchised non professional rescuers to reverse VF. Current evidence supports the value of a well-organized program of bystanders initiated CPR and, in some settings, public access defibrillation [6]. Within the past year, the Chain of Survival has been amended to include an additional link, namely post-resuscitation management [7]. The therapeutic management of patients that recover spontaneous circulation, based on life support measures and a series of actions based on "clinical judgment," might not be the best way to treat patients with post-cardiac arrest syndrome. The use of the goal-guided protocols to manage these patients including therapeutic measures of proven efficacy, such as mild therapeutic hypothermia and early revascularization, when indicated, can improve the prognosis considerably in these patients [8].

In this sense, the term cardiopulmonary and cerebral resuscitation proposed by scientists and practitioners might be more appropriate.

An alternative approach to improve survival from SCA is to use the continuous quality improvement (CQI) approach, a process often used to address public health problems. CQI advocates that one obtains baseline survival rate for his/her field of action and uses this baseline data to achieve improvements under a continuous re-evaluation process. Using CQI, significant improvement in survival of patients with out-of-hospital cardiac arrest has been achieved. For example, Drs. Ewy and Sanders from Arizona recommended that all emergency medical systems determined their baseline survival rates from cardiac arrest and considered implementing the CQI approach if the community did not obtain a neurologically intact survival rate of at least 30 % [9].

The translation of basic science into everyday clinical practice may be difficult and it still remains a major issue in contemporary medicine. For this purpose, a new discipline has been created, the translational research, which has been trying to assess the discrepancies between research and clinical field. Translational research is a continuum of research in which basic science discovering is integrated into clinical applications and clinical observations are used to generate scientific topics of basic science [10]. Research to advance cardiac arrest knowledge is a difficult task. Experts set up a series of guidelines that represent a keystone for educational needs and evolving technology.

23.3 Decalogue of Translation Research

The official definition of translational research as stated by the National Institute of Health (NIH) is as follows: "Translational research transforms scientific discoveries arising from laboratory, clinical or population studies into new clinical tools and applications that improve human health by reducing disease incidence, morbidity and mortality" (modified from "Transforming Translation—Harnessing Discovery for Patient and Public Benefit"—Report of the Translational Research Working Group of the National Cancer Advisory Board, US NIH, 2007).

Translational research moves in a bidirectional manner from one type of research to another—from basic research to patient-oriented research, to population-based research, and back—and involves collaboration among scientists from multiple disciplines. Research in resuscitation training should be considered an example of translational science, where rigorous studies of skill acquisition with outcome measures serve to transfer the results to the clinical environment for analysis of their impact upon patient care [11]. Medicine moves basic biological discoveries from the research bench to the patient-care setting and uses clinical observations to inform basic biology. It focuses on patient care, including the creation of new diagnostics, prognostics, prevention strategies, and therapies based on biological discoveries. Bioinformatics involves algorithms to represent, store, and analyze basic biological data, including DNA sequence, RNA expression, and

Table 23.1 Decalogue of translation research

Pharmacology, regenerative medicine, and tissue engineering
Inflammation during resuscitation
Oxygenation during and after cardiopulmonary resuscitation
Cardioprotection
Vasopressor agents for cardiopulmonary resuscitation
Amplitude Spectrum Area (AMSA)
Na^+/H^+ channelpathies and pharmacological defibrillation
Brain ischemia/reperfusion
Therapeutic hypothermia
Kynurenine pathway

protein and small-molecule abundance within cells. Translational bioinformatics spans these two fields; it involves the development of algorithms to analyze basic molecular and cellular data with an explicit goal of affecting clinical care. In this section of the book the authors summarize some experimental and clinical aspects of translation research in the field of resuscitation (Table 23.1).

23.3.1 Pharmacology, Regenerative Medicine, and Tissue Engineering

Regenerative medicine is a rapidly evolving multidisciplinary, translational research field whose explicit purpose is to advance technologies for the repair and replacement of damaged cells, tissues, and organs [12]. Scientific progress in the field has been steady and expectations for its robust clinical application continue to rise. Indeed, in 2007, the phrase "regenerative pharmacology" was coined to describe the enormous possibilities that could occur at the interface between pharmacology, regenerative medicine, and tissue engineering. The operational definition of regenerative pharmacology is "the application of pharmacological sciences to accelerate, optimize, and characterize (either in vitro or in vivo) the development, maturation, and function of bioengineered and regenerating tissues." Thus, regenerative pharmacology seeks to cure disease through restoration of tissue/organ function. This strategy is distinct from standard pharmacotherapy, which is often limited to the amelioration of symptoms. The goal here is to get pharmacologists more involved in this field of research by exposing them to the tools, opportunities, challenges, and interdisciplinary expertise that will be required to ensure awareness and galvanize involvement. Christ and coworkers reported that science can drive future innovations in regenerative medicine and tissue engineering and thus help to revolutionize the discovery of curative therapeutics [13]. In the setting of cardiac arrest, Dr. Wang and colleagues have reported that administration of allogeneic bone marrow mesenchymal stem cells improved myocardial function and survival after cardiopulmonary resuscitation in myocardial infarcted rats [14].

23.3.2 Inflammation During Resuscitation

Proinflammatory mediators such as tumor necrosis factor-alpha (TNFα) have been implicated in the pathophysiology of a number of acute disease states. TNFα can contribute to cell death, apoptosis, and organ dysfunction. It can be generated during sepsis or ischemia-reperfusion by activation of cell mitogen-activated protein kinases and nuclear factor kappa B. A number of strategies to modulate TNF have been recently explored, including factors directed toward mitogen-activated protein kinases, TNFα transcription, anti-inflammatory ligands, heat shock proteins, and TNF-binding proteins. However, TNFα may also play an important role in the adaptive response to injury and inflammation. Control of the deleterious effects of TNFα and other proinflammatory cytokines represents a realistic goal for clinical emergency medicine [15]. Indeed, an important inflammatory response, similar to a sepsis-like syndrome, occurs after resuscitation from cardiac arrest [16]. Interactions among pleiotropic mediators, coagulation abnormalities, activation of the inflammatory cytokine cascade, chemokine upregulation, and ultimately recruitment of inflammatory leukocytes and reactive astrogliosis have been reported after cardiac arrest and are major players in the final outcome [16, 17]. Several translational approaches have been investigated in animal models of cardiac arrest and proposed to the clinical scenario such to mitigate the post-resuscitation inflammation, i.e., hypothermia and/or therapeutic gases [18, 19].

23.3.3 Oxygenation During and After Cardiopulmonary Resuscitation

Reversal of tissue hypoxia, particularly in the heart and brain, is a fundamental goal of cardiopulmonary resuscitation. However, a growing body of evidence suggests that hyperoxia, especially after return of spontaneous circulation, may worsen outcome. Therefore, the concept of controlled oxygenation during and after cardiac arrest has become determinant [20, 21].

Animal studies over the last two decades have built a compelling case that arterial hyperoxemia during the first hours after resuscitation causes increased oxidative damage, increased neuronal death, and worse neurological function. In a meta-analysis of animal studies, treatment with 100 % oxygen resulted in a significantly worse neurological deficit score than oxygen administered at lower concentrations, with a standardized mean difference of -0.64 (95 % CI -1.06 to

−0.22). In four of five studies, histological evidence of increased neuronal damage was present in animals that received 100 % oxygen therapy. The administration of 100 % oxygen therapy was therefore associated with worse neurological outcome than lower oxygen concentrations in animal models of cardiac arrest [21].

However, human data are limited [22–24]. There are conflicting findings from observational studies regarding the nature of the association between hyperoxia and risk of mortality in patients admitted to intensive care following cardiac arrest. The only prospective randomized clinical trial comparing different inspired oxygen concentrations in post-cardiac arrest patients was underpowered to detect a difference in survival or neurologic outcome. More recently, a retrospective analysis of data from a multicenter registry found that initial arterial hyperoxemia (paO2 $\geq$ 300 mmHg) was associated with increased mortality and worse functional outcome in patients admitted to the intensive unit care after cardiac arrest. The existing evidence, though limited, has contributed to new guidelines for oxygen therapy in patients resuscitated from cardiac arrest. The benefit of supplemental oxygen during cardiopulmonary resuscitation remains uncertain. However, in patients who achieve resuscitation after cardiac arrest, available evidence supports adjusting inspired oxygen content to avoid arterial hyperoxemia while providing adequate arterial oxyhemoglobin saturation. This strategy is likely to be most effective when initiated as soon as possible and appears to be most important during the first hours after resuscitation. Definitive clinical trials are needed to determine the ultimate impact on outcome.

23.3.4 Cardioprotection

The National Heart, Lung, and Blood Institute convened a Workshop on September 20–21, 2010, called "New Horizons in Cardioprotection," to identify future research directions for cardioprotection against ischemia and reperfusion injury. Since the early 1970s, there has been evidence that the size of a myocardial infarction (MI) could be altered by various interventions. Early coronary artery reperfusion has been an intervention that consistently reduces myocardial infarct size in animal models as well as in humans. Pharmacological adjunctive therapies have failed to either reduce infarct size or improve clinical outcome. However, some adjunctive therapies have shown promise in data subanalyses or subpopulations of clinical trials (adenosine, therapeutic hypothermia, and hyperoxemic reperfusion) or in small clinical trials (atrial natriuretic peptide, ischemic postconditioning, and cyclosporine, the mitochondrial permeability transition pore inhibitor) [25]. Indeed, over the past 30 years, hundreds of experimental interventions (both pharmacological and nonpharmacological) have been reported to protect the ischemic myocardium in experimental animals; however, with the exception of early reperfusion, none of them has been translated succesfully into the clinical practice.

The National Heart, Lung, and Blood Institute convened a working group to discuss the reasons for the failure to translate potential therapies for protecting the heart from ischemia and reperfusion and to recommend new approaches to accomplish this goal. The Working Group concluded that cardioprotection in the setting of acute myocardial infarction, cardiac surgery, and cardiac arrest was at a crossroad. Present basic research approaches to identify cardioprotective therapies are inefficient and counterproductive. For three decades, significant resources have been invested in single-center studies that have often yielded inconclusive results. A new paradigm is needed to obviate many of the difficulties associated with translation of basic science findings. The Working Group urged a new focus on translational research that emphasizes efficacy and clinically relevant outcomes, and recommended the establishment of a system for rigorous preclinical testing of promising cardioprotective agents with clinical trial-like approaches (i.e., blinded, randomized, multicenter, and adequately powered studies using standardized methods). Accordingly, a national preclinical research consortium would enable rational translation of important basic science findings into clinical use [26].

23.3.5 Vasopressor Agents for Cardiopulmonary Resuscitation

The primary goal of cardiopulmonary resuscitation is to reestablish blood flow to vital organs until spontaneous circulation is restored. Adrenergic vasopressor agents produce systemic vasoconstriction. This increases aortic diastolic pressure, and consequently, coronary and cerebral perfusion pressures. The pharmacologic responses to the adrenergic agents are mediated by a group of receptors that are classified as alpha (alpha), including alpha1 and alpha2, and beta (beta), including beta1 and beta2. Epinephrine, which has each of these adrenergic actions, has been the preferred adrenergic agent for the management of cardiac arrest for almost 40 years. Its primary efficacy is due to its alpha-adrenergic vasopressor effects. This contrasts with its beta-adrenergic actions, which are inotropic, chronotropic, and vasodilator. Accordingly, beta-adrenergic actions prompt increases in myocardial oxygen consumption, ectopic ventricular arrhythmias, and transient hypoxemia due to pulmonary arteriovenous shunting. This may account for the failure to demonstrate that epinephrine improves ultimate outcome in human victims of cardiac arrest. Accordingly, epinephrine, the primary pharmacological intervention in the treatment of cardiac arrest, improves only the immediate outcome [27]. Major interest has more recently been focused on selective alpha-adrenergic agonists [28]. Both alpha1-agonists and alpha2-agonists are peripheral vasopressors. However, rapid desensitization of alpha1-adrenergic receptors occurs during cardiopulmonary resuscitation. Moreover, alpha1-adrenergic receptors are present in the myocardium, and beta1-agonists, like beta-adrenergic agonists, increase myocardial oxygen consumption. If they cross the blood–brain barrier, alpha2-adrenoceptor agonists also have centrally acting vasodilator effects. In the absence of central nervous system access, alpha2-adrenergic agonists have selective peripheral vasoconstrictor effects. Experimentally, these selective alpha2-agonists have been reported to be as effective as epinephrine for initial cardiac resuscitation and have the additional advantage of minimizing myocardial oxygen consumption during the global myocardial ischemia of cardiac arrest. The effects of selective alpha[2]-adrenergic agonist alpha-methylnorepinephrine (alpha-MNE) on the initial success of resuscitation and post-resuscitation myocardial function were compared with nonselective alpha- and beta-adrenergic epinephrine in a swine model of cardiac arrest. Ejection fraction was reduced by 35 % and 14 % by epinephrine and alpha-MNE, respectively, after resuscitation. Epinephrine and alpha-MNE increased post-resuscitation heart rate by 38 % and 15 %, respectively. Accordingly, significantly less post-resuscitation impairment followed the administration of alpha-MNE [29]. The combination of epinephrine and vasopressin may be effective, but has been incompletely studied. Clinical trials of vasopressor agents, which minimize direct myocardial effects are needed [30].

23.3.6 Na$^+$/H$^+$ Channelpathies and Pharmacological Defibrillation

Voltage-gated Na(+) channels are essential for the amplitude and upstroke velocity of the cardiac action potential, which are important determinants for impulse propagation and impulse conduction velocity throughout the working myocardium. Mutations in the major cardiac Na(+) channel gene SCN5A have been implicated in rare, familial forms of cardiac arrhythmias, namely LQT3, Brugada syndrome, progressive cardiac conduction disorder, and sudden infant death syndrome. Indeed, it is now recognized that mutations that increase Na$^+$ current (INa) delay cardiac repolarization, prolong action potential duration, and cause long QT syndrome, while mutations that reduce INa decrease cardiac excitability, reduce electrical conduction velocity, and induce Brugada syndrome, progressive cardiac conduction disease, sick sinus syndrome, or combinations thereof. Recently, mutation-induced INa dysfunction was also linked to dilated cardiomyopathy, atrial fibrillation, and sudden infant death syndrome. It is increasingly recognized that such mutations, apart from changing channel gating characteristics, may also be related to changes in channel protein trafficking and expression. Regulation of ion channel protein expression depends on a fine-tuned balance among various processes, such as gene transcription, RNA processing, protein synthesis, assembly and post-translational modification, the transport to the cell surface, the anchoring to the cytoskeleton, and regulation of endocytosis and controlled degradation of the protein [31]. While clinical and genetic studies have laid the foundation for our understanding of cardiac sodium channelopathies by establishing links between arrhythmogenic diseases and mutations in genes that encode various subunits of the cardiac sodium channel, biophysical studies (particularly in heterologous expression systems and transgenic mouse models) have provided insights into the mechanisms by which INa dysfunction causes disease in such channelopathies.

Amin and coworkers described the structure and function of the cardiac sodium channel and its various subunits, summarizing major cardiac sodium channelopathies and the current knowledge concerning their genetic background and underlying molecular mechanisms, and discussing recent advances in the discovery of mutation-specific therapies in the management of these channelopathies [32, 33]. Indeed, the concept of Na^+-H^+ exchange (NHE) involvement in cardiac pathology has been exposed for decades and supported by a plethora of experimental studies demonstrating salutary effects of NHE inhibition in protecting the myocardium against ischemic and reperfusion injury as well as attenuating myocardial remodeling and heart failure. NHE is actually a family of sodium and proton transporting proteins of which 10 isoforms have been identified. Myocardial NHE is represented primarily by the ubiquitous NHE-1 subtype which is expressed in most tissues. The robust positive results seen with NHE-1 inhibitors in experimental studies have led to a relatively rapid development of these pharmacological agents for clinical assessment, especially as potential cardioprotective therapies. Episodes of VF and myocardial dysfunction commonly occur after cardiac resuscitation compromising the return of stable circulation. Gazmuri and coworkers investigated in a pig model of VF whether limiting $Na(+)$-induced cytosolic $Ca(2+)$ overload using the sarcolemmal (NHE-1) inhibitor cariporide. Cariporide administered at the start of chest compression helped to restore electrically and mechanically stable circulation after resuscitation from cardiac arrest [34].

The EXPEDITION study addressed the efficacy and safety of inhibiting the NHE-1 by cariporide in the prevention of death or MI in patients undergoing coronary artery bypass graft surgery. The premise was that inhibition of NHE-1 limits intracellcular Na^+ accumulation and thereby limits Na/Ca-exchanger-mediated calcium overload to reduce infarct size. Surprisingly, the incidence of death or MI was reduced from 20.3 % in the placebo group to 16.6 % in the treatment group ($p = 0.0002$). Paradoxically, MI alone declined from 18.9 % in the placebo group to 14.4 % in the treatment group ($p = 0.000005$), while mortality alone increased from 1.5 % in the placebo group to 2.2 % with cariporide ($p = 0.02$). The increase in mortality was associated with an increase in cerebrovascular events. Unlike the salutary effects that were maintained at 6 months, the difference in mortality at 6 months was not significant. As a result of the increased mortality associated with an increase in cerebrovascular events, it was considered unlikely that cariporide would have been used clinically [35].

23.3.7 Amplitude Spectrum Area

High quality cardiopulmonary resuscitation and prompt defibrillation when appropriate (i.e., in VF and pulseless ventricular tachycardia) are currently the best early treatment for cardiac arrest. In cases of prolonged cardiac arrest due to shockable rhythms, it is reasonable to presume that a period of CPR before defibrillation could partially revert the metabolic and hemodynamic deteriorations imposed on the heart by the no flow state, thus increasing the chances of successful defibrillation. Despite supporting early evidences in cardiac arrest cases in which Emergency Medical System response time was longer than 5 min, recent studies have failed to confirm a survival benefit of routine CPR before defibrillation. These data have imposed a change in guidelines from 2005 to 2010. Taking into account all the variables encountered when treating cardiac arrest (heart condition before cardiac arrest, time elapsed, metabolic and hemodynamic changes, efficacy of CPR, responsiveness to defibrillation attempt), it would be helpful to have a real-time and noninvasive tool able to predict the chances of defibrillation success [36].

In a recent study by Ristagno and coworkers the efficacy of an electrocardiographic parameter, "amplitude spectrum area" (AMSA), to predict the likelihood that any one electrical shock would restore a perfusing rhythm was investigated during cardiopulmonary resuscitation in human victims of out-of-hospital cardiac arrest [37]. AMSA analysis is not invalidated by artifacts produced by chest compression and thus it can be performed during CPR, avoiding detrimental interruptions of chest compression and ventilation. Analysis was performed on a database of electrocardiographic records, representing lead 2 equivalent recordings from AEDs including 210 defibrillation attempts from 90 victims of out-of-hospital cardiac arrest. AMSA values were significantly greater in successful defibrillation (restoration of a perfusing rhythm), compared to unsuccessful defibrillation ($P < 0.0001$). An AMSA value of 12 mV Hz was able to predict the success of each defibrillation attempt with high sensitivity and specificity. AMSA, indeed, represents a clinically applicable method, which provides a real-time prediction of the success of defibrillation attempts. AMSA may minimize the delivery of futile and detrimental electrical shocks, reducing thereby post-resuscitation myocardial injury. Recent evidences have suggested that ECG waveform analysis of VF, such as the derived Amplitude Spectrum Area, can fit the purpose of monitoring the CPR effectiveness and predicting the responsiveness to defibrillation. While awaiting clinical studies confirming this promising approach, CPR performed according to high quality standard and with minimal interruptions together with early defibrillation are the best immediate ways to achieve resuscitation [38].

23.3.8 Brain Ischemia and Reperfusion

Brain damage accompanying cardiac arrest and resuscitation is frequent and devastating. Neurons in the hippocampal CA1 and CA4 zones and cortical layers III and V are selectively vulnerable to death after an ischemia and reperfusion injury. Ultrastructural evidence indicates that most of the structural damage is associated with reperfusion, during which the vulnerable neurons develop disaggregation of polyribosomes, peroxidative damage to unsaturated fatty acids in the plasma membrane, and prominent alterations in the structure of the Golgi apparatus that is responsible for membrane assembly. Reperfusion is also associated with prominent production of messenger RNAs for stress proteins and for the proteins of the activator protein-1 complex, but vulnerable neurons fail to efficiently translate these messages into the proteins. The inhibition of protein synthesis during reperfusion involves alteration of translation initiation factors, specifically serine phosphorylation of the alpha-subunit of eukaryotic initiation factor-2 (elF-2 alpha). Growth factors—in particular, insulin—have the potential to reverse phosphorylation of elF-2 alpha, promote effective translation of the mRNA transcripts generated in response to ischemia and reperfusion, enhance neuronal defenses against radicals, and stimulate lipid synthesis and membrane repair. There is now substantial evidence that the insulin-class growth factors have neuron-sparing effects against damage by radicals and ischemia and reperfusion. This new knowledge may provide a fundamental basis for a rational approach to "cerebral resuscitation" that will allow substantial amelioration of the often dismal neurologic outcome now associated with resuscitation from cardiac arrest [39].

Recommendations represent the most extensive and rigorous systematic review of the resuscitation literature to date. Current guideline recommendations include the induction of mild therapeutic hypothermia for comatose cardiac arrest survivors. Accordingly, constituent national member associations of International Liaison Committee on Resuscitation (ILCOR), including the American Heart Association, incorporated the recommendation for therapeutic hypothermia into their respective guidelines. Despite these endorsements there is a concern that therapeutic hypothermia is not being used consistently in the clinical practice. Data from a number of surveys in Europe and the United States suggest that rates of use of hypotermia may be as low as 30–40 % of instances. Despite the cost and effort associated with the production of guidelines and the potential impact on patient care, current efforts in implementing the guideline have not achieved widespread success [40].

23.3.9 Therapeutic Hypothermia

The estimated number of out-of-hospital care arrest cases is about 300,000 per year in the United States. Two landmark studies published in 2002 demonstrated that the use of therapeutic hypothermia after cardiac arrest decreased mortality and improved neurologic outcome. Based on these studies, the ILCOR and the American Heart Association recommended the use of therapeutic hypothermia after cardiac arrest. Therapeutic hypothermia is defined as a controlled lowering of core body temperature to 32–34 °C. This temperature goal represents the optimal balance between clinical effect and cardiovascular toxicity. Therapeutic hypothermia does require resources to be implemented, including device, close nursing care, and monitoring. It is important to select patients who have potential for benefit from this technique which is a limited resource and carries potential complications.

Good neurologic outcome after cardiac arrest is hard to achieve. Interventions during the resuscitation phase and treatment within the first hours after the event are critical. Therapeutic hypothermia following return of spontaneous circulation has been advocated for decades prior to its clinical acceptance [41]. More than a decade ago it has been reported that young and healthy people underwent accidental deep hypothermia with cardiac arrest were able to survive with no or minimal cerebral impairment even after prolonged cardiac arrest. The concept of hypothermia for reducing either or both ischemic and reperfusion injury of the brain represents a pioneering contribution of the late Professor Peter Safar and the persistence of his efforts through his students, and especially Professor Fritz Sterz [42–44]. In 1996, Professor Safar induced hypothermia by instilling Ringer's solution maintained at a temperature of 4 °C into the abdominal cavity of dogs after resuscitation from cardiac arrest. Cooling was maintained for 12 h. Functional recovery was associated with minimal histological brain damage [41]. More recent investigations provided evidence that even better neurological and cardiac outcomes may be achieved if hypothermia is begun during CPR. Rapid and selective head cooling has been specifically investigated by our group. Head cooling reduced jugular venous temperature by 3.7 °C over an interval of 5 min during experimental CPR and significantly increased the likelihood of resuscitation, minimized post-resuscitation neurological deficit and myocardial dysfunction, and resulted in significantly greater 96 h functional survival [44].

More recently, a collaborative team approach involving physicians and nurses is critical for successful development and implementation of therapeutic hypothermia. In 2004, the "Advanced Cardiac Admission Program" was launched at the St. Luke's Roosevelt Hospital Center of Columbia University in New York. The program consisted of a series of projects, which have been developed to bridge the gap between published guidelines and implementation during "real world" patient care. The pathway was divided into three steps: Step I, from the field through the emergency department into the cardiac catherization laboratory and to the critical care unit; Step II, induced invasive hypothermia protocol in the critical care unit (this step was divided into three phases: 1, invasive cooling for the first 24 h; 2, rewarming; 3, maintenance); Step III, management post the rewarming phase, including the recommendation for out-of-hospital therapy and the ethical decision to define goal of care [45].

Arrich and coworkers performed a systematic review and meta-analysis to assess the effectiveness of therapeutic hypothermia in patients after cardiac arrest. The authors searched the following databases: the Cochrane Central Register of Controlled Trials (CENTRAL) (The Cochrane Library, 2007 Issue 1); MEDLINE (1971 to January 2007); EMBASE (1987 to January 2007); CINAHL (1988 to January 2007); PASCAL (2000 to January 2007); and BIOSIS (1989 to January 2007). The authors included all randomized controlled trials assessing the effectiveness of the therapeutic hypothermia in patients after cardiac arrest without language restrictions. Studies were restricted to adult populations cooled with any cooling method applied within 6 h of cardiac arrest. Overall, four trials and one abstract reporting on 481 patients were included in the systematic review. Quality of the included studies was good in three out of five included studies. For the three comparable studies on conventional cooling methods all authors provided individual patient data. With conventional cooling methods patients in the hypothermia group were more likely to reach a best cerebral performance categories score of one or two (CPC, five-point scale; 1 = good cerebral performance, to 5 = brain death) during hospital stay (individual patient data; RR, 1.55; 95 % CI 1.22–1.96) and were more likely to survive to hospital discharge (individual patient data; RR, 1.35; 95 % CI 1.10–1.65) compared to standard post-resuscitation care. Across all studies there was no significant difference in reported adverse events between hypothermia and control. The authors concluded that conventional cooling methods to induce mild therapeutic hypothermia seemed to improve survival and neurologic outcome after cardiac arrest. The review supported the current best medical practice as recommended by the International Resuscitation Guidelines [46].

23.3.10 Kynurenine Pathway

Post-stroke inflammation may induce upregulation of the kynurenine (KYN) pathway for tryptophan (TRP) oxidation, resulting in neuroprotective (kynurenic acid, KA) and neurotoxic metabolites (3-hydroxyanthranillic acid, 3-HAA). Brouns and coworkers investigated whether activity of the kynurenine pathway in acute ischemic stroke was related to initial stroke severity, long-term stroke outcome, and the ischemia-induced inflammatory response. Plasma concentrations of TRP and its metabolites were measured in 149 stroke patients at admission, at 24 h, at 72 h, and at day 7 after stroke onset. Indeed, the activity of the kynurenine pathway for TRP degradation in acute ischemic stroke correlated with stroke severity and long-term stroke outcome. Accordingly, TRP oxidation was related to the stroke-induced inflammatory response [47].

More recently, Ristagno and coworkers measured TRP and KYN metabolites concentrations in plasma from rats, pigs, and humans after cardiac arrest in order to assess KYN pathway activation and its potential role in post-resuscitation outcome [48]. KYN pathway was activated after cardiac arrest in rats, pigs, and humans. Decreases in TRP occurred during the post-resuscitation period and were accompanied by significant increases in its major metabolites, 3-hydroxyanthranilic acid (3-HAA) and kynurenic acid in each species, that persisted up to 3–5 days post-cardiac arrest ($p < 0.01$). In rats, changes in KYN metabolites reflected changes in post-resuscitation myocardial function. In pigs, changes in TRP and increases in 3-HAA were significanlty related to the severity of cerebral histopathogical injuries. In humans, KYN pathway activation was observed, together with systemic inflammation. Post-cardiac arrest increases in 3-HAA were greater in patients that did not survive. In this fully translational investigation, the authors concluded that the KYN pathway was activated early following resuscitation from cardiac in rats, pigs, and humans, and might have contributed to post-resuscitation outcome.

23.4 Future Direction and Perspectives

The quality of education and frequency of training retraining are critical factors in improving the effectiveness of resuscitation. Resuscitation programs should systematically monitor cardiac arrests, the quality of resuscitation care provided, and the outcome. This information is necessary to optimize resuscitation care and improve the resuscitation performance [49].

Teaching strategies should be evaluated and compared on the basis of how well learners achieve predefined teaching outcomes. Unfortunately, there is not a single method suitable for all circumstances. CPR consists of cognitive as well as team and psychomotor skills. Hence, it might be beneficial to learn and train the different aspects of CPR in different modes and at different times.

Moreover, health education specialists have the training and the experience to engage in and facilitate translational research, as well as the opportunity to learn from the translational efforts of other professions and enhance research, practice, and community partnerships through translational efforts [50].

References

1. van Berlo JH, Maillet M, Molkentin JD (2013) Signaling effectors underlying pathologic growth and remodeling of the heart. J Clin Invest 123:37–45
2. Wang X (2012) A new vision of definition, commentary, and understanding in clinical and translational medicine. Clin Transl Med 1:5
3. Chugh SS, Reinier K, Teodorescu C et al (2008) Epidemiology of sudden cardiac death: clinical and research implications. Prog Cardiovasc Dis 51:213–222
4. Spooner PM (2009) Sudden cardiac death: the larger problem… the larger genome. J Cardiovasc Electrophysiol 20:585–596
5. Jacobs I, Nadkarni V, Bahr J et al (2004) Cardiac arrest and cardiopulmonary resuscitation outcome reports: update and simplification of the Utstein templates for resuscitation registries: a statement for healthcare professionals from a task force of the International Liaison Committee on Resuscitation (American Heart Association, European Resuscitation Council, Australian Resuscitation Council, New Zealand Resuscitation Council, Heart and Stroke Foundation of Canada, InterAmerican Heart Foundation, Resuscitation Councils of Southern Africa). Circulation 110:3385–3397
6. Weisfeldt ML, Sitlani CM, Ornato JP et al (2010) Survival after application of automatic external defibrillators before arrival of the emergency medical system: evaluation in the resuscitation outcomes consortium population of 21 million. JAMA 55:1713–1720
7. American Heart Association (2005) Guideline for cardiopulmonary resuscitation and emergency cardiovascular care. Part 7.5: postresuscitation support. Circulation 112(Suppl I):IV-84–IV-88
8. Nolan JP, Neumar RW, Adrie C et al (2008) Post-cardiac arrest syndrome: epidemiology, pathophysiology, treatment, and prognostication a scientific statement from the international

liaison committee on resuscitation; the American Heart Association Emergency Cardiovascular Care Committee; the Council on Cardiovascular Surgery and Anesthesia; the Council on Cardiopulmonary, Perioperative, and Critical Care; the Council on Clinical Cardiology; the Council on Stroke. Resuscitation 79:350–379

9. Ewy GA, Sanders AB (2013) Alternative approach to improving survival of patients with out-of-hospital primary cardiac arrest. J Am Coll Cardiol 61:113–118

10. Keramaris NC, Kanakaris NK, Tzioupis C et al (2008) Translational research: from benchside to bedside. Injury 39:643–650

11. López-Messa JB, Martín-Hernández H, Pérez-Vela JL et al (2011) Novelities in resuscitation training methods. Med Intensiva 35:433–441

12. Yannas IV (2013) Emerging rules for inducing organ regeneration. Biomaterials 34:321–330

13. Christ GJ, Saul JM, Furth ME et al (2013) The pharmacology of regenerative medicine. Pharmacol Rev 65:1091–1133

14. Wang T, Tang W, Sun S et al (2009) Mesenchymal stem cells improve outcomes of cardiopulmonary resuscitation in myocardial infarcted rats. J Mol Cell Cardiol 46:378–384

15. Cairns CB, Panacek EA, Harken AH et al (2000) Bench to bedside: tumor necrosis factor-alpha: from inflammation to resuscitation. Acad Emerg Med 7:930–941

16. Adrie C, Adib-Conquy M, Laurent I et al (2002) Successful cardiopulmonary resuscitation after cardiac arrest as a "sepsis-like" syndrome. Circulation 106:562–568

17. Meybohm P, Gruenewald M, Albrecht M et al (2009) Hypothermia and postconditioning after cardiopulmonary resuscitation reduce cardiac dysfunction by modulating inflammation, apoptosis and remodeling. PLoS ONE 4:e7588

18. Fries M, Brücken A, Çizen A et al (2012) Combining xenon and mild therapeutic hypothermia preserves neurological function after prolonged cardiac arrest in pigs. Crit Care Med 40:1297–1303

19. Meybohm P, Gruenewald M, Albrecht M et al (2011) Pharmacological postconditioning with sevoflurane after cardiopulmonary resuscitation reduces myocardial dysfunction. Crit Care 15:R241

20. Neumar RW (2011) Optimal oxygenation during and after cardiopulmonary resuscitation. Curr Opin Crit Care 17:236–240

21. Pilcher J, Weatherall M, Shirtcliffe P et al (2012) The effect of hyperoxia following cardiac arrest—a systematic review and meta-analysis of animal trials. Resuscitation 83:417–422

22. Janz DR, Hollenbeck RD, Pollock JS et al (2012) Hyperoxia is associated with increased mortality in patients treated with mild therapeutic hypothermia after sudden cardiac arrest. Crit Care Med 40:3135–3139

23. Kilgannon JH, Jones AE, Shapiro NI et al (2010) Association between arterial hyperoxia following resuscitation from cardiac arrest and in-hospital mortality. JAMA 303:2165–2171

24. Bellomo R, Bailey M, Eastwood GM et al (2011) Arterial hyperoxia and in-hospital mortality after resuscitation from cardiac arrest. Crit Care 15:R90

25. Kloner RA, Schwartz Longacre L (2011) State of the science of cardioprotection: challenges and opportunities. J Cardiovasc Pharmacol Ther 16:223–232

26. Bolli R, Becker L, Gross G et al (2004) Myocardial protection at a crossroads: the need for translation into clinical therapy. DANHLBI working group on the translation of therapies for protecting the heart from ischemia. Circ Res 95:125–134

27. Tang W, Weil MH, Sun S et al (1995) Epinephrine increases the severity of postresuscitation myocardial dysfunction. Circulation 92:3089–3093

28. Pellis T, Weil MH, Tang W et al (2003) Evidence favoring the use of an alpha2-selective vasopressor agent for cardiopulmonary resuscitation. Circulation 108:2716–2721

29. Klouche K, Weil MH, Tang W et al (2002) A selective alpha(2)-adrenergic agonist for cardiac resuscitation. J Lab Clin Med 140:27–34

30. Zhong JQ, Dorian P (2005) Epinephrine and vasopressin during cardiopulmonary resuscitation. Resuscitation 66:263–269

31. Herfst LJ, Rook MB, Jongsma HJ (2004) Trafficking and functional expression of cardiac Na+ channels. J Mol Cell Cardiol 36:185–193
32. Wann SR, Weil MH, Sun S et al (2002) Cariporide for pharmacologic defibrillation after prolonged cardiac arrest. J Cardiovasc Pharmacol Ther 7:161–169
33. Amin AS, Asghari-Roodsari A, Tan HL (2010) Cardiac sodium channelopathies. Pflugers Arch 460:223–237
34. Ayoub IM, Kolarova J, Gazmuri RJ (2010) Cariporide given during resuscitation promotes return of electrically stable and mechanically competent cardiac activity. Resuscitation 81:106–110
35. Mentzer RM Jr, Bartels C, Bolli R et al (2008) EXPEDITION study investigators (2008) sodium-hydrogen exchange inhibition by cariporide to reduce the risk of ischemic cardiac events in patients undergoing coronary artery bypass grafting: results of the EXPEDITION study. Ann Thorac Surg 85:1261–1270
36. Povoas HP, Bisera J (2000) Electrocardiographic waveform analysis for predicting the success of defibrillation. Crit Care Med 28:N210–N211
37. Ristagno G, Gullo A, Berlot G et al (2008) Prediction of successful defibrillation in human victims of out-of-hospital cardiac arrest: a retrospective electrocardiographic analysis. Anaesth Intensive Care 36:46–50
38. Scapigliati A, Ristagno G, Cavaliere F (2013) The best timing for defibrillation in shockable cardiac arrest. Minerva Anestesiol 79:92–101
39. White BC, Grossman LI, O'Neil BJ et al (1996) Global brain ischemia and reperfusion. Ann Emerg Med 27:588–594
40. Brooks SC, Morrison LJ (2008) The 2005 International Liaison Committee on Resuscitation (ILCOR) Consensus on Science and Implementation of therapeutic hypothermia guidelines for post-cardiac arrest syndrome at a glacial pace: seeking guidance from the knowledge translation literature. Resuscitation 77:286–292
41. Safar P, Xiao F, Radovsky A et al (1996) Improved cerebral resuscitation from cardiac arrest in dogs with mild hypothermia plus blood flow promotion. Stroke 27:105–113
42. The Hypothermia After Cardiac Arrest Study Group (2002) Mild therapeutic hypothermia to improve the neurologic outcome after cardiac arrest. N Engl J Med 346:549–556
43. Fritz HG, Bauer R (2004) Secondary injuries in brain trauma: effects of hypothermia. J Neurosurg Anesthesiol 16:43–52
44. Guan J, Barbut D, Wang H et al (2008) A comparison between head cooling begun during cardiopulmonary resuscitation and surface cooling after resuscitation in a pig model of cardiac arrest. Crit Care Med 36:S428–S433
45. Herzog E, Shapiro J, Aziz EF et al (2010) Pathway for the management of survivors of out-of-hospital cardiac arrest. Crit Pathw Cardiol 9:49–54
46. Arrich J, Holzer M, Herkner H et al (2010) Cochrane corner: hypothermia for neuroprotection in adults after cardiopulmonary resuscitation. Anesth Analg 110:1239
47. Brouns R, Verkerk R, Aerts T et al (2010) The role of tryptophan catabolism along the kynurenine pathway in acute ischemic stroke. Neurochem Res 35:1315–1322
48. Ristagno G, Fries M, Brunelli L et al (2013) Early kynurenine pathway activation following cardiac arrest in rats, pigs, and humans. Resuscitation. Jun 15 Epub. pii: S0300-9572(13)00309-2
49. Nielsen AM, Isbye DL, Lippert FK et al (2013) Can mass education and a television campaign change the attitudes towards cardiopulmonary resuscitation in a rural community? Scand J Trauma Resusc Emerg Med 21:39
50. Mata HJ, Davis S (2012) Translational health research: perspectives from health education specialists. Clin Transl Med 1:27

Index